BMA

SECOND EDITION

Refractive Cataract Surgery

Best Practices and Advanced Technology

SECOND EDITION

Refractive Cataract Surgery

Best Practices and Advanced Technology

EDITED BY
JOHN A. HOVANESIAN, MD, FACS
HARVARD EYE ASSOCIATES
LAGUNA BEACH, CALIFORNIA
CLINICAL FACULTY
JULES STEIN EYE INSTITUTE
UNIVERSITY OF CALIFORNIA
LOS ANGELES, CALIFORNIA

SLACK
INCORPORATED

www.Healio.com/books

ISBN: 978-1-63091-197-3

Note: Materials from Chapter 2 and Chapter 6 have previously appeared in *Mastering Refractive IOLs: The Art and Science*, 2008 and *Presbyopic Lens Surgery: A Clinical Guide to Current Technology*, 2007, respectively, from SLACK Incorporated.

Cover design concept: Joseph Hovanesian

The procedures and practices described in this publication should be implemented in a manner consistent with the professional standards set for the circumstances that apply in each specific situation. Every effort has been made to confirm the accuracy of the information presented and to correctly relate generally accepted practices. The authors, editors, and publisher cannot accept responsibility for errors or exclusions or for the outcome of the material presented herein. There is no expressed or implied warranty of this book or information imparted by it. Care has been taken to ensure that drug selection and dosages are in accordance with currently accepted/recommended practice. Off-label uses of drugs may be discussed. Due to continuing research, changes in government policy and regulations, and various effects of drug reactions and interactions, it is recommended that the reader carefully review all materials and literature provided for each drug, especially those that are new or not frequently used. Some drugs or devices in this publication have clearance for use in a restricted research setting by the Food and Drug and Administration or FDA. Each professional should determine the FDA status of any drug or device prior to use in their practice.

Any review or mention of specific companies or products is not intended as an endorsement by the author or publisher.

SLACK Incorporated uses a review process to evaluate submitted material. Prior to publication, educators or clinicians provide important feedback on the content that we publish. We welcome feedback on this work.

Published by: SLACK Incorporated
6900 Grove Road
Thorofare, NJ 08086 USA
Telephone: 856-848-1000
Fax: 856-848-6091
www.Healio.com/books

Contact SLACK Incorporated for more information about other books in this field or about the availability of our books from distributors outside the United States.

Names: Hovanesian, John A., 1967- editor.
Title: Refractive cataract surgery : best practices and advanced technology / edited by John A. Hovanesian.
Other titles: Premium cataract surgery.
Description: Second edition. | Thorofare, NJ : Slack Incorporated, [2017] | Preceded by Premium cataract surgery : a step-by-step guide / edited by John A. Hovanesian. c2012. | Includes bibliographical references and index.
Identifiers: LCCN 2016057973 (print) | LCCN 2016059372 (ebook) | ISBN 9781630911973 (alk. paper) | ISBN 9781630911980 (epub) | ISBN 9781630911997 (web)
Subjects: | MESH: Cataract Extraction--methods | Lens Implantation, Intraocular | Practice Management, Medical | Physician-Patient Relations
Classification: LCC RE451 (print) | LCC RE451 (ebook) | NLM WW 260 | DDC 617.7/42059--dc23
LC record available at https://lccn.loc.gov/2016057973

Printed in the United States of America.

Last digit is print number: 10 9 8 7 6 5 4 3 2 1

Dedication

This book is dedicated to our patients, who entrust us surgeons with their most precious resource, their vision.

Contents

Dedication .... *v*
Acknowledgments .... *ix*
About the Editor .... *xi*
Contributing Authors .... *xiii*
Preface .... *xix*
Foreword to the Second Edition by Robert K. Maloney, MD, MA .... *xxiii*
Foreword to the First Edition by David F. Chang, MD .... *xxv*
Introduction .... *xxvii*

Section I Setting the Stage for Premium Cataract Surgery 1

Chapter 1 How to Get Started in Premium Cataract Surgery 3
John A. Hovanesian, MD, FACS

Chapter 2 Refractive Intraocular Lenses: Everyday Ethical Issues 9
David F. Chang, MD and Bryan S. Lee, MD, JD

Chapter 3 Prognostic Predictors for Premium Intraocular Lenses 15
George O. Waring IV, MD; R. Luke Rebenitsch, MD, PCEO; and Jason E. Stahl, MD

Chapter 4 Preparing the Ocular Surface for Cataract and Refractive Surgery 27
Jodi Luchs, MD, FACS

Chapter 5 Preoperative Testing for Refractive Cataract Surgery 41
Kevin Jwo, MD; William F. Wiley, MD; Ji Won Kwon, MD, PhD; and Jimmy Lee, MD

Chapter 6 Practice Management Considerations of Refractive Cataract Surgery 61
Kevin J. Corcoran, COE, CPC, CPMA, FNAO

Chapter 7 Advertising and Public Relations for Premium Cataract Surgery 75
Paul Stubenbordt, BS

Chapter 8 Educating Patients About Refractive Cataract Surgery 87
John A. Hovanesian, MD, FACS

Section II Surgical Technique and Implants 93

Chapter 9 Femtosecond Laser-Assisted Cataract Surgery 95
Kendall E. Donaldson, MD, MS

Chapter 10 Intraoperative Wavefront Aberrometry 115
Joel M. Solano, MD and John P. Berdahl, MD

Chapter 11 Microincisional Cataract Surgery 123
Mujtaba A. Qazi, MD; Abu-Bakar Zafar, MD; and Jay S. Pepose, MD, PhD

Chapter 12 Micro-Invasive Glaucoma Surgery 141
Savak "Sev" Teymoorian, MD, MBA

Chapter 13 The Toric Intraocular Lens: Successful Strategies 157
Adi Abulafia, MD and Warren E. Hill, MD

Chapter 14 Limbal Relaxing Incisions 167
R. Bruce Wallace III, MD and John A. Hovanesian, MD, FACS

Chapter 15 Integrating Monovision Into Presbyopic Intraocular Lens Surgery 177
J. E. "Jay" McDonald II, MD and Garth Rotramel, BA, SPHR

Chapter 16 Multifocal Implants 189
Farrell (Toby) Tyson, MD, FACS

Chapter 17 Accommodating Implants: The Crystalens 199
Robert J. Weinstock, MD

Section III Postoperative Considerations and Enhancements 213

Chapter 18 Refractive Intraocular Lenses: Managing Unhappy Patients...... 215
Eric Donnenfeld, MD; Alanna Nattis, DO; Eric Rosenberg, DO; and Allon Barsam, MD, MA, MRCOphth

Chapter 19 Enhancement With Piggyback or Intraocular Lens Exchanges.. 225
Adi Abulafia, MD and Warren E. Hill, MD

Chapter 20 Excimer Laser Enhancements After Intraocular Lens Surgery.. 233
Jay Bansal, MD and Arun C. Gulani, MD, MS

Chapter 21 Enhancements With Micro-Radial Keratotomy/Astigmatic Keratotomy 245
Frank A. Bucci Jr, MD

Financial Disclosures...257
Index...261

Acknowledgments

In this, the second edition of this book, we have altered the title from the first edition, which was called *Premium Cataract Surgery: A Step By Step Guide*. This second edition is called *Refractive Cataract Surgery: Best Practices and Advanced Technology* to reflect that advanced cataract surgery is now a mainstream offering rather than a premium alternative, as it once was. However, in both editions, credit for the content belongs mostly to the chapter authors, who made it possible. Each carefully constructed a stepwise path to success for relative beginners in refractive cataract surgery. Each author is a recognized leader in the field and a noted teacher. Despite many other demands, each enthusiastically took on the task of writing and met a tight editorial deadline to produce this text in a timely manner.

David Chang must be credited with the idea for this book. Shortly after the publication of his wonderfully edited and comprehensive textbook, *Mastering Refractive IOLs: The Art and Science*, he suggested the need for a somewhat more manageable length text targeted at an audience of surgeons who were new to premium cataract surgery and giving a step-by-step approach to success. It was my honor to answer this challenge and assemble the material that made up the first and now second editions of this book.

David Hardten and Kevin Corcoran deserve special mention. Each has participated for many years in a course we teach together at the American Academy of Ophthalmology annual symposium as well as the annual American Society of Cataract and Refractive Surgery meeting. Each has taught me many lessons about how a premium practice should treat patients.

Dick Lindstrom, my dear friend and one of the most generous people I know, has given me mentorship and guidance in so many areas. This book has been no exception.

My partners in practice, Roger Ohanesian, Ed Kim, Diana Kersten, Savak Teymoorian, and Brian Kim have built a truly premium practice since well before premium implants existed. Thanks to them, Harvard Eye Associates in Laguna Hills, California has been a truly wonderful place to practice medicine. Interestingly, Roger, who implanted the world's first foldable intraocular lens in a human subject as part of the Staar Surgical study many years ago, reviewed the introduction on history of premium surgery. He was, I thought, highly qualified to review this history since he personally lived it.

Robert Maloney, more than any other mentor, has shaped the way I think about both refractive surgery and the treatment of refractive patients. His mentorship at UCLA, and that of Bartly Mondino and Gary Holland, taught me that we should run toward, not away from, our most challenging patients. His willingness to write the foreword to this book honors me greatly.

Those who were my early teachers at Henry Ford Health System in Detroit all deserve much credit and include Con McCole, David Carey, Dan Steen, Howard Neff, Dave Bogorad, Julian Nussbaum, Bob Lesser, Murray Christianson, Uday Desai, Paul Edwards, Tom Byrd, Barry Skarf, Brian Bachynski, Pat Dennehy, and others.

I have also had the pleasure of working on medical advisory boards and symposium panels with countless leaders in the field of cataract surgery who have shaped our collective understanding of this subject matter and deserve our gratitude.

John Bond, Tony Schiavo, Katherine Rola, April Billick, Emily Densten, Michelle Gatt, and Jennifer Kilpatrick from SLACK Incorporated have provided advice, support, many hours of work, and patience while I made changes to this book over and over. Pete Slack, Joan-Marie Stiglich, Pat Nale, Nancy Hemphill, and Dave Mullin also have my gratitude for their collaboration since 2005 in publishing educational materials for eye care professionals. Working with them has been continuously enjoyable and personally rewarding.

A thousand thank yous to my wife Tanya. As always, she has been unselfishly supportive of work on this book and other teaching efforts, even when it took me away (again and again) from helping her manage our 3 young children.

Speaking of my kids, I'm very proud of my thirteen-year-old son, Joseph Hovanesian, who designed the cover of this book. He drew the image by hand, and the fine graphic artists at SLACK Incorporated turned it into publishable vector art. I may be biased, but I think his first "professional" art assignment turned out quite well.

Finally, it is appropriate to thank the patients of all this book's contributors. Their continued trust and confidence, their referrals, and their willingness to participate in research studies has made all of our learning possible, and to them we dedicate not just this book but also our lives' work.

About the Editor

John A. Hovanesian, MD, FACS is a member of the clinical faculty at the UCLA Jules Stein Eye Institute and is in private ophthalmic practice in Laguna Hills, California with Harvard Eye Associates. He completed his undergraduate training in 3 years in the Honors Chemistry program at the University of Michigan, where he was a James B. Angell Scholar and was inducted into the Phi Beta Kappa honor society as a sophomore. After graduating summa cum laude, he earned his medical degree from the University of Michigan Medical School and completed his residency training at Henry Ford Hospital, where he was named Resident of the Year and was selected by his faculty to serve as chief resident. He then completed a 2-year fellowship in cornea and external disease at the UCLA Jules Stein Eye Institute. In his private practice in Southern California, he directs one of the country's most recognized Food and Drug Administration study centers, evaluating new eye care technologies. He serves as a board member or consultant for over 20 eye technology companies.

As the son of 2 teachers, Dr. Hovanesian enjoys contributing to ophthalmic education and serves the American Academy of Ophthalmology as editor or the Online News and Education network's cataract and anterior segment section. He is a regular contributor and member of the editorial board for *Ocular Surgery News*, *Cataract and Refractive Surgery Today*, *The Premier Surgeon*, *Advanced Ocular Care*, and *Primary Care Optometry News*. He blogs at www.healio.com.

In his spare time, Dr. Hovanesian enjoys spending time with his wife and 3 children. An Eagle Scout, he is also a volunteer leader with the Boy Scouts of America, serving both of his sons' Scout groups and also as chairman of the board of directors of the Orange County, California Council. He also volunteers with Armenian EyeCare Project, a non-profit focused on eliminating preventable blindness in the former Soviet Union. He and his wife also teach Sunday school at his church in Costa Mesa, California.

Contributing Authors

Adi Abulafia, MD (Chapters 13, 19)
Ophthalmology Department
Shaare Zedek Medical Center
The Hebrew University of Jerusalem
Hadassah Medical School
Jerusalem, Israel

Jay Bansal, MD (Chapter 20)
Medical Director
LaserVue Eye Center
Santa Rosa, California

Allon Barsam, MD, MA, MRCOphth (Chapter 18)
Medical Director
AB Vision
London, United Kingdom

John P. Berdahl, MD (Chapter 10)
Vance Thompson Vision
Sioux Falls, South Dakota

Frank A. Bucci Jr, MD (Chapter 21)
Founder and Director
Bucci Laser Vision Institute
Wilkes Barre, Pennsylvania

David F. Chang, MD (Chapter 2)
Clinical Professor of Ophthalmology
University of California, San Francisco
San Francisco, California

Private Practice
Los Altos, California

Kevin J. Corcoran, COE, CPC, CPMA, FNAO (Chapter 6)
President
Corcoran Consulting Group
San Bernadino, California

Kendall E. Donaldson, MD, MS (Chapter 9)
Associate Professor of Ophthalmology
Bascom Palmer Eye Institute
Miami, Florida

Eric Donnenfeld, MD (Chapter 18)
Partner
Ophthalmic Consultants of Long Island
Rockville Centre, New York

Clinical Professor of Ophthalmology
New York University
New York, New York

Trustee
Dartmouth Medical School
Hanover, New Hampshire

Arun C. Gulani, MD,MS (Chapter 20)
Founding Director & Chief Surgeon
Gulani Vision Institute
Jacksonville, Florida

Warren E. Hill, MD (Chapters 13, 19)
Medical Director
East Valley Ophthalmology
Mesa, Arizona

Kevin Jwo, MD (Chapter 5)
Department of Ophthalmology and Visual Sciences
Montefiore Medical Center
Albert Einstein College of Medicine
Bronx, New York

Ji Won Kwon, MD, PhD (Chapter 5)
Associate Professor
Department of Ophthalmology
Seonam University Myongji Hospital
Goyang, South Korea

Bryan S. Lee, MD, JD (Chapter 2)
Altos Eye Physicians
Los Altos, California

Adjunct Clinical Assistant Professor of Ophthalmology
Stanford University
Stanford, California

Jimmy Lee, MD (Chapter 5)
Director of Cornea and Refractive Surgery
Division of Cornea Cataract and External Diseases
Department of Ophthalmology and Visual Science
Montefiore Medical Center
Assistant Professor
Albert Einstein College of Medicine
Bronx, New York

Jodi Luchs, MD, FACS (Chapter 4)
Associate Clinical Professor
Hofstra Northwell School of Medicine
Hempstead, New York

J. E. "Jay" McDonald II, MD (Chapter 15)
Assistant Clinical Professor
University of Arkansas Medical Sciences
Department of Ophthalmology
McDonald Eye Associates
Fayetteville, Arkansas

Alanna Nattis, DO (Chapter 18)
Ophthalmic Consultants of Long Island
Rockville Centre, New York

Jay S. Pepose, MD, PhD (Chapter 11)
Director
Pepose Vision Institute
Professor of Clinical Ophthalmology and Visual Sciences
Washington University School of Medicine
St. Louis, Missouri

Mujtaba A. Qazi, MD (Chapter 11)
Director, Clinical Studies
Pepose Vision Institute
St. Louis, Missouri

R. Luke Rebenitsch, MD, PCEO (Chapter 3)
ClearSight Center
Oklahoma City, Oklahoma

Executive Committee Member
Refractive Surgery Alliance
Scottsdale, Arizona

Eric Rosenberg, DO (Chapter 18)
Ophthalmology Resident
New York Medical College
Valhalla, New York

Garth Rotramel, BA, SPHR (Chapter 15)
Ictus Solutions
Fayetteville, Arizona

Joel M. Solano, MD (Chapter 10)
Acuity Eye Specialists
Palm Desert, California

Jason E. Stahl, MD (Chapter 3)
Durrie Vision
Overland Park, Kansas

Assistant Clinical Professor of Ophthalmology
Kansas University Medical Center
Prairie Village, Kansas

Paul Stubenbordt, BS (Chapter 7)
President and Founder
Stubenbordt Consulting, Inc
Roanoke, Texas

Savak "Sev" Teymoorian, MD, MBA (Chapter 12)
Specialist in Glaucoma and Cataract Surgery
Harvard Eye Associates
Laguna Hills, California

Farrell (Toby) Tyson, MD, FACS (Chapter 16)
Medical Director
Cape Coral Eye Center
Cape Coral, Florida

R. Bruce Wallace III, MD (Chapter 14)
Clinical Professor of Ophthalmology
Louisiana State University
Tulane University
New Orleans, Louisiana

George O. Waring IV, MD (Chapter 3)
Associate Professor of Ophthalmology
Director of Refractive Surgery
Medical University of South Carolina
Charleston, South Carolina

Adjunct Assistant Professor of Bioengineering
College of Engineering and Science
Clemson University
Clemson, South Carolina

Robert J. Weinstock, MD (Chapter 17)
Director of Cataract and Refractive Surgery
Eye Institute of West Florida
Largo, Florida

William F. Wiley, MD (Chapter 5)
University Hospitals
Cleveland, Ohio

Abu-Bakar Zafar, MD (Chapter 11)
Carle Foundation Hospital
Urbana, Illinois

Preface

A History of Premium Cataract Surgery in the United States

Premium cataract surgery is a concept that probably dates to the late 1980s, when progressive surgeons in many United States metropolitan areas, much to the chagrin of their counterparts in more traditional medical circles, began advertising in the media their skills performing small-incision, no-stitch cataract removal. They positioned themselves as "premium" providers of eye care, offering free rides to and from surgery in fancy buses and limousines. In an era of high reimbursement from Medicare and with minimal oversight of what have since been deemed inappropriate inducements, these high-volume surgeons seemed a world away from the mainstream of ophthalmologists, who referred to them as "cataract cowboys" for their bravado. Limited by the imprecision of contact A-scan biometry and monofocal implants, these surgeons targeted emmetropia, but their primary concern was the correction of cataract with little promise to patients of a spectacle-free life.

Fifteen years later, with a steady decline in Medicare reimbursement for cataract surgery and a growing aging population, most cataract surgeons around the developed world adopted new minimally traumatic, topical anesthetic, sutureless clear corneal incision techniques. These allowed faster surgery and induced a predictable and minimal amount of astigmatism. Coupled with these techniques, advances in lens implant calculations through optical biometry allowed prediction of the refractive outcome of cataract surgery to easily within one diopter and often much less. This set the stage nicely for products and techniques for refractive cataract surgery.

In 1997, Advanced Medical Optics (now Abbott Medical Optics) introduced a radical new concept—an intraocular lens (IOL) with multiple focal points called the Array. This unusual lens promised patients the hope of restoring a small part of their youth. It offered surgeons a new definition of refractive cataract surgery—one in which correcting presbyopia no longer meant monovision. Succeeding with the lens, though, required much attention to details like patient selection and counseling, lens centration, and management of astigmatism. Charging patients for extra counseling time and attention to detail was not an option, and introducing fees for noncovered extra testing and follow-up exams was not common practice. Moreover, anecdotal reports emerged of lens exchanges performed because of disabling glare and halo symptoms. In other words, use of the Array entailed more work, more risk, and yet no additional income. Sales fizzled. Despite its relative failure, the Array lens introduced the world to a concept that would change eye surgery forever—refractive cataract surgery.

STAAR Surgical's toric IOL was approved in the United States in 1998, allowing simultaneous correction of astigmatism and cataract surgery. Surgeons were cautious in adopting these lenses not only because of the same reimbursement issues that were faced by the Array lens but also because of reports of rotational instability with the early versions of this lens. Meanwhile, incisional techniques for correcting astigmatism (astigmatic keratotomy and limbal relaxing incisions) naturally gained attention during this period because many surgeons were already familiar with similar concepts (most commonly radial keratotomy) for the correction of myopia.

In 2003, the Food and Drug Administration approved the first ever accommodating IOL, the Crystalens AT-45, made by southern California startup Eyeonics, Incorporated. Within a few months, the Alcon ReSTOR and Advanced Medical Optics ReZoom implants were almost simultaneously approved. These multifocal lenses differentiated themselves from the earlier Array by claiming more advanced design to offer truly physiologic multifocality. Each of these new lenses had its technical limitations but offered meaningful near vision for patients.

The biggest challenge faced by surgeons during the first months after approval of these lenses was the inability to offer them to Medicare beneficiaries because Medicare did not allow any greater reimbursement for presbyopia-correcting IOLs (PC-IOLs), which cost between $800 and $1000 for the lens alone, than it did for traditional, monofocal lenses (about $100). Furthermore, Medicare did not allow surgeons to "balance bill" the patient for the added cost of the PC-IOL, since every IOL was regarded as a fully covered service. There was no differentiation in reimbursement among traditional and presbyopia-correcting lens implants. Only the most altruistic surgeons could consider offering these lenses at a substantial personal financial loss to Medicare beneficiaries, who represented a majority of their cataract patients. For an awkward period of nearly 2 years, these lenses were used primarily in the non-Medicare population, where balance billing was not expressly forbidden.

In May 2005, everything changed when the Centers for Medicare and Medicaid Services announced a ruling on PC-IOLs, acknowledging that they provided a different kind of visual result than monofocal lenses. The ruling further recognized that the cost of these lenses was higher than the reimbursement provided by the Centers for Medicare and Medicaid Services for a traditional lens and that their use required additional physician services that were not covered as part of the global fee for cataract surgery. Now surgeons could offer PC-IOLs to virtually any patient considering cataract surgery.

First Experience With Presbyopia-Correcting IOLs

How did ophthalmologists respond to this new freedom? As with most new technologies, the majority of cataract surgeons, unfamiliar with the challenge of refractive cataract surgery, simply followed the news in journals and podium presentations. Others embraced the new technology and put it to work for their patients, along the way learning how to best make these lenses work.

The early days of presbyopia-correcting implants were fraught with challenges, as surgeons around the country learned a number of lessons about the limitations of these lenses. Patients receiving the first Crystalens accommodating implants occasionally developed capsular fibrosis inducing tilting of the lens (capsular contraction syndrome), which caused irregular astigmatism. Those receiving the first multifocal implants were occasionally disturbed by glare that required explantation. The importance of early yttrium aluminum garnet laser capsulotomies and enhancements for residual refractive error for these patients were not well understood. With time and experience, surgeons learned "rules of the road" to stay out of trouble. Though none of these first lenses are still in use (Crystalens AT-45, ReSTOR +4 nonaspheric, and ReZoom), the importance of these rules endures.

Future Technologies

As the popularity and availability of femtosecond laser-assisted cataract surgery increases, a new standard of precision for refractive cataract surgery is being set, creating an opportunity for novel lens implant designs and other surgical devices whose designs couldn't be conceived and whose use couldn't be considered without the precision of these lasers. Resourceful surgeons and creative industry personnel now have a new frontier to explore. As consumers increasingly are asked to shoulder the burden of cost of their nonelective health care, price sensitivity will also become more acute and will require these new technologies to offer meaningful additive benefits if they are to succeed in the growing medical marketplace.

Foreword to the Second Edition

We humans are very good at adapting to limitations the environment places on us. Walk long enough with a pebble in your shoe, and you won't feel it. Walk even longer, then remove the pebble, and it feels like your shoe is too loose. So it is with the correction of refractive errors. Patients got used to glasses and contact lenses and viewed it as a normal part of life. Ophthalmologists thought it was normal too. It became so normal, in fact, that those of us who argued otherwise several decades ago were labeled "cowboys" or "wild men." When I started my career at a university medical center, I remember the other faculty looking at me in puzzlement, silently asking themselves the question, "Why do we need a refractive surgeon here?" It was the same sense of puzzlement that one of the cardinals might have if the pope had invited a lawyer to set up a divorce practice in the Vatican. Their puzzlement wasn't completely misplaced. The results of radial keratotomy were mediocre at best, but radial keratotomy led to the development of LASIK, a spectacularly effective procedure that is safer and more effective than contact lenses by a number of measures.

Cataract surgeons have not been unaware of the refractive benefits of cataract surgery, but they have historically been equally resistant. When Ridley proposed placing polymethylmethacrylate intraocular lenses (IOL) in the eye, he was roundly criticized, and he remained an outsider to the ophthalmology establishment for decades. His first academic honor came 40 years after he placed the first IOL in a human eye, when he received an honorary degree from the Medical University of South Carolina. In contrast, Robert Machemer, the inventor of the vitrectomy, was named chairman at Duke University just 8 years after his first vitrectomy in a human. Just as ophthalmologists came to see the benefits of refractive surgery, so too did cataract surgeons come to see the benefits of IOLs. Phacoemulsification faced similar resistance: one United States department chairman called it "a tornado inside the eye." He wasn't far off with early phaco machines, but the technology evolved. Now, it's hard to imagine returning to extracapsular cataract surgery for any reason other than expense. Phacoemulsification has become an essential component of refractive cataract surgery.

We now have a profusion of new IOLs that dramatically increase our ability to limit spectacle dependence postoperatively. This is driving a revolution in refractive surgery, as we recognize that the crystalline lens may be the optimal site for refractive correction. Yet, a surprising number of our colleagues have not adopted refractive cataract surgery. Today, perhaps half of cataract surgeons do not use advanced lenses. Even misery can seem preferable to change. In the Philippines in World War II, Allied prisoners who had been interned under brutal conditions were liberated at the end of the war. They looked out when the gates were thrown open and then went back to their barracks rather than risk the unknown. So, too, it has happened with many cataract surgeons: the gates to refractive cataract surgery have been thrown open, and they turned around and went back to their old habits.

But not you, Dear Reader. By picking up this book, you have shown your commitment to embracing the future rather than the past. What a journey you are in for. Success in refractive cataract surgery requires expertise in informed consent, a bit of sales skills, and discerning preoperative evaluation, all of which and more you will learn about in Section I. Section II will introduce you to advanced techniques, including femtosecond laser cataract surgery and various intraocular implants. And Section III will persuade you, if you aren't already persuaded, that you can't be a refractive cataract surgeon without also being a refractive surgeon. By the end of this book, you will have the knowledge and confidence to largely free your patients from their dependence on optical devices. I promise you'll have a lot of fun doing it too. If you are over 50 years old, I salute you. It's hard to adapt to new ideas. For those of you who are young, this book will give you the foundation you need to embark on a long and successful career. It is said that you can always recognize the pioneer, because he is the one with the arrows in his back. This book will also give you the foundation you need to be an innovator of the next generation of advancements, a cowboy and a wild man or woman of the future. As you feel the arrows hit you in the back, take heart in knowing that many have come before you and many will come after.

Robert K. Maloney, MD, MA
Clinical Professor of Ophthalmology
Jules Stein Eye Institute
UCLA David Geffen School of Medicine
Los Angeles, California

Foreword to the First Edition

If you think about it, the evolution toward what we now call "refractive" cataract surgery began more than 60 years ago when Harold Ridley implanted the first artificial intraocular lens (IOL) implant. Until the IOL, avoiding cataract blindness meant wearing aphakic spectacles and effectively becoming a refractive high ametrope. With the subsequent application of biometry and regression formulae for IOL power calculations, surgeons could actually target a desired postoperative spherical refractive error. The next major step was the reduction of surgically induced astigmatism. The adoption of phacoemulsification spurred the development of foldable IOLs, and the resulting small temporal incisions became astigmatically neutral. This allowed surgeons to simultaneously address pre-existing astigmatism at the time of surgery using first incisional keratotomy and later toric IOLs.

Many of us remember the excitement surrounding Food and Drug Administration approval of the first multifocal IOL (Array, Abbott Medical Optics) in 1997 and the first accommodating IOL (Eyeonics Crystalens, Bausch & Lomb) in 2003. Both times, the initial optimism and enthusiasm was significantly tempered with the clinical realization that these technologies often did not meet patient expectations, and the low market share for these IOLs reflected this reality. Many cataract surgeons chose to remain on the sidelines while awaiting better technologies.

As LASIK became a household word in the 1990s, we found that patients increasingly expected cataract surgery to eliminate their eyeglasses and for their health insurance to cover everything. The historic 2005 Centers for Medicare and Medicaid Services ruling allowing patients to pay out of pocket for presbyopia-correcting IOLs dramatically ushered in a new era—cataract patients now had the opportunity to elect and pay separately for refractive IOL technologies and services. Now, in 2012, there is no turning back. Refractive IOLs and adjunctive refractive procedures are interwoven with the modern practice of cataract surgery, and it is an ethical responsibility to at least educate cataract patients about these options. Many promising IOL technologies are in the investigational pipeline, including toric multifocal, new concept accommodating, and light-adjustable IOLs. Finally, femtosecond laser–assisted cataract surgery is a potentially revolutionary technology that will be paid for by patients as an optional refractive service.

Market surveys indicate that many cataract surgeons have yet to embrace this new paradigm of offering refractive IOLs and services. The challenges are understandably daunting. As I proposed to readers in the preface of my book, *Mastering Refractive IOLs: The Art and Science*, "We must all improve our surgical proficiency, our understanding of clinical optics, our communication skills, our clinical judgment, and our expertise in avoiding and managing complications." This textbook provides a practical and manageable roadmap for the transitioning refractive cataract surgeon. Dr. Hovanesian has assembled a notable group of authors with both the clinical expertise and an understanding of the obstacles facing those who are just starting to implant refractive IOLs.

Those of you reading this textbook are taking an important next step along the path that pioneers such as Ridley and Kelman first started us all on. Refractive cataract surgery has a bright future as both a medical and functional procedure that we should all embrace. The penultimate goal in lens replacement surgery—clear vision with minimal spectacle dependence—requires excellence in all aspects of the procedure. This includes not only the surgery and the IOL technology, but also the perioperative evaluation, counseling, and care. Congratulations on embracing the challenge of becoming a better refractive cataract surgeon.

David F. Chang, MD
Clinical Professor of Ophthalmology
University of California, San Francisco
San Francisco, California

Private Practice
Los Altos, California

Introduction

This book was written for cataract surgeons who wish to begin offering premium surgery or expand their premium surgery offerings. These include the reduction of astigmatism with limbal relaxing incisions and toric lens implants as well as the full range of accommodating and multifocal lens options. Each author, a recognized leader in refractive cataract surgery, has designed his or her chapter(s) as a stand-alone, how-to guide for the subject matter covered, so readers can learn about a particular subject of interest or can peruse chapters sequentially to gain a broader view of refractive cataract surgery.

Refractive cataract surgery should be both a challenge and a joy. Just as we raise the bar on what refractive cataract surgery patients can expect, we also raise their gratitude at receiving the hoped-for result. Happy patients refer friends, who grow the surgeon's reputation of expertise; yet, while a happy patient may tell 3 friends, an unhappy one seems to tells 10.

Newcomers to refractive surgery have a natural tendency to overemphasize the technical aspects of performing procedures and under-recognize the emotional and psychological aspects that are far more important to patients. While technique is highly important, it is usually the easiest part of refractive surgery to master. Far more difficult for many surgeons, who are not accustomed to the higher demands of refractive surgery patients, are managing expectations, dealing with disappointment, and maintaining the patient's confidence and trust throughout the process. Missing the mark in these matters is usually far more damaging to a patient's perceived outcome and to the surgeon's reputation than most technical subtleties. For this reason, we have devoted considerable space to the psychological aspects of premium cataract surgery in Section I of this book (Chapters 1, 2, and 8) and addressed practice organization, billing issues, and marketing strategies in Chapters 6 and 7.

Section II is where surgeons will find highly practical and stepwise information on approaching surgery, beginning with femtosecond laser cataract surgery (Chapter 9), intraoperative aberrometry (Chapter 10), and microincision cataract surgery (Chapter 11). While not an absolute necessity for performing today's refractive cataract surgery, these advanced techniques are likely to grow and increase refractive accuracy in the future, and learning these skills now will only benefit any surgeon.

We include a chapter on minimally invasive glaucoma surgery because this add-on procedure adds value to cataract surgery for as many as 15% of patients who have both cataract and glaucoma. Offering the most advanced cataract surgery necessarily involves understanding these techniques.

Astigmatic correction with either toric implants (Chapter 13) or limbal relaxing incisions (Chapter 14) is probably the best way to get started in refractive cataract surgery, as these techniques are much less technically challenging than presbyopia correction and less likely to require enhancement. These chapters give readers a complete and easy-to-follow approach to these 2 methods.

Because true spectacle independence can only be achieved by correcting both refractive error and presbyopia, Section II also details the steps necessary to succeed with all methods for presbyopic intraocular lens surgery, including monovision (Chapter 15), multifocal (Chapter 16), and accommodating lens implants (Chapter 17).

Section III helps us solve the least pleasant reality of refractive cataract surgery—that not all results are exactly as planned. The management of unhappy patients (Chapter 18) and enhancements with piggyback lenses, intraocular lens exchanges, excimer laser enhancements, and even micro-radial and astigmatic keratotomy (Chapters 19 to 21) are described in sufficient stepwise detail that every surgeon should find a technique that fits the style and setting of his or her practice.

While new technologies and implants will emerge that enhance the precision, safety, and results of surgery, they will bring new challenges that grow beyond the scope of this text. However, it is the hope of this book's contributors that surgeons who follow their step-by-step approach will feel both confidence to take on new techniques successfully and satisfaction at giving patients a better life through visual freedom.

Section I

Setting the Stage for Premium Cataract Surgery

Chapter 1

How to Get Started in Premium Cataract Surgery

John A. Hovanesian, MD, FACS

What Is Premium or Refractive Cataract Surgery?

First, let's define *premium* or *refractive* cataract surgery as happening any time the surgeon takes extra steps in a cataract procedure beyond the *covered services* defined by Medicare, with the aim of achieving a specific refractive result, usually to achieve some degree of spectacle independence. Some of these extra steps are diagnostic, such as corneal topography to define corneal astigmatism beyond the more limited information given by keratometry alone. Some are therapeutic, such as performing limbal relaxing incisions (LRI) intraoperatively. Either way, these extra steps require more work (by the surgeon and his or her staff) than routine cataract surgery; and, more importantly, they require us to deliver to the patient on a promise of better vision.

How to Get Started With Premium Cataract Surgery

Walking the Walk

Surgical Confidence

The first step in offering refractive cataract surgery is a consistent ability to perform uncomplicated surgery to achieve predictable results (ie, "walking the walk"). This means fairly atraumatic surgery through a small incision, a round capsulotomy of desired size (just under 6 mm for most lenses) and leaving behind a clean, intact capsule. For surgeons who are not completely comfortable delivering uncomplicated small-incision phacoemulsification, the prospect of offering refractive cataract surgery is likely to become an exercise in frustration for patient and physician alike.

Hovanesian JA.
Refractive Cataract Surgery: Best Practices and Advanced Technology, Second Edition (pp 3-8). © 2017 SLACK Incorporated.

Equipping the Office

Here, we will examine equipment that is commonly used in the preoperative assessment and postoperative treatment of patients and categorize these devices as *essential, highly useful*, and *nice to have*. Individual practice preferences apply, of course.

Essential

Preoperative biometry is, from a refractive standpoint, the most critical preoperative step toward premium cataract surgery. In recent years, contact ultrasound has given way to optical interferometry–based methods of keratometry, axial length, and anterior chamber depth measurements using the IOLMaster (Carl Zeiss Meditec) or Lenstar (Haag-Streit) instruments. Both instruments depend on patient fixation and are limited in their ability to perform biometry in highly opaque cataracts, but both instruments offer much greater resolution and accuracy in axial length measurements than ultrasound methods, assuming they can produce an adequate signal-to-noise ratio. In cases of dense cataract, immersion ultrasound biometry provides the most accurate axial length measurement. A number of ultrasound devices can provide consistent results using immersion ultrasound, though this technique is somewhat more demanding and operator-dependent.

Lens calculation software incorporating new-generation formulas like Holladay II, Haigis-L, and Barrett is usually a worthwhile investment, even if extra costs are involved in obtaining these modern formulas. Especially in long and short eyes and those with prior refractive surgery, these formulas allow much more accurate prediction of intraocular lens (IOL) power than their early generation counterparts. For eyes with prior refractive surgery, an especially useful, free web-based calculator is available at www.ascrs.org. This calculator allows input of pre-refractive surgery keratometry and refraction (when available) and uses all the modern formulas described previously.

Corneal topography or tomography provides critical information on the eye's only remaining structure that meaningfully refracts light after the lens is removed. Beyond keratometry, which measures only 2 points on the cornea, topography and tomography give both qualitative and quantitative information on thousands of points on the ocular surface. This aids in identifying an unhealthy ocular surface with areas of lost data or irregularity. These instruments pick up keratoconus, can detect which patients have had prior refractive surgery, and generally give a more accurate representation of cylinder axis than other instruments.

Most commercially available topography or tomography units can fill the need to provide an image of corneal surface power, but an additional useful feature is an estimate of the effective central power. The following devices can report values that can be used with the online calculator from the American Society of Cataract and Refractive Surgery[1] for calculating IOL powers in eyes that have had previous keratorefractive surgery:

- ATLAS (Carl Zeiss Meditec): Average powers in the central 0, 1, 2, and 3 mm of the cornea (numerical view)
- EyeSys Corneal Analysis System (EyeSys Vision): Effective refractive power
- Tomey Topographic Modeling System (Tomey Corporation): Average central corneal power
- Ziemer Galilei (Ziemer Ophthalmic Systems): Total corneal power

Additionally, measurement of posterior corneal astigmatism may increase the predictability of astigmatic correction. The Ziemer Galilei, Pentacam (Oculus), and Cassini (i-Optics) instruments all claim to measure and report posterior corneal astigmatism.

Diamond LRI blades and associated markers (essential) allow correction of astigmatism during surgery and are absolutely necessary, unless a surgeon plans on using only toric implants. In Chapter 14, Dr. R. Bruce Wallace describes in detail how to plan and perform these procedures. Diamond LRI knives come in a variety of designs and from many manufacturers, including those of fixed incision depth, usually 600 microns, and those with a micrometer, allowing customized incision depth. The choice between these depends on which type of nomogram the surgeon will use and whether the same blade may also be used for more central (mini-radial keratotomy) incisions. Another feature to consider is the design of the metal guards adjacent to the diamond blade tip; some designs allow easier visibility of the blade tip than others during cutting. Finally, handle length can be important, as shorter blade handles are less awkward to use when performing enhancements at the slit lamp. Longer blade handles can interfere with the slit lamp swinging light source.

Optical coherence tomography (essential) has become an extremely valuable tool for the premium refractive surgery patient. When the presence of cataract precludes a clear view of the fundus, subtle abnormalities like epiretinal membranes, diabetic macular edema, and macular traction can be impossible to detect through examination alone. Identifying these abnormalities before surgery is essential to setting proper expectations. In general, the presence of any macular pathology that affects contrast sensitivity would be a contraindication to a multifocal implant. We also generally avoid accommodating lenses when macular pathology reduces potential visual acuity before surgery (or is expected to do the same soon after surgery) to less than 20/25. Naturally, exceptions exist; occasionally, highly motivated patients with mild macular pathology will appreciate the benefits of an accommodating lens. However, it is incumbent upon the surgeon to convey an appropriate expectation, taking into account all the information available, which usually includes an optical coherence tomography scan.

Highly Useful

Femtosecond laser cataract surgery automates those steps of cataract surgery—capsulotomy, lens fragmentation, and incision creation—during which the inherent variability of manual techniques can reduce refractive predictability. Multiple peer-reviewed studies have now shown that these devices do indeed lessen endothelial cell loss and reduce anterior chamber inflammation after surgery.[2,3] Many surgeons believe more precise refractive outcomes are also achieved with these instruments because, in theory, a more precisely created, more stable incision will allow fewer wound leaks after surgery and a more predictable capsulotomy will allow better consistency of the effective lens position.

Intraoperative aberrometry allows a surgeon to measure refractive error during surgery in the aphakic or newly pseudophakic state. A measurement performed after the lens is removed and corneal incisions are created will theoretically offer greater accuracy than one performed before surgery. Indeed, the growing sentiment among users of these devices is that they reduce the incidence of postoperative refractive "surprises" and the frequency of enhancements, especially for challenging patients with previous refractive surgery.

Surgical alignment systems (highly useful) assist in ensuring that toric implants and astigmatic incisions are aligned with the patient's preoperative astigmatism. When a patient moves from an upright to a supine position, the extraocular muscles may induce several degrees of cyclotorsion. Additionally, inaccuracy of head alignment relative to its normal, upright position can cause meaningful error in placing treatment on the intended axis. Alignment systems measure landmarks on the eye with the patient upright, then, using those landmarks as a reference point, register the proper axis of astigmatic correction while the patient is lying down.

Nice to Have

Specular microscopy can be very helpful in assessing endothelial cell count in patients with Fuchs endothelial corneal dystrophy and the less common nonguttate corneal endothelial dystrophies. Some refractive cataract surgeons perform these tests routinely on all patients before surgery, though this is not considered the standard of care. Naturally, the corneal endothelium can and should be assessed clinically at the slit lamp with specular reflection, and visual inspection will generally identify the presence of central guttate that can reduce contrast sensitivity even when endothelial function is preserved. The added benefit of a specular microscope is the ability to calculate cell density. This calculation, when combined with corneal thickness measured by a pachymeter, can be useful.

Ultrasound pachymetry can provide predictive value, helping identify patients who are more likely to have corneal decompensation. Generally, patients with central endothelial cell density less than 1000 cells/mm^2 with corneal thickness greater than 600 microns are in a high-risk group, especially if the lens nucleus is brunescent or other comorbidities (such as pseudoexfoliation) make surgery challenging or risky.

Dry eye diagnostics, such as tear film osmolarity and testing for matrix metalloproteinases, allow objective measurement of a patient's dry eye. Many clinicians choose to perform these tests to identify patients at risk for postoperative dry eye, and some use the test outcomes to educate patients as to why strict adherence to dry eye treatment regimens is necessary for the desired outcome. In Chapter 4, Dr. Jodi Luchs will further explore this topic and a proven approach to managing dry eye in these special patients.

Excimer laser surgery is a simple and effective way to correct residual refractive error after cataract surgery. It allows precision that cannot be matched by other methods of enhancement like piggyback lens placement or incisional enhancements and permits correction of residual astigmatism. Naturally, investing in an excimer laser only makes sense for a practice that offers laser refractive surgery as a revenue stream to defray the cost of the instrument. Having access to a laser in some manner helps make enhancements easy to recommend and perform. This is highly important, because the most common cause of patient dissatisfaction with refractive cataract surgery is residual refractive error—a problem that is generally easily remedied.

Talking the Talk

The second prerequisite to succeeding with premium cataract surgery is mastering personal communication with patients about expected and delivered results. This task is far more challenging and uncomfortable than the first for most surgeons, who are already able to perform predictable procedures. Why is this? The traditional doctor-patient relationship is governed by what psychologists call a *social norm*, yet when a patient pays out-of-pocket for an outcome of reduced spectacle independence, we introduce into the relationship elements of a *market norm*.[4]

To better understand social norms and market norms, consider what happens when an ophthalmic technician—let's call her Amy—overwhelmed with an overbooked clinic schedule, works extra hard to perform workups in a timely manner, turns on extra charm with patients so they will remain calm despite delays, and stays late to make sure everyone is taken care of. Exhausted, before going home, she asks the doctor if there is anything else he needs. The doctor says, "Amy, I know you were really a trooper today. Thank you so much for looking out for our patients and taking a personal interest in them." No matter how well Amy is paid, she feels she worked above the call of duty. She genuinely appreciates the praise and will most certainly repeat the same good behavior the next time the schedule is so overbooked.

What if the doctor, instead of praising her at the end of the day, handed the technician a $20 bill and unappreciatively said, "This is for staying late." Most of us know (hopefully not from making this mistake!) that Amy would not feel the least bit rewarded for her good behavior. Her attitude would more likely be, "Is *that* what he thinks my extra effort is worth? I saved his practice today, and all he gives me is $20?"

Why is the first response, verbal praise, which has no material value, much more desirable than a monetary reward? Because when a boss gives praise, the interchange is governed by a social norm, where the technician's hard work is a "gift" to her boss—a courtesy. It is returned in kind with a courtesy—a gift of praise and thanks. When the boss gives $20, the interchange puts a numeric value on her "gift." The boss expresses no appreciation. Their relationship is suddenly governed by market forces, or a market norm. Predictably, Amy has a feeling of underappreciation.

In the traditional doctor-patient relationship, a patient seeks a physician's aid for relief from a medical problem, placing all his or her confidence in the doctor and trusting that he or she will choose the best medicines and materials for curing the ailment. To the best of his or her ability, the doctor renders treatment, and the patient understands that, whatever the result, it is the best that nature will allow. In traditional cataract surgery, even though the patient pays the doctor for the service, this payment is usually through a third-party payer, which isolates the patient from quantification of the payment. In fact, the financial aspect of the exchange is almost never discussed between doctor and patient. The physician performs his or her age-old duty, and the patient is grateful. This relationship is, therefore, governed by a social norm.

Enter refractive cataract surgery. No longer is the doctor merely curing an ailment. He or she is offering some degree of spectacle independence, a result that insurance carriers deem *medically unnecessary*. In doing so, he or she is seeking to profit from these added costs. There are counselors who function in a sales capacity and color brochures. This shifts the psychology of at least this part of the doctor-patient exchange to a market norm.

This shift in mental rules from those of social to those of market norms explains why refractive cataract patients are so much more demanding than those electing traditional results. Simply put, they expect to get what they've paid for.

This does *not* mean that offering refractive cataract surgery reduces the trust and admiration between doctor and patient. The most successful refractive cataract surgeons do not find their relationships with patients diminished by this dynamic but, rather, enhanced. Those surgeons who convey through words and body language a desire to deliver superior vision generally find that patients respond with appreciation and acceptance of this new concept despite the added costs.

Conveying genuine interest and confidence that the patient's expectations will be exceeded is not a communication process that can be faked. Those surgeons who don't completely believe their added services are worth the cost would do better not to offer them. A surgeon who will be annoyed by Mrs. Jones questioning the quality of her uncorrected vision after surgery of 20/25 and Jaeger 2 needs to rethink whether he or she is prepared for managing the psychology of refractive surgery patients. Mrs. Jones is most likely not an unreasonable person. She needs education in what to expect.

In Chapter 8, I will present 10 principles for communicating with patients before surgery. In Chapter 18, Drs. Eric Donnenfeld, Alanna Nattis, Eric Rosenberg, and Allon Barsam will give *7 Cs* as reasons why postoperative patients can be unhappy and explore techniques for communicating that don't erode the physician-patient relationship. Moreover, a growing number of courses and symposia at national and regional eye meetings are beginning to teach these principles using video and live role-playing, which demonstrate these concepts in a way that cannot be captured in this or any textbook. The successful refractive cataract surgeon seeks out these opportunities to learn better communication skills and continuously evaluates his or her own words from the perspective of the sometimes-unhappy patient. It's not enough to just operate. We must also educate.

References

1. American Society of Cataract and Refractive Surgery. IOL power calculation in eyes that have undergone LASIK/PRK/RK. http://iolcalc.ascrs.org/. Updated 2015. Accessed January 4, 2017.
2. Conrad-Hengerer I, Al Juburi M, Schultz T, Hengerer FH, Dick HB. Corneal endothelial cell loss and corneal thickness in conventional compared with femtosecond laser-assisted cataract surgery: three-month follow-up. *J Cataract Refract Surg.* 2013;39(9):1307-1313.
3. Abell RG, Allen PL, Vote BJ. Anterior chamber flare after femtosecond laser-assisted cataract surgery. *J Cataract Refract Surg.* 2013;39(9):1321-1326.
4. Ariely D. *Predictably Irrational: The Hidden Forces That Shape Our Decisions.* New York, NY: HarperCollins; 2008.

Chapter 2

Refractive Intraocular Lenses
Everyday Ethical Issues

David F. Chang, MD and Bryan S. Lee, MD, JD

The availability of presbyopia-correcting intraocular lenses (IOL) and the Centers for Medicare and Medicaid Services ruling allowing patients to pay for them out of pocket as noncovered refractive services have dramatically altered the practice of every cataract and refractive surgeon. Ready or not, the availability of these options has made every cataract patient a potential refractive patient. Furthermore, presbyopic patients who believed laser vision correction to be the only refractive procedure available now have entirely different surgical alternatives to consider. These myriad new options and the premium remuneration that they command create a number of ethical issues for ophthalmologists. In a profession in which the IOL industry spends a great deal of money to market products to us, we have the challenge and the important responsibility of educating patients as objectively as possible.

Offering and explaining the option of reduced spectacle dependence would be far easier if we had an IOL technology that consistently eliminated the need for eyeglasses in every patient. The benefit would be easy to understand, and qualified candidates would decide what they wanted based upon the affordability of this option. Lacking such an elegant solution, we and our patients must analyze and understand the potential benefits and tradeoffs of current refractive IOLs, knowing that the results will vary from one individual to the next.

Patients consulting a plastic surgeon already understand that their interest in elective cosmetic surgery is not because of a health need or recommendation. This concept may not be clear, however, to patients hearing about refractive IOLs for the first time prior to scheduling cataract surgery. Already somewhat confused about cataracts and IOLs, many patients won't understand the distinction between what is the refractive treatment and what is the cataract treatment. They may not understand that the financial decision

Hovanesian JA.
Refractive Cataract Surgery: Best Practices and Advanced Technology, Second Edition (pp 9-14). © 2017 SLACK Incorporated.

they are being asked to make concerns lifestyle benefits, such as convenience, rather than what is "best" for their eyes.

The nature of medical ethics is such that reasonable minds may have differing opinions and philosophies about a particular issue. However, we probably all agree that the essence of ethical practice means treating our patients in the same way that we and our families would want to be treated in an identical situation. With that in mind, what are some common ethical issues that cataract and refractive surgeons now face with respect to refractive IOLs?

Should Every Patient Undergoing Cataract Surgery Be Informed of These Options?

We believe that most patients want to hear about all of their options prior to cataract surgery. Even if they are not a good multifocal IOL candidate, they would prefer to have the surgeon explain why rather than to learn about this option later from a boastful friend. The question "Why wasn't I told about this option?" may arise long after the patient was discharged from the surgeon's care. If left unanswered, this doubt may be a nagging source of confusion or disappointment. What if the surgeon does not offer these IOLs? If you are worried about the drawbacks of these implants, you can share your concerns with your patients. However, you should then be willing to refer that patient if, after your discussion, you determine that he or she is an excellent candidate who wants a presbyopia-correcting or other refractive IOL.

Another issue might be one that we call *financial profiling*. Based upon their attire or their home address, it is tempting to assume that certain individuals would not be able to afford a premium IOL. Such assumptions are often but not always accurate. We believe that patients would be disappointed to learn that certain options were not explained to them because it was assumed that they could not afford them. Instead, we should still explain the choices, but in a way that is sensitive to their needs and means.

What About New Technology in the Pipeline?

This is an important question, as we have all read about improved IOL technologies being developed for the future. For instance, one practice consultant in the early 1990s recommended that with the anticipated approval of the excimer laser and the ensuing competitive free-for-all, now was the time to establish one's reputation as a refractive surgeon by learning to perform radial keratotomy. But how would a patient feel seeing all of the ads touting the new laser's advantages less than 1 year after having had bilateral radial keratotomy?

For cataract patients, the decision is often simple. Unless a better technology is imminently available, we would want our own family member to enjoy the benefits of cataract surgery now rather than later. Some of our current refractive IOLs took 10 or more years following initial human implantation to gain Food and Drug Administration approval. Even after it was finally approved, it took widespread clinical use of the Array IOL (Abbott Medical Optics) to truly understand its capabilities and limitations. Meanwhile, postponing cataract surgery that is otherwise functionally indicated may increase the risk of falls or traffic accidents.

Refractive lens exchange (RLE) patients are a different story. We all acknowledge that current refractive IOL technology is imperfect, and this is why so many of us are reluctant to perform RLE for a presbyopic emmetrope. RLE is a legitimate option for hyperopes and myopes who are presbyopic. However, if we were myopic, we would want to be told about the uncertain but higher risk of retinal detachment in pseudophakes. We would also want to know if there were a better technology on the foreseeable horizon worth waiting for. This might not influence a frustrated high hyperope who has become contact lens–intolerant and increasingly presbyopic. On the other hand, consider a presbyopic myope who is reasonably happy with contact lenses but came in for a LASIK consultation only to learn that this won't eliminate reading glasses. Although he or she may be a multifocal IOL-RLE candidate, this patient might prefer to wait for better IOL technology if this possibility were explained.

How Aggressively Should our Practice Promote This Option to Patients?

Compared to radial keratotomy, LASIK is a great procedure. In appropriate candidates, there are very few risks and downsides, the benefit is stable, and the satisfaction rate is extremely high. Marketing not only spreads the word about this exciting procedure but can help to justify the significant cost by defining the potential benefits. In our opinion, presbyopia-correcting IOLs are not yet on par with laser vision correction in terms of patient satisfaction. Costs aside, there are inherent optical drawbacks with multifocal IOLs that must be counterbalanced by that patient's strong motivation to see without glasses. In a significant percentage of patients, the potential upside to multifocal IOLs outweighs the downside; in many other patients, it does not.

The manner by which patients are informed about these options is therefore very important. In most cataract practices, the majority of patients will still receive a monofocal IOL. Over-touting presbyopia-correcting IOLs through internal marketing may leave those who cannot have or afford them feeling shortchanged. It is also very easy for patients to misunderstand and think that the more expensive lens is better for their eyes. If they could afford to, most patients would pay extra for a technology that benefited their ocular health, particularly if they perceived that the doctor favored it. "My eyes are important to me," we so often hear. Historically, this was the concern that the Centers for Medicare and Medicaid Services had with allowing surgeons to balance-bill patients for noncovered services. Would some surgeons take advantage of less sophisticated patients by selling them on costly upgrades that they didn't need? It is important that patients who choose these premium technologies understand the real nature of the refractive benefits.

Can I Maintain Objectivity Despite Strong Financial Incentives?

The higher the reimbursement, the more important this question becomes. As physicians, we have enormous power to influence elective decisions that our patients make. This is only true because patients trust us to make treatment recommendations without regard to which choice is more profitable to us. The tradition of implicit patient trust in this fundamental responsibility has been forged throughout the long course of modern medical history. Putting ourselves in our patient's shoes should guide each of us with respect to issues such as co-management, specialist referrals, and recommendations for testing and procedures.

In the end, being constantly mindful of this responsibility provides us with good guidance. Patients can accept that you tried your best on their behalf, even if they are disappointed with their postoperative vision. However, by virtue of the high out-of-pocket premium that they paid, unhappy refractive IOL patients may look back and view what they perceive to have been promotion or sales pressure with suspicion. Your unhappiest refractive IOL patients will be those who are dissatisfied and believe that someone in your practice talked them into choosing the more expensive IOL.

Should Surgery Be Billed to the Insurance Company?

For insurance purposes, if the decision to have lens replacement surgery is because of visually significant cataract symptoms, then it should be billed as cataract surgery. On the other hand, if the patient's primary motivation for surgery is the correction of refractive error, then it should be billed as an RLE, which is not medically necessary. Insurance companies rely upon the surgeon to make this distinction. The reason why the operation is or is not covered by insurance should also be explained to the patient. This decision is similar to that involved in other elective surgeries, such as ptosis, in which the functional indications must be distinguished from the cosmetic motivation.

What Is a Fair Price for a Noncovered Service?

Are patients currently being overcharged? Unlike prescription medications and gasoline, refractive surgery and refractive IOLs are luxury items. As long as patients understand the optional and elective nature of this service, they can ultimately judge the value of the service and whether the cost is fair. We certainly don't profess to know what the correct premium charge should be. However, we believe that additional surgical time is not the deciding factor. For instance, the charge for elective astigmatic keratotomy is based on the knowledge of when and how to correct astigmatism at the time of cataract surgery, not the additional operative time. Refractive IOL surgery undeniably raises the bar, both in terms of patient expectations and necessary surgical precision. Offering these IOLs requires an entirely different level of preoperative evaluation, counseling, and education. The necessary commitment to excellence is significant, and the value of the professional component of reducing spectacle dependence should not be calculated based on the additional surgical time or preoperative testing necessary to implant these IOLs. For a patient, it is what lies between the surgeon's 2 ears that matters most: knowledge, experience, preparation, clinical judgment, compassion, and the ethical commitment to do what is best.

How Should I Handle Residual Postoperative Refractive Error?

Some physicians include the potential cost for laser vision enhancement to correct residual refractive error in their charge for a multifocal IOL. Others choose not to increase their price for the premium IOL, but they should be prepared for the need to discuss the cost of laser keratorefractive surgery after cataract surgery. Patients may understandably be upset to be asked to make an additional out-of-pocket payment postoperatively; surgeons taking the latter approach should therefore discuss this possibility before the cataract operation, especially in patients at higher risk of having residual refractive error.

Other alternatives to address refractive error include intraocular lens exchange and astigmatic keratotomy. Cataract surgeons who do not perform laser vision correction may utilize these procedures effectively but should be willing to refer patients elsewhere if surface ablation or LASIK is a superior option.

How Do I Communicate About Surgical Complications?

According to the Institute of Medicine, transparency is an essential characteristic of quality care. It is difficult to discuss any type of bad outcome or complication with a patient, and this may be even harder when that patient has paid extra to receive a refractive IOL or has been referred by another provider. However, this type of honest communication is necessary both before and after surgery.

The patient has the right to know what has occurred, what the prognosis is, and what the plan is for optimal outcome. Second, there is evidence that this type of discussion decreases the likelihood of a lawsuit. Third, disclosing physicians may experience less guilt and emotional distress. We are fortunate that cataract surgery has such a high success rate and is so beneficial to our patients, but the saying "The only surgeon without complications is one who doesn't operate" is true. In these rare situations, we should be prepared to act ethically and compassionately and treat our patient as we would want our own family member treated in the same situation.

How Should I Discuss the Femtosecond Laser With Patients?

Advertising for femtosecond laser should adhere to the relevant legal and ethical restrictions. Broad claims that this is superior to conventional cataract surgery are not supported by the peer-reviewed literature at this time. As with presbyopia-correcting

IOLs, strong promotion may cause patients not having this technology to feel short-changed.

Preoperatively, surgeons who do use the femtosecond laser for cataract surgery should discuss the laser with patients honestly and using the best available scientific evidence. In the United States, this discussion should recognize the fact that Medicare patients are only permitted to pay out of pocket for the femtosecond laser technology's refractive benefits. In situations and cases in which surgeons feel that the femtosecond laser would improve outcomes, this should be explained to the patient in a way that clarifies the elective and noncovered status of the laser. Large studies involving several thousands of patients do not currently support a general claim of increased safety. As with any new technology, the risk-benefit and cost-benefit analyses may evolve over time and with a patient's or surgeon's individual situation.

Medical decisions require balancing the benefits vs the risks. There are arguably stronger ethical considerations when presenting elective options requiring out-of-pocket payment. The added expense may pose a financial burden to many patients, who must rely on their surgeon's advice regarding the importance or advisability of these options. Cataract surgeons should therefore avoid being overly promotional of any refractive IOL technology and should be especially careful regarding the femtosecond laser because the implications of using a laser are easily misunderstood by patients.

Most of us are reluctant to place a price on safety, but the value of refractive enhancement is very personal and subjective. Patients need our unbiased help to understand the difference between medical and refractive benefits when deciding whether they should spend the extra fees. They trust us to place our own financial conflicts of interest aside and to advise and act in their best interest. This is the essence of ethical practice.

Chapter 3

Prognostic Predictors for Premium Intraocular Lenses

George O. Waring IV, MD;
R. Luke Rebenitsch, MD, PCEO;
and Jason E. Stahl, MD

The advent of toric and presbyopia-correcting intraocular lenses (IOLs) has minimized the distinction between refractive and cataract surgeons. With refractive IOLs, however, it is no longer possible to choose a single go-to lens for all patients. Instead, the lens must be matched to the patient's lifestyle. As no IOL is perfect, it is necessary to understand the patient's comprehension and tolerance for the trade-offs involved with any IOL. Tracking patient outcomes can help identify important factors that determine level of satisfaction with a premium IOL.

The arena of premium IOLs continues to change rapidly. New concepts in presbyopia-correcting IOLs, such as chromatic aberration-reducing, extended depth-of-focus IOLs (Symfony, Abbott Medical Optics [AMO]), dual-optic accommodating IOLs (AMO), IOL optics that can change their curvature with accommodation (NuLens; FluidVision Lens, PowerVision Inc), and electroactive optics (Elenza, PixelOptics) are in clinical trials, currently available outside the United States, or in development. Even monofocal IOLs are seeing breakthroughs, such as the Calhoun Light Adjustable Lens (Calhoun Vision), which will allow for post-implantation changes in refraction. As the variety of premium IOLs and the understanding of how to match the patient to these lenses increase, patient groups that were once considered unsuitable for premium IOLs, such as post-LASIK patients or anisometropic patients,[1] are now starting to achieve successful results with premium IOLs.[2,3]

The current choices in refractive IOLs include toric IOLs, multifocal IOLs (including refractive and diffractive IOLs), and accommodating IOLs. Each of the presbyopia-correcting IOLs has different strengths and weaknesses. As a result of light splitting with multifocal IOLs, eyes tend to have diminished contrast sensitivity in dim light and more reports of halos and glare than accommodating IOLs, which produce only a single image at the retina

Hovanesian JA.
Refractive Cataract Surgery: Best Practices and Advanced Technology, Second Edition (pp 15-25).

Table 3-1
Food and Drug Administration–Approved Presbyopia-Correcting Refractive IOLs, Their Spectacle Plane Add Power, and Design

Company	*IOL*	*Spectacle Plane Add Power*	*Presbyopia-Correcting Design*
Alcon	ReSTOR +3	+2.5	Diffractive multifocal
Alcon	ReSTOR +2.5	+2	Diffractive multifocal
AMO	Tecnis MF +4	+3	Diffractive multifocal
AMO	Tecnis MF +3.25	+2.37	Diffractive multifocal
AMO	Tecnis MF +2.75	+2.01	Diffractive multifocal
AMO	ReZoom	+2.85	Refractive zonal multifocal
Bausch & Lomb	Crystalens AO	N/A	Accommodating
Bausch & Lomb	Trulign	N/A	Accommodating and astigmatic
Tecnis	Symfony IOL	N/A	Extended depth of focus

without splitting of light. The induction of higher-order aberrations and perception of halos is proportional to the separation of focal point with lower add powers having less-perceived halos and easier neuroadaptation; although this is being diminished with improved engineering.[4] Multifocal IOLs are also sensitive to decentration, which can impact visual acuity and quality.[5,6] Currently available accommodating IOLs are subject to variance in effective lens position and the resultant variance in postoperative refractive target.

Multifocal IOLs now have a much broader range of near points than in the past. In the United States, all Food and Drug Administration–approved multifocal lenses are bifocal. Trifocal IOLs with distance, intermediate, and near focal points are available elsewhere. For patients with the greatest near vision requirement, there is the Tecnis MF +4 (AMO). The trade-off is weaker intermediate visual acuity. For patients with more intermediate vision requirements, there are many more options. Currently available multifocal IOLs are the ReSTOR +3 (Alcon), ReSTOR +2.5 (Alcon), Tecnis MF +3.25 (AMO), Tecnis MF +2.75 (AMO), and ReZoom (AMO). Accommodating IOLs include the Crystalens AO IOL (Bausch & Lomb) and astigmatism-treating Trulign (Bausch & Lomb), which provide better intermediate visual acuity but less near acuity. These presbyopia-correcting IOLs, along with their spectacle plane, add powers, and method of presbyopia correction can be seen in Table 3-1. Presbyopia-correcting IOLs can also be combined, one in each eye, to increase a patient's range of near-intermediate vision, although caution needs to be taken due to the difference in IOL design, optics, and neuroadaptation processes.

Toric Intraocular Lenses

Until recently there has only been one toric presbyopia-correcting IOL available in the United States: the accommodating Trulign; although toric, multifocal, and accommodating IOLs have been available outside the United States and in US clinical trials. The Symfony Toric IOL, which works through extending depth of focus, is the newest astigmatism correcting premium IOL. These IOLS are an excellent lens choice for patients desiring astigmatism correction and a presbyopia correction IOL. In refractive cataract or refractive lens exchange patients with astigmatism, a decision must be made whether to use one of these toric presbyopia-correcting IOLs, to use a multifocal IOL with corneal astigmatic correction, or to correct just the astigmatism with a monofocal toric IOL. First, toric IOLs may not be appropriate for patients with high degrees of irregular astigmatism. For patients not desiring presbyopia correction, we usually recommend a toric IOL for those patients with significant astigmatism (> 2.0 diopters [D]) over limbal relaxing incisions (LRI). Toric IOLs with monovision are also a reasonable choice for people with high astigmatism who wish to reduce dependency on spectacles. For high astigmatism patients who are committed to having a presbyopia-correcting IOL, we make sure they understand that a second corneal procedure (LASIK, photorefractive keratectomy [PRK], or LRIs) will be necessary to correct the astigmatism and allow them to receive the full benefit of the IOL.

Toric IOLs are an excellent introduction to implementing a refractive style approach in a cataract practice. They require a little more chair time and some education on how a toric IOL can improve vision, but not as much as for the presbyopia-correction patient. When using the Trulign, patients are also usually less demanding, as they expect some spectacle wear after surgery.

Presbyopia-Correcting Intraocular Lenses

Astigmatism Correction

Greater than 0.50 D of astigmatism should be surgically addressed when implanting any presbyopia-correcting IOL. A database survey by Kezirian[7] demonstrated the decrease in uncorrected distance visual acuity with residual cylinder of greater than 0.75 D (Figure 3-1).

LASIK or other corneal procedures can be combined with implantation of a presbyopia-correcting IOL. Low levels of astigmatism (≤ 1.75 D) can be managed with LRIs.[8]

Refractive Cataract Patient Assessment

The preoperative examination for refractive cataract surgery should include, but may not be limited to, determination of eye dominance, visual acuity, refraction, and keratometry. Corneal topography is necessary for all patients to detect highly aberrated eyes that do not do well with multifocal IOLs, or any other corneal abnormality, to check ocular surface quality, and to plan for astigmatism management. There should be agreement between topographic and keratometric cylinder magnitude. If not, carefully repeat measurements and plan for lenticular astigmatism that may be additive or subtractive

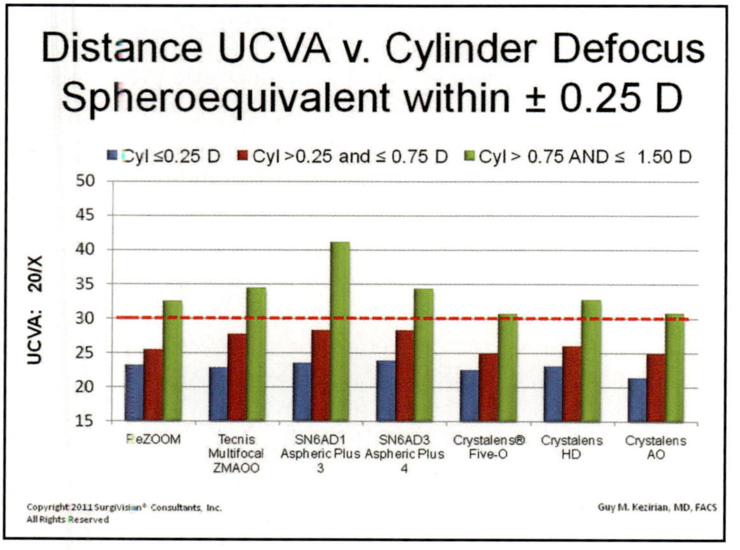

Figure 3-1. Uncorrected distance visual acuity (UCDVA) vs cylinder defocus. All eyes have spherical equivalent ± 0.25 D. Increase in cylinder decreases UCDVA for all presbyopia-correcting IOLs. (Reprinted with permission from Guy Kezirian, MD, FACS.)

depending on the relative meridians. Pupil size should be measured in bright and dim light. A careful dilated fundus examination and macular optical coherence tomography can help identify retinal pathology that may affect outcomes.

The popularity of corneal refractive surgical procedures such as PRK and LASIK has raised patient expectations for excellent vision without spectacles or contact lenses. In our practice, we have found a significant increase of patients in their 50s and 60s coming in for LASIK because of a decrease in quality of their vision. They have good Snellen acuity, although they have decreased contrast sensitivity and are losing accommodative amplitude. We find that the crystalline lens in these patients frequently has lenticular opacities that increase forward light scatter, decrease contrast sensitivity, and increase spherical aberration (Figure 3-2). We term this *dysfunctional lens syndrome* (DLS).

The Dysfunctional Lens Syndrome and Refractive Lens Exchange Patient Assessment

Not all patients have a loss of Snellen visual acuity sufficient to meet the medical diagnostic criteria of cataract. However, the increase in light scatter, loss of contrast sensitivity, and sensitivity to glare can impact a patient's quality of life. DLS can be measured with advanced diagnostics such as Scheimpflug imaging and Hartmann-Shack aberrometry as well as double pass aberrometry, ray tracing, and contrast sensitivity measures. The double pass AcuTarget HD (Visiometrics) displays point spread function and a simulated loss of clarity of the retinal image. The ray tracing, iTrace (Tracey Technologies), separates corneal aberrations from crystalline lens aberrations, allowing the surgeon to locate the cause of the visual disturbances along the visual axis as well as objectively determine whether the cornea is too aberrated to allow for good vision with a multifocal IOL. Both the double pass and ray tracing system help patients understand that a refractive procedure such as LASIK may not address these changes due to degradation of the crystalline lens. Patients with DLS may also be good candidates for lens

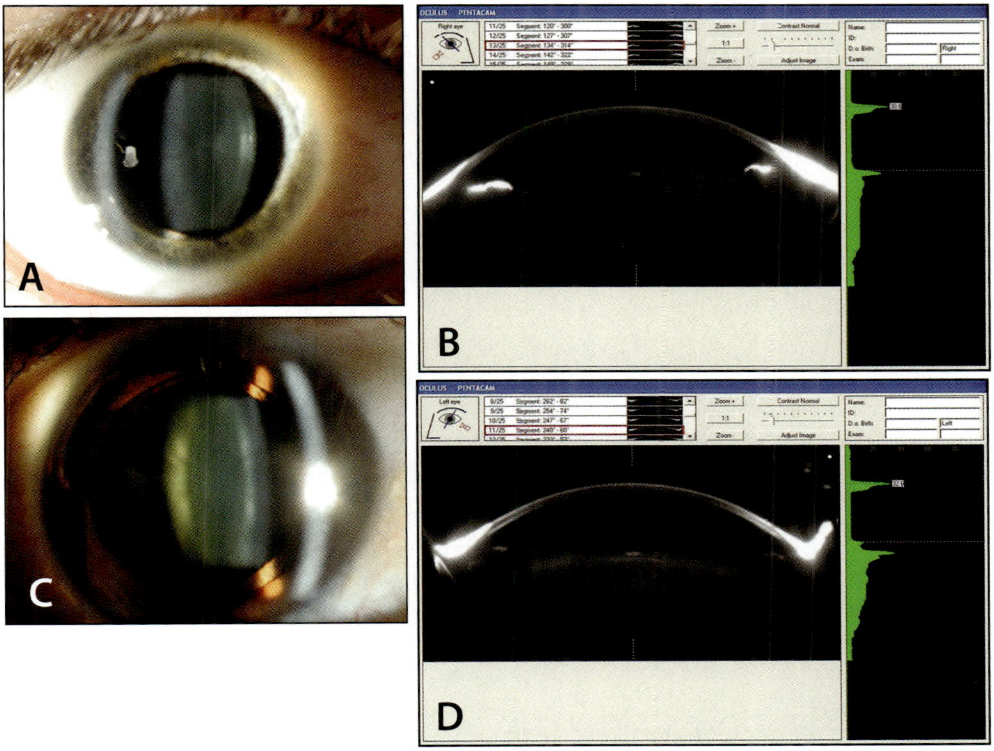

Figure 3-2. (A) Slit-lamp photograph and (B) the Pentacam densitometry chart of a clear lens. (C) Slit-lamp photograph and (D) the Pentacam densitometry chart of a lens with early nuclear sclerosis.

extraction followed by implantation of a presbyopia-correcting IOL. The clinical assessment and approach to these patients is the same as for a cataract patient interested in a presbyopia-correcting IOL.

Lens Position

Toric and multifocal IOLs must be centered on the patient's estimated line of sight for maximum effect. IOL decentration can result in blurred vision or photic phenomena.[5] Conditions such as a high Chang-Waring (CW) axis and reflex or exotropia are contraindications for implanting a multifocal IOL.[9] A high CW, the angle between the visual and the optical axes, makes it difficult to center a multifocal IOL on the eye's line of site. As a result, preoperative planning and intraoperative attention to centration of a multifocal IOL on the estimated line of sight with a coaxially fixated light source is recommended. Diagnostic equipment such as the iTrace and OPD-Scan III (Marco) objectively measure a variation of CW. Accommodating IOLs that are designed to be aspherically neutral are more tolerant of decentration and are a better choice in patients with conditions in which alignment of the visual axis and the pupil with the IOL is difficult, such as high angle alpha and anomalous fixators.

One of the factors that remains unpredictable is the final position of the lens in the capsular bag, or effective lens position. For those patients with a large capsule or other anatomic variation that suggests an unpredictable lens position, we avoid accommodating

IOLs. Capsular fibrosis can have a large impact on effective lens position and, as a result, a low threshold for early yttrium-aluminum-garnet capsulotomy is recommended with the currently available accommodating IOLs.

Pupil Size

Small pupils (<3 mm) can lead to decreased near visual acuity in refractive IOLs such as the ReZoom. The ReZoom has concentric alternating distance and near optical zones. With a small pupil, a greater percentage of the overall light passes through the central, distance-dominant zone, with less light available for the more peripheral near zone. In ReSTOR IOLs, small pupils may be unable to take advantage of the peripheral concentric zone for distance vision designed to minimize photic phenomena. Patients with larger pupils are more likely than those with smaller pupils to experience photic phenomena[10] and to notice existing higher-order aberrations, which may manifest as night-vision problems.[11] For these patients, an accommodating IOL may be more appropriate. In Tecnis MF IOLs, light is split equally between near and distance at all pupil sizes, making them essentially pupil-independent. This allows them to have improved mesopic near vision over the ReSTOR, but it also increases the risk of halos from higher-order aberrations.[12,13]

Patient Needs

The primary question for patients who may be suitable for implantation of a multifocal IOL is, "Would you like to be less dependent on your glasses?" For those patients motivated to decrease their need for spectacles, a premium IOL may be indicated. Further assessment of the patient's vision needs, such as driving at night, favorite sports or crafts, and computer and reading habits, will determine which premium IOL is appropriate. A patient who frequently drives at night may prefer an accommodating IOL rather than a multifocal IOL, as the multifocal IOLs tend to produce more glare and lower contrast sensitivity than the single-focus accommodating IOLs.[14] Conversely, a heavy reader or someone with a hobby demanding good near visual acuity may be better served by a multifocal IOL. Young patients with clear lenses who are not experiencing loss of contrast from early nuclear sclerosis tend to be heavily reliant on computers (immediate vision) and should be counseled appropriately that no perfect lens exists. The Symfony IOL provides more halos than an accommodating IOL, but fewer than a multifocal IOL. Naturally, there is no universally accepted set of rules for pairing patients and lenses, but these kinds of considerations are worth thinking about in this process. A patient questionnaire can be helpful in identifying each individual's visual needs. Many surgeons have developed their own questionnaires tailored to their practice. One developed by Steven Dell, MD[15] is available at http://crstoday.com/articles/2015-sep/monovisions-role-in-cataract-surgery (Figure 3-3).

Managing Patient Expectations

Taking the time to talk to the patient is essential. It is important that it is the patient, not the surgeon, who makes the decision to move to a premium IOL. We typically tell patients interested in presbyopia-correcting IOLs that spectacles of some variety are in

Date__________ Name__________________________

Cataract and Refractive Lens Exchange Questionnaire

The term "cataract" refers to a cloudy lens within the eye. When a cataract is removed, an artificial lens is placed inside the eye to take the place of the human lens that has become the cataract. Occasionally, clear lenses that have not yet developed cataracts are also removed to reduce or eliminate the need for glasses or contacts. If it is determined that surgery is appropriate for you, this questionnaire will help us provide the best treatment for your visual needs. It is important that you understand that many patients still need to wear glasses for some activities after surgery. Please fill this form out completely and give it to the doctor. If you have questions, please let us know and we will assist you with this form.

1. After surgery, would you be interested in seeing well **without glasses** in the following situations?

Distance vision (driving, golf, tennis, other sports, watching TV)
___Prefer no **Distance** glasses. ___ I wouldn't mind wearing **Distance** glasses.

Mid-range vision. (computer, menus, price tags, cooking, board games, items on a shelf)
___Prefer no **Mid-range** glasses. ___ I wouldn't mind wearing **Mid-range** glasses.

Near vision (reading books, newspapers, magazines, detailed handwork)
___Prefer no **Near** glasses. ___ I wouldn't mind wearing **Near** glasses.

2. Please check the **single** statement that best describes you in terms of **night vision**:
___ a. Night vision is extremely important to me, and I require the best possible quality night vision.
___ b. I want to be able to drive comfortably at night, but I would tolerate some slight imperfections.
___ c. Night vision is not particularly important to me.

3. If you **had** to wear glasses after surgery for one activity, for which activity would you be **most** willing to use glasses? ____**Distance Vision.** ____**Mid-range Vision.** ____**Near Vision.**

4. If you could have good **Distance Vision during the day without glasses**, and good **Near Vision for reading without glasses**, but the compromise was that you might see some **halos or rings** around lights at night, would you like that option? ____Yes ____No

5. If you could have good **Distance vision during the day and night** without glasses, and good **Mid-range Vision** without glasses, but the compromise was that you might need glasses for reading the finest print at near, would you like that option? ____Yes ____No

6. Surgery to reduce or eliminate your dependence upon glasses for **Distance, Mid-range and Near Vision** may be partially covered by insurance if you have a cataract that is covered by insurance. Would you be interested in learning more about this option?
____Yes ____No ____Maybe, it depends on how much is covered by insurance.

7. Please place an "X" on the following scale to describe your personality as best you can:

[--I--]
Easy going Perfectionist

Please Sign Here

Figure 3-3. Patient survey developed by Steven Dell, MD. (Reprinted with permission from Steven Dell.)

their future, but we explain that the real goal is to reduce their need for glasses to a bare minimum. Technology is not yet capable of replicating the action of a young, clear, accommodating crystalline lens. Patients who seem unhappy with the concept that they may not be 100% spectacle-free need special counseling and may not be good candidates for a premium IOL.[15] Patients may also need to understand that they may need some fine-tuning of their vision with a corneal refractive procedure to get the maximum benefit from a premium IOL. In other circumstances, a piggyback IOL may be preferred for residual refractive error. The patients should understand that a lens exchange may be indicated if they are truly unable to tolerate a premium IOL.

Finally, the maxim for successful management of patient expectations with premium IOLs, as with any refractive procedure, is, “under promise and over deliver.”

Patient Personality

A good premium lens candidate takes a realistic approach and understands the limitations of corneal IOL technology. Patients who understand and accept the trade-offs of each type of premium IOL are usually happy with a good outcome. Beware of patients who are very demanding; they may be poor candidates for presbyopia-correcting IOLs, as well as patients who are uncooperative. Other unlikely candidates for presbyopia-correcting IOLs are individuals who are depressive, obsessive, or compulsive. Although extremely observant, detail-oriented individuals are usually considered poor candidates for presbyopia-correcting IOLs, they may be good candidates if they are counseled correctly on the trade-offs of these IOLs.

Preoperative Refractive Error

Spherical hyperopes are a good group to start with for presbyopia-correcting IOLs. Since middle adulthood, they have worn glasses for near vision and will appreciate the decreased need for spectacle wear. At the other end of the spectrum, low myopes may be less impressed with their near vision with a presbyopia-correcting IOL.[16] They can require extra chair time to make sure they have appropriate expectations. Individuals who have been very happy with contact lenses and monovision may notice somewhat less clarity with multifocal IOLs, due to the multiple focal planes of the IOL.

For those patients whose refractive error was previously treated by LASIK or other corneal procedures, multifocal IOLs may not be recommended, although small treatments and/or more recent technologies may not result in a cornea with too many higher-order aberrations. Due to compounding higher-order aberrations, an accommodating IOL with an aspherically neutral optic is an excellent choice for patients with questionably aberrated corneas. For the greatest benefit, accurate targeting of multifocal IOLs is essential. Due to errors in keratometric measures, IOL power calculation is more difficult in patients who have undergone a refractive procedure. However, recent studies have shown that good visual outcomes in patients previously treated for myopia with LASIK can be achieved.[2,3]

Dry Eye

We strongly recommend ocular surface optimization prior to implant of a premium IOL. Accurate topography is an essential diagnostic tool for surgical planning, particularly when addressing astigmatism. Significant topographic errors as well as inaccurate optical biometry may result from dryness. Many patients have undiagnosed dry eye syndrome. Many perimenopausal women also need to be treated for dry eye prior to surgery. Critical vital dye evaluation, osmolarity testing (TearLab), AcuTarget HD dry eye testing (Visiometrics), Schirmer test, or tear breakup time may help identify patients with dry eye. Patients with dry eye may be put on artificial tears, topical steroids, oral omega-3 fatty acids, topical azithromycin, and topical cyclosporine prior to surgery. Punctal plugs are also effective in relieving some forms of dry eye. In patients with more moderate dry eyes primarily due to meibomian gland dysfunction, LipiFlow (Tear Science) can be considered. In patients with severe dry eye, a piggyback IOL is preferable to a corneal procedure if a postoperative touch-up is needed. Finally, accommodating IOLs may be the best option for dry eye patients, due to the light-splitting effect of multifocal IOLs.

Contraindications

Multifocal and extended depth of focus IOLs are generally not recommended in patients with moderate or severe dry eye, significant wavefront higher-order aberrations, previous corneal refractive procedures (LASIK, PRK, radial keratotomy, or conductive keratoplasty), significant Fuchs dystrophy, significant corneal scarring, pseudoexfoliation, or ocular conditions such as age-related macular degeneration and epiretinal membrane. Accommodating IOLs are not recommended in patients with weak ciliary muscles, damaged or loose zonules, or ruptures or tears of the posterior capsule. Caution with accommodating IOLs should be used in high axial myopes due to the possibility of an abnormally large capsule and less accurate and effective lens position.

New and Other Considerations

Refractive IOL surgery of course does not end after the consultation and in-office diagnostics. The surgery itself is undergoing rapid innovation. Given the necessity to hit the refractive target with refractive IOL surgery, intraoperative aberrometry has been developed. Although more systems are in development, the only system currently available is ORA with VerifEye+ (Alcon). It has been shown to be beneficial in improving both spherical and astigmatic outcomes in virgin eyes, but especially in post-refractive eyes, in which traditional IOL calculations become more complex.[17,18] One of the primary benefits of this system is the ability to take into full account the posterior cornea.

Another consideration is the advent of femto-IOL surgery, which is becoming increasingly popular. Depending on the system, femtosecond lasers are able to create corneal incision, perform LRIs, create free-floating capsulotomies, and do lens fragmentation. Although refractive accuracy and safety over traditional IOL surgery is controversial, femto refractive IOL surgery has been shown to increase the reproducibility of the corneal incision, decrease the required ultrasound energy, and decrease the strength of the remaining capsule.[19-21] It has been shown to be safe and likely preferable in mature crystalline lenses, Fuchs endothelial dystrophy, previous trauma, and pseudoexfoliation syndrome.

Finally, with the recent approval of the KAMRA inlay (AcuFocus Inc), the treatment of presbyopia in patients with either a cataract or a dysfunctional lens has expanded to a combined cornea and IOL approach. An increased depth of focus can be attained with placement of a monofocal or toric IOL with placement of the KAMRA inlay in the cornea.[22-24]

Conclusion

Premium IOLs can provide improvements in the quality and range of patients' visual function and improve their quality of life in the process. For those starting to implement advanced IOLs in a refractive practice, toric IOLs may be a good place to start. Once comfortable with toric IOLs, the surgeon can move to presbyopia-correcting IOLs, which require more patient assessment to match the patient to the IOL. For all premium IOLs, hitting the refractive target is key, as is optimizing the ocular surface. Armed with a proper assessment of patient visual needs, ocular health, and patient personality, implanting premium IOLs can be an effective and rewarding procedure for both patient and surgeon.

References

1. Petermeier K, Gekeler F, Spitzer MS, Szurman P. Implantation of the multifocal ReSTOR apodised diffractive intraocular lens in adult anisometropic patients with mild to moderate amblyopia. *Br J Ophthalmol.* 2009;93:1296-1301.
2. Fernández-Vega L, Madrid-Costa D, Alfonso JF, Montés-Micó R, Poo-López A. Optical and visual performance of diffractive intraocular lens implantation after myopic laser in situ keratomileusis. *J Cataract Refract Surg.* 2009;35:825-832.
3. Muftuoglu O, Dao L, Mootha VV, et al. Apodized diffractive intraocular lens implantation after laser in situ keratomileusis with or without subsequent excimer laser enhancement. *J Cataract Refract Surg.* 2010;36:1815-1821.
4. Kim JS, Jung JW, Lee JM, Seo KY, Kim EK, Kim TI. Clinical outcomes following implantation of diffractive multifocal intraocular lenses with varying add powers. *Am J Ophthalmol.* 2015;160(4):702-709
5. Hayashi K, Hayashi H, Nakao F, Hayashi F. Correlation between pupillary size and intraocular lens decentration and visual acuity of a zonal-progressive multifocal lens and a monofocal lens. *Ophthalmology.* 2001;108(11):2011-2017.
6. Woodward MA, Randleman JB, Stulting RD. Dissatisfaction after multifocal intraocular lens implantation. *J Cataract Refract Surg.* 2009;35:992-997.
7. Kezirian GM. Qualifying visual performance with the Crystalens. *Cataract and Refractive Surgery Today.* 2010;May(Suppl):3-4.
8. Muftuoglu O, Dao L, Cavanagh HD, McCulley JP, Bowman RW. Limbal relaxing incisions at the time of apodized diffractive multifocal intraocular lens implantation to reduce astigmatism with or without subsequent laser in situ keratomileusis. *J Cataract Refract Surg.* 2010;36:456-464.
9. Chang DH, Waring GO IV. The subject-fixated coaxially sighted corneal light Reflex: a clinical marker for centration of refractive treatments and devices. *Am J Ophthalmol.* 2014;158(5):863-874.
10. Salati C, Salvetat ML, Zeppieri M, Brusini P. Pupil size influence on the intraocular performance of the multifocal AMO-Array intraocular lens in elderly patients. *Eur J Ophthalmol.* 2007;17:571-578.
11. Feinbaum CG. Patient selection for presbyopic refractive surgery. *Cataract and Refractive Surgery Today Europe.* 2010;April:40-42.
12. Cillino G, Casuccio A, Pasti M, Bono V, Mencucci R, Cillino S. Working-age cataract patients: visual results, reading performance, and quality of life with three diffractive multifocal intraocular lenses. *Ophthalmology.* 2014;121(1):34-44.
13. Pepose JS, Wang D, Altmann GE. Comparison of through-focus image quality across five presbyopia-correcting intraocular lenses (an American Ophthalmological Society thesis). *Trans Am Ophthalmol Soc.* 2011;109:221-231.
14. Hofmann T, Zuberbuhler B, Cervino A, Montés-Micó R, Haefliger E. Retinal straylight and complaint scores 18 months after implantation of the AcrySof monofocal and ReSTOR diffractive intraocular lenses. *J Refract Surg.* 2009;25:485-492.
15. Dell S. Screening and evaluating presbyopic patients. *Cataract and Refractive Surgery Today.* 2007;March:81-82.

16. Bucci FA Jr. Patient selection, preoperative evaluation critical for success. www.healio.com/ophthalmology/practice-management/news/online/%7B36258382-305f-49bd-8586-872d394c644e%7D/patient-selection-preoperative-evaluation-critical-for-success. Published October 15, 2006. Accessed January 4, 2017.
17. Canto AP, Chhadva P, Cabot F, et al. Comparison of IOL power calculation methods and intraoperative wavefront aberrometer in eyes after refractive surgery. *J Refract Surg*. 2013;29(7):484-489.
18. Ianchulev T, Hoffer KJ, Yoo SH, et al. Intraoperative refractive biometry for predicting intraocular lens power calculation after prior myopic refractive surgery. *Ophthalmology*. 2014;121(1):56-60.
19. Menapace RM, Dick HB. Femtosecond laser in cataract surgery. A critical appraisal. *Ophthalmologe*. 2014;111(7):624-637.
20. Conrad-Hengerer I, Schultz T, Jones JJ, Hengerer FH, Dick B. Cortex removal after laser cataract surgery and standard phacoemulsification: a critical analysis of 800 consecutive cases. *J Refract Surg*. 2014;30(8):516-520.
21. Conrad-Hengerer I, Hengerer FH, Joachim SC, Schultz T, Dick HB. Femtosecond laser-assisted cataract surgery in intumescent white cataracts. *J Cataract Refract Surg*. 2014;40(1):44-50.
22. Huseynova T, Kanamori T, Waring GO IV, Tomita M. Outcomes of small aperture corneal inlay implantation in patients with pseudophakia. *J Refract Surg*. 2014;30(2):110-116.
23. Vilupuru S, Lin L, Pepose JS. Comparison of contrast sensitivity and through focus in small-aperture inlay, accommodating intraocular lens, or multifocal intraocular lens subjects. *Am J Ophthalmol*. 2015;160(1):150-162.
24. Hatch KM, Talamo JH. Laser-assisted cataract surgery: benefits and barriers. *Curr Opin Ophthalmol*. 2014;25(1):54-61.

Chapter 4

Preparing the Ocular Surface for Cataract and Refractive Surgery

Jodi Luchs, MD, FACS

Cataract surgery is one of the most common surgical procedures performed in the United States.[1,2,3] Over the past several decades, there have been major advances in technology surrounding cataract surgery: from newer, more advanced pharmaceuticals and topical anesthesia, to femtosecond laser–assisted cataract surgery and advanced technology toric and presbyopic lens implants. These advances, and others, have elevated cataract surgery to the level of precision and recovery commonly associated with refractive surgery.

Similarly, there are approximately 700,000 refractive surgical procedures performed annually in the United States.[4] Refractive surgery, like cataract surgery, has evolved significantly over the years with the advent of eye tracking, custom wavefront-guided/wavefront-optimized procedures, iris registration, and femtosecond laser flap creation. These advances have greatly enhanced the precision, optical outcome, and speed of recovery from refractive surgery.

With patients now expecting to recover from ocular surgery and be glasses-free within hours of their procedure, it has become essential to pay close attention to every aspect of the surgical process, beginning with the preoperative evaluation. Critically important are the health and integrity of the tear film and ocular surface.

The tear film is the very first refracting surface of the eye. Incoming light must pass through a pristine, uniform, and undisturbed tear film as a first step toward proper focus on the retina. Approximately two-thirds of the eye's optical power is derived from the cornea—including the tear film—and the greatest change in refractive index occurs between air and the tear film.[5] Any disruption to the uniformity, optical clarity, spreadability, and longevity of the tear film on the ocular surface will disturb this process, often with untoward effects on vision and recovery from ocular surgery.

Hovanesian JA.
Refractive Cataract Surgery: Best Practices and Advanced Technology, Second Edition (pp 27-39). © 2017 SLACK Incorporated.

When the tear film becomes unstable or irregular, variations in optical power may occur, which can induce significant higher-order aberrations. Patients may report symptoms of diplopia, starbursts, glare, and shadowing.[5] While blinking can temporarily restore the tear film in these cases, between blinks the tear film degrades and once again becomes irregular. Studies have demonstrated that increased light scatter in patients with dry eye worsens image quality.[6] Similarly, image quality has been shown to be highest immediately after a blink, and image quality degradation and higher-order aberrations develop more quickly between blinks in dry eyes compared with normal eyes.[7,8]

In an era when patients spend more time viewing handheld mobile devices, tablets, and computer monitors—all of which reduce blink rate—dry eye has become more prevalent.

An unstable tear film and ocular surface poses a wide range of potential problems for the surgical patient and can negatively impact multiple aspects of the surgical process including preoperative measurements, intraocular lens selection, the surgical procedure itself, postoperative recovery, and the development of symptomatic postoperative dry eye.

Accordingly, it is crucial to focus on the health and integrity of the ocular surface and tear film in our patients about to undergo ocular surgery.

Causes of an Unstable Tear Film

Ocular surface diseases such as dry eye, blepharitis, and ocular allergy are the most common causes of an unstable tear film, which can affect ocular surgery.

Dry Eye

Aqueous-deficiency dry eye reduces the tear volume and spreadability and is associated with increased osmolarity. Both reduced tear volume and increased osmolarity can produce ocular surface damage, which can disrupt the normal smooth contour of the ocular surface. Clinically, this is evidenced by fluorescein and lissamine green staining as a marker for ocular surface damage and irregularity. Dry eye has been associated with increased light scatter within the eye, which can be improved with lubrication.[9]

Blepharitis

Blepharitis commonly presents in anterior and posterior forms. Anterior blepharitis is often associated with an overgrowth of gram-positive bacteria on the lid margins. Clinically, this condition is associated with crusting at the base of the lashes (colarettes), and even ulceration of the lid margin in severe cases. The excessive gram-positive bacteria on the lid margins triggers inflammation on lids and ocular surface, which may result in the release of inflammatory cytokines in the tear film, producing instability or ocular surface damage. In addition, the increased bacterial load on the lid margins may increase the risk of postoperative infection[10] if not addressed preoperatively.

Posterior blepharitis is associated with inflammation within and surrounding the meibomian glands, which can alter the composition and clinical characteristics of the meibomian gland secretions. These secretions form the lipid layer of the tear film, which is responsible for promoting proper spreading of the tears on the ocular surface as well as retarding evaporation. In the presence of posterior blepharitis, both the quality and the quantity of these lipid secretions is altered, thereby producing an unstable tear film that may not spread properly and evaporates rapidly. This can be identified clinically by a rapid tear film breakup time. In addition, the evaporative tear loss can increase tear film osmolarity and directly and indirectly lead to ocular surface damage.

Allergy

Ocular allergy, along with dry eye and blepharitis, is a common ocular surface disease. When allergens in the air dissolve in the tear film of susceptible individuals, they initiate an inflammatory cascade within the conjunctiva that begins with the release of histamine and other inflammatory mediators from mast cells. These inflammatory mediators in the tear film produce destabilization and facilitate the recruitment of additional inflammatory cells into the conjunctiva which then release additional inflammatory mediators. This cycle of inflammation, especially in those who suffer from chronic ocular allergy, may produce an unstable tear film and lead to ocular surface staining. Patients suffering from ocular allergy have been shown to have a higher incidence of dry eye,[11,12] contact lens intolerance,[13] diffuse lamellar keratitis after LASIK,[14] and haze and regression following photorefractive keratectomy.[15] In addition, patients suffering from ocular allergies often take oral antihistamine medications, which can worsen dry eye, further destabilizing the ocular surface.

Surgical Patients Are at Risk

Patients seeking cataract and refractive surgery are already at higher risk for ocular surface disease. Refractive surgical patients are self-selected for dry eye and ocular surface disease, often seeking refractive surgery because they are unable to tolerate contact lenses. Many of these patients have been long-term contact lens wearers, which increases the risk of concomitant dry eye and meibomian gland dysfunction.[16-18] Patients seeking cataract surgery are usually older and experiencing hormonal changes, whether they are perimenopausal women or men with reduced testosterone levels. Patients in this demographic are generally taking more systemic medications, many of which may dry the ocular surface, further increasing their risk. These patients are often marginally compensated prior to surgery, and the increased corneal anesthesia produced by the surgical procedure may convert them into overtly symptomatic disease.

However, it is easy to overlook ocular surface disease in these patients, as our attention is primarily focused on the refractive error (in the case of refractive surgical patients) or the cataract as the cause of the patients' visual complaints. After surgery, however, the ocular surface disease will remain, and may be potentially exacerbated, thereby impacting surgical recovery and the patient's ultimate outcome and satisfaction. One study by Luchs et al found that up to 59% of patients evaluated at the time of their biometry for cataract surgery had clinical signs of blepharitis, and 36% of those with blepharitis had tear film breakup time of 5 seconds or less.[19] Another study by Trattler et al[20] found that 80% of patients presenting for cataract surgery had clinical signs of International Task Force on Dry Eye level 2 or higher, with only 22% of patients having a previously known diagnosis of dry eye. Both of these studies suggest that dry eye and blepharitis are very common in our cataract surgical patients, often producing a clinically significant tear film disturbance, yet are frequently overlooked by clinicians.

Both refractive surgery and cataract surgery can produce dry eye postoperatively,[15-17] even without the presence of ocular surface disease preoperatively. However, the presence of any of these conditions preoperatively will worsen any postoperative dry eye, illustrating the importance of identifying and treating the condition preoperatively.

Specific Effects of Ocular Surface Disease on Ocular Surgery

Preoperative Measurements

The irregular and unstable tear film from ocular surface diseases can significantly impact the accuracy, repeatability, and reliability of many of the instruments we use to evaluate our patients preoperatively and upon whose data we make surgical decisions. Keratometry and Placido-based corneal topography rely upon reflections from a stable tear film on the ocular surface in order to generate their data. Tear film instability can significantly impact the reliability of these results. Similarly, unstable tear film will alter the accuracy of manual or automated refractometry, optical biometry, and the wavefront analysis of optical aberrations within the eye. Wavefront aberrations have been demonstrated to increase in the presence of dry eye and increasing tear film osmolarity.[9-11]

The consequences of these inaccurate measurements can be significant. Errors in preoperative keratometry or optical biometry can lead to errors in intraocular lens calculations, which may produce an off-target, postoperative refractive "miss." This can be particularly problematic in patients receiving a multifocal implant when the defocus curves drop off significantly with uncorrected refractive errors above 0.5 diopters. Similarly the magnitude or axis of toric intraocular lenses may be affected by inaccuracies of preoperative keratometry. Errors in preoperative wavefront or topography measurements may alter refractive surgical planning, thus affecting refractive outcomes in these patients as well.

Intraoperative Surgical Implications

While most of the ramifications of untreated ocular surface disease are realized in the preoperative evaluation and postoperative recovery from surgery, there are some intraoperative considerations as well. Any significant corneal surface irregularity, especially centrally, can affect the surgical view during cataract surgery. Similarly, heavy meibomian gland debris in the tear film from untreated posterior blepharitis can interfere with the surgical view or end up under the flap following LASIK surgery. An unhealthy corneal epithelial surface is more likely to be further damaged by multiple preoperative medications, dilating drops, intraoperative irrigation/manipulation, or applanation from cataract or refractive surgical femtosecond laser interfaces, thereby increasing the risk of intraoperative or perioperative epithelial defects.

Postoperative Considerations

While both cataract and refractive surgery can produce dry eye postoperatively,[16] pre-existing disease can significantly increase the likelihood of symptomatic disease postoperatively. Postoperative dry eye can produce significant symptoms for our patients, which can be very difficult to treat. In addition, the ocular surface damage can produce significant discomfort as well as interfere with vision, producing significant light scattering, glare, halos, delays in visual recovery, and/or reduced best-corrected visual acuity. These effects may be particularly prominent in patients receiving a multifocal intraocular lens implant or a presbyopic corneal inlay. Identification and treatment of these conditions preoperatively allows a proactive approach, which can help to reduce the likelihood of these complications or allow better management should they occur. Identification of these conditions preoperatively also facilitates a conversation with the patient alerting them to the pre-existing condition prior to surgery, potentially avoiding a situation where the patient believes that the condition was caused by the surgery or a surgical complication.

How to Diagnose Ocular Surface Diseases Preoperatively

History

Ocular surface diseases, while common in surgical patients, are frequently overlooked by clinicians. In order to avoid the pitfalls described previously, it is important to have a high index of suspicion. Careful attention to the patient history is required. Complaints of dryness, itch, irritation, burning, grittiness, or foreign body sensation all suggest ocular surface diseases and should be taken seriously. If patients do not volunteer this information spontaneously, specific questions should be asked in order to determine whether they have experienced these symptoms. Validated instruments, such as the Ocular Surface Disease Index (OSDI)[21] and Standard Patient Evaluation of Eye Dryness (SPEED) questionnaires[22] are also helpful and may indicate functional difficulties associated with ocular surface disease. A patient history of fluctuating vision also suggests an unstable tear film. Fixed visual problems such as a cataract or refractive error tend to produce fixed visual problems or complaints. However, a fluctuating problem such as an unstable tear film will produce fluctuating vision, especially in the presence of another fixed deficit in the visual pathway, such as a cataract. A history of artificial tear use suggests that they are self-medicating their condition and strongly points to the presence of ocular surface disease. Many years of contact lens wear and/or contact lens intolerance also suggests the diagnosis. It is equally important to look at the patient's list of systemic medications for those that may produce or worsen dry eye.

Point-of-Care Diagnostics

Once a careful history is taken, there are several point-of-care diagnostic tests that can be helpful indicators of the presence of dry eye. Many of these tests can easily be performed by technicians as part of their patient workup and are useful adjuncts to the workup of presurgical patients.

Tear Film Osmolarity

Osmolarity is a measurement of the concentration of dissolved solutes in a solution. In the tear film, the osmolarity is generally expressed in units of milliosmoles/liter (mOsm/L). Hyperosmolarity of the tear film is a recognized and validated marker of dry eye. Hyperosmolarity of the tear film occurs through decreased flow of the aqueous component of the tear film from the lacrimal gland, and/or through increased evaporation and instability of the tear film. Increased osmolarity of the tear film stimulates the release of inflammatory cytokines, enhances the rate of cell apoptosis, and results in a decrease in the number of goblet cells.[23,24] Tear film osmolarity can be easily tested with a handheld device that is touched to the tear film and provides a digital readout of tear film osmolarity within seconds.

Patients with a normal tear film typically have a stable tear film osmolarity. A higher degree of fluctuation in tear film osmolarity is observed in patients with dry eye. Fluctuations occur both between measurements taken from the same eye and measurements concurrently taken between eyes of a patient. In general, an elevated tear film osmolarity is correlated with dry eye; the normal tear film osmolarity in patients without dry eye ranges from 270 to 308 mOsm/L (mean of 302 mOsm/L). A threshold of 308 mOsm/L has been found to be indicative of early/mild dry eye, while a tear film osmolarity of 316 mOsm/L or higher is correlated with moderate to severe dry eye. Based on the stability of the tear film in the eyes of normal patients, a difference in the tear film osmolarity of patients > 8 mOsm/L between eyes is indicative of dry eye disease.[25-27]

The evaluation of osmolarity should be conducted prior to disturbance of the eye in order to obtain accurate results, as any disturbance to the ocular surface may stimulate reflex tearing, which can falsely lower the reading. While an elevated measurement of tear film osmolarity is a strong indicator for dry eye, the presence of an elevated osmolarity reading may not correlate with a patient's symptoms or other clinical signs, due to the nature of the disease and fluctuations observed in these patients; trends observed through repeated osmolarity assessments are beneficial in the diagnosis of individual patients.[25,26]

Matrix Metalloproteinase-9 Detectors

Recent research has evaluated matrix metalloproteinase-9 (MMP-9), an enzyme that is produced by corneal epithelial cells, as a biomarker for dry eye. The MMP family of enzymes plays an important role in wound healing and inflammation through the ability to degrade collagen. Elevated levels of MMP-9 have been observed in the tears of patients with dry eye.[26,27] The presence of MMP-9 over 40 ng/mL in the tear film has been correlated with the presence of the inflammatory component of dry eye disease. MMP-9 testing of the tear film can now be easily performed with a handheld disposable device that produces results within minutes. A positive test strongly suggests ocular surface disease–related inflammation on the ocular surface and should prompt the initiation of anti-inflammatory therapy.

Lactoferrin and Immunoglobulin E Analysis

Levels of several protein components of the lacrimal secretions have been found to be altered in the tear film of patients with ocular surface diseases, allowing these proteins to be used as biomarkers.[28,29]

Lactoferrin is one of the most abundant protein components of the healthy tear film. Lactoferrin, through the sequestration of iron, acts as an antimicrobial agent and plays a role in the immunological and anti-inflammatory properties of the tear film. The concentration of lactoferrin in the tear film has been observed to be reduced in patients with aqueous-deficient dry eye.[30] A point-of-care diagnostic for the measurement of the concentration of lactoferrin in the tear film of suspected dry eye patients is currently available. Lactoferrin levels below 0.9 mg/mL suggest the patient has aqueous-deficient dry eye, with the severity of the disease correlated with lower levels of the biomarker.[24,31]

Immunoglobulin E (IgE) proteins, antibodies specific for particular allergens, are found in the tear film of patients with ocular allergic conditions. Exposure to allergen particles results in binding of IgE and interaction with mast cells in the conjunctiva, initiating the inflammatory response of the allergic cascade.[22,32]

The same point-of-care test commercially available to measure tear film lactoferrin concentrations can also evaluate the level of IgE in tear samples. IgE levels ≥ 80 ng/mL suggest a diagnosis of allergic conjunctivitis, with the level of IgE present in the tear film correlating with the severity of the allergic condition.[33]

Tear film IgE testing will also be available in the near future, coupled to the same device that currently performs MMP-9 analysis.

Meibomography

Meibomography, which is now readily available through the use of several devices, may also be a helpful adjunct in the diagnosis of meibomian gland disease. These non-invasive photographic devices visually display the meibomian gland architecture, revealing tortuosity, shortening or dropout—all of which are diagnostic of meibomian gland disease. The visual demonstration of the shortening or loss of meibomian glands is often very impactful and helps invest the patient in his or her diagnosis and treatment.

Tear Film Interferometry

The lipid layer of the tear film can also be directly visualized using interferometry, aiding in the diagnosis of evaporative dry eye, and allowing direct visualization of tear film stability. Colored images of the superficial layer of the tear film, the lipid layer, can be generated and evaluated to assess the thickness across the ocular surface.[31,34] A reduction in the thickness of the lipid layer (< 60 nm) has been correlated with meibomian gland dysfunction and symptoms of dry eye.

Conjunctival Impression Cytology

Conjunctival impression cytology, once reserved primarily for research centers, can now be performed easily in the office through the use of a new diagnostic device. While useful to demonstrate goblet cell loss and squamous metaplasia associated with dry eye, the results are not immediately available, unlike the other point-of-care diagnostics. A modification of this device to collect ocular surface disease biomarkers is also under development.

Slit-Lamp Examination

Once the preliminary history and technician workup is complete, it is important to perform a careful slit-lamp examination looking for the presence of ocular surface diseases. This examination begins as soon as you enter the room. Observation of the patient's natural blink rate, presence of lid retraction, inferior scleral show, incomplete blink, or lagophthalmos can be helpful. External examination under the slit lamp should involve a thorough examination of the lids and lid margins. Look for signs of crusting, collarettes, or lid margin ulceration suggesting anterior blepharitis. Also look for lid margin thickening, telangiectasia, and meibomian gland pouting, inspissation, plugging, or obliteration, which indicate posterior blepharitis. Care should be taken to press on the lid margins to express meibum from the meibomian glands. Normal meibum should have a clear, "cooking oil" type of consistency and should be easily expressible. Abnormal secretions can be yellow, cloudy, granular, or even "toothpaste-like" in consistency. Any abnormal meibomian secretions may produce an unstable tear film. In severe cases, the meibomian glands may be inexpressible or even obliterated.

The height of the tear film meniscus should be inspected to evaluate the overall volume of tears on the ocular surface. Normal tear-film meniscus height is approximately 0.15 to 0.3 mm. Automated methods for evaluation of the tear film meniscus height and volume are now available and can be helpful. Fluorescein and lissamine green staining of the ocular surface are essential to evaluate tear film stability and to screen for ocular surface damage. Tear film breakup time is easily evaluated with a fluorescein stained tear film, and a breakup time of less than 10 seconds is considered abnormal.[24] Automated tear film breakup time analysis is now also available. The fluorescein stained tear film may also reveal *negative staining*, in which subtle elevations on the ocular surface become evident as the fluorescein rolls off the high points and pools in the lower areas. This can be extremely helpful to reveal subtle ocular surface irregularities such as those seen with anterior basement membrane dystrophy, corneal degenerations, or scarring. Such irregularities can produce significant optical aberrations and can potentially have a profound effect on cataract and refractive surgery. It is important to be aware of these conditions preoperatively in order to properly counsel the patient and properly plan for the upcoming surgical procedure.

Ocular surface damage can be evaluated by looking at the fluorescein and lissamine green staining patterns. Ideally, there should be no staining. The presence of staining suggests the presence of ocular surface injury/damage from ocular surface disease. It is important to wait at least 2 minutes after instilling fluorescein or lissamine green prior to evaluating the staining patterns, as they can take time to develop; a casual, rushed examination may miss important diagnostic clues. Schirmer testing can also be useful in these patients, although it may not be routinely performed. Schirmer testing without anesthesia is particularly useful, because it demonstrates reflex tearing due to the irritation produced by the strips. If a patient only produces 5 mm or less of wetting after 5 minutes on this test, it strongly suggests the presence of dry eye.

Corneal topography is also an extremely useful tool to help diagnose ocular surface disease as well as corneal shape abnormalities and should be part of the workup of any patient undergoing ocular surgery. The incidence of keratoconus in the general population is approximately 1/2000,[35] although there are many more individuals with undiagnosed, mild, or forme fruste disease. Those patients often present for refractive surgery evaluation, and corneal topography and/or tomography is essential to help identify those patients who would otherwise be at high risk for ectasia postoperatively. Similarly, patients with mild disease may present for cataract surgery later in life, having never been diagnosed with the condition. Corneal topography can reveal the characteristic pattern, which would have otherwise gone unrecognized, thereby providing essential information for the patient and the clinician. The patient can now be counseled as to the presence of the condition, and the surgeon can make better choices regarding intraocular lens selection. The use of a multifocal lens in these patients is generally contraindicated, and the refractive response to toric lenses may be unpredictable.

Previously unrecognized corneal irregularities can also be diagnosed with corneal topography. A pattern of irregular astigmatism may be seen in corneal dystrophies, such as anterior basement membrane dystrophy, and stromal dystrophies, such as granular, lattice, or Avellino dystrophy. While the stromal dystrophies tend to be easily observable on slit-lamp evaluation, basement membrane dystrophy can be extremely subtle and easy to miss. Map-dot-fingerprint basement membrane changes are common, affecting up to 76% of the population over age 50 years and between 6% and 42% of the general population,[36,37] and can produce subtle irregular astigmatism that can affect vision. Subtle grayish "maps" or fine fingerprint lines can be seen under the slit lamp with careful observation. However, often these findings are missed. Instillation of fluorescein in the tear film often reveals negative staining indicative of the underlying condition and underscoring the surface irregularity. Corneal topography can similarly reveal the irregular pattern, and the finding of irregular astigmatism without a known cause should prompt a second look at the ocular surface to rule out abnormalities.

Corneal topography is also an excellent screening tool for unstable tear film and ocular surface disease. Since Placido-based corneal topography depends on analysis of reflected rings projected onto the ocular surface, irregularities of the tear film or ocular surface will distort those rings, producing areas of uninterpretable data. These areas with no interpretable data are graphically represented on the color printout as white spots within the color map (Figure 4-1). These white spots of missing data may be considered similar to *dry spots* on the ocular surface and should raise the suspicion of ocular surface disease. The presence of these white spots should prompt a second look at the patient and a thorough evaluation for the presence of ocular surface disease.

The presence of irregular astigmatism on corneal topography is another diagnostic clue, not only suggesting the possibility of a corneal shape abnormality as discussed previously, but also potentially indicating an unstable tear film. The irregular tear film with a rapid breakup time distorts the reflected corneal rings producing a computer interpretation of an irregular shape. This irregular shape is graphically represented by an asymmetrical distribution of color on the corneal topography printout (Figure 4-2). The presence of these topographic irregularities without a previously known cause of irregular astigmatism should prompt a second look at the cornea to rule out a structural cause, such as anterior basement membrane dystrophy, as mentioned previously. In the absence

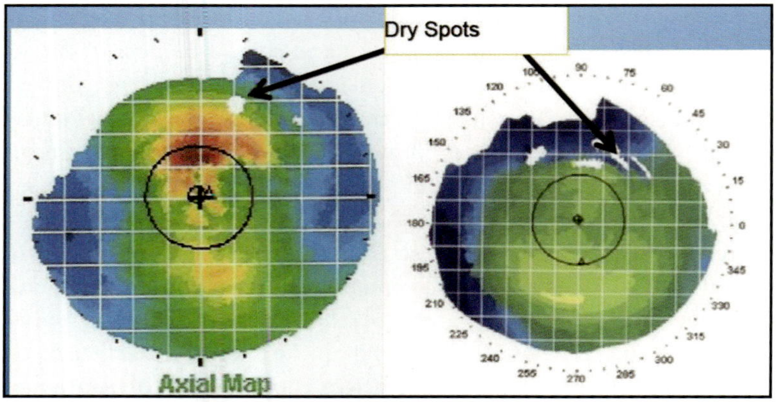

Figure 4-1. White spots on topography maps indicating areas of no data, often corresponding to dry spots on the cornea. (Reprinted with permission from William Trattler, MD.)

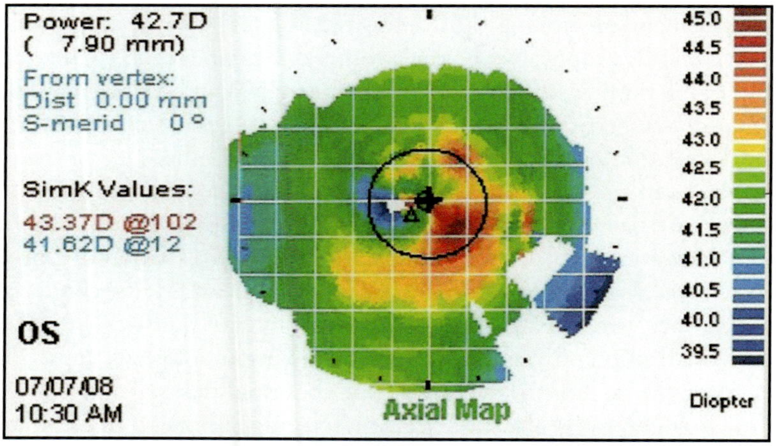

Figure 4-2. Case 1: A 58-year-old man seeking cataract surgery. A very irregular pattern consistent with irregular astigmatism and multiple white spots of missing data is present. (Reprinted with permission from William Trattler, MD.)

of any structural cause of irregular astigmatism, an unstable tear film due to the presence of ocular surface disease must be considered.

Treatment of Ocular Surface Disease

Once ocular surface diseases are discovered, it is important to treat them in order to optimize our patients' surgical outcomes. While there is always a concern on the part of the surgeon that any delay in surgery may discourage the patient and incite them to seek care elsewhere, most of the time, proper treatment can effect a significant improvement within a few weeks, thereby avoiding any significant surgical delay. Furthermore, patients will be grateful for the extra attention and time that you took in order to make the diagnosis. The extra time taken to diagnose and treat these conditions preoperatively generally pays dividends in avoiding untoward outcomes, lengthy explanations, unsatisfactory results, and unhappy patients.

When treating ocular surface disease in presurgical patients, it is important to remember that many patients may exhibit more than one condition. Multiple ocular surface diseases are often present in the same patient. In order to effectively stabilize the tear film in these patients, it is crucial to identify and treat all of the conditions present. For example, a patient with dry eyes and posterior blepharitis may require a regimen of warm compresses, lid massage, artificial tears, topical cyclosporine, and a short course of topical steroids in order to rehabilitate their ocular surface.

Once treatment for ocular surface disease is initiated, patients should be re-examined in 1 to 2 weeks. Repeat evaluation should include osmolarity (if available), careful examination of the lid margin with manual expression of the meibomian glands, careful slit-lamp examination of the ocular surface, tear film breakup time, evaluation of fluorescein and lissamine green staining patterns, and corneal topography. Often, improvement will be seen at this time, allowing repeat biometry and surgery to proceed as originally scheduled. Even if surgery needs to be postponed for a few weeks, the delay is time well spent, and patients will be appreciative of the extra attention.

Intraoperative Considerations

In patients with known ocular surface disease, it can be helpful to choose surgical techniques that may help to minimize postoperative dry eye. During the surgery, attempt to minimize topical agents containing benzalkonium chloride and minimize topical anesthetics. Lubricate frequently with balanced salt solution and consider the use of a viscoelastic on the ocular surface. For patients with astigmatism, consider toric lens implantation rather than limbal relaxing incisions or femtosecond arcuate incisions. For low cylindrical corrections, intrastromal femtosecond incisions can be considered because they are generally placed below the nerve plexus.

Postoperative Considerations

Postoperative care in patients with known ocular surface disease should focus on maintaining the integrity of a smooth epithelial surface after it has been stressed by the surgical procedure. Furthermore, corneal sensation is temporarily reduced in these patients, which further increases the risk of keratopathy. Preoperative measures to treat ocular surface diseases, such as preservative-free lubrication, topical cyclosporine, and lid massage, should be maintained. In addition, an effort should be made to minimize any preservative-containing medication. Topical steroids and nonsteroidal anti-inflammatory drugs should be used in the lowest effective dose and discontinued when no longer necessary. Punctal plugs, if not already placed preoperatively, may also be helpful adjuncts in patients with reduced tear production postoperatively.

Conclusion

In this era of advanced cataract and refractive surgical techniques, with advanced technology surrounding every aspect of the preoperative, intraoperative, and postoperative procedure, patients expect a quick, painless procedure with a rapid recovery of vision and the ability see clearly at distance and near, without the need for spectacle correction. In order to deliver upon these types of expectations, it is crucial for ophthalmic surgeons to focus on the health of the ocular surface in our surgical patients. We must make an extra effort to screen for, diagnose, and treat an unstable tear film and ocular surface disease *before* we operate in order to avoid the pitfalls associated with untreated, worsened ocular surface disease postoperatively. Fortunately, we have many tools now available to help us diagnose these conditions and avoid these potential complications. Corneal topography, as demonstrated earlier, is one of those tools and should be an integral part of every preoperative evaluation for cataract and refractive surgery. Tear film osmolarity, MMP-9 testing, and other point-of-care diagnostics currently available and in development will continue to aid us in this process. Nothing, however, substitutes for a careful ocular history, with appropriate questions regarding symptoms of ocular surface diseases, as well as a careful, thorough slit-lamp evaluation.

Careful attention to these details will help provide accurate data upon which to make informed surgical decisions and achieve optimized surgical outcomes. Patients will appreciate the extra time spent, and the few extra minutes of chair time will reap valuable rewards in terms of postoperative results and patient satisfaction.

References

1. Williams A, Sloan FA, Lee PP. Longitudinal rates of cataract surgery. *Arch Ophthalmol.* 2006;124(9):1308-1314.
2. Harmon D. Q1 2010 US IOL procedures climb 4.6 percent. *Ophthalmic Market Perspectives.* June 16, 2010. St. Louis, MO: Market Scope, LLC.
3. Congdon N, Vingerling JR, Klein BE, et al; Eye Diseases Prevalence Research Group. Prevalence of cataract and pseudophakia/aphakia among adults in the United States. *Arch Ophthalmol.* 2004;122(4):487-494.
4. Statista. Number of LASIK surgeries in the United States from 1996 to 2020 (in thousands). www.statista.com/statistics/271478/number-of-lasik-surgeries-in-the-us/. Published 2016. Accessed January 4, 2017.
5. Tutt R, Bradley A, Begley C, Thibos LN. Optical and visual impact of tear breakup in human eyes. *Invest Ophthalmol Vis Sci.* 2000;41:4117-4123.
6. Benito A, Perez GM, Mirabet S, et al. Objective optical assessment of tear-film quality dynamics in normal and mildly symptomatic dry eyes. *J Cataract Refract Surg.* 2011;37:1481-1487.
7. Goto E, Yagi Y, Masumoto Y, Tsubota K. Impaired functional visual acuity of dry eye patients. *Am J Ophthalmol.* 2002;133:181-186.
8. Montés-Micó R. Role of the tear film in the optical quality of the human eye. *J Cataract Refract Surg.* 2007;33:1631-1635.
9. Diaz-Valle D, Arriola-Villalobos P, García-Vidal SE, et al. Effect of lubricating eyedrops on ocular light scattering as a measure of vision quality in patients with dry eye. *J Cataract Refract Surg.* 2012;38(7):1192-1197.
10. Speaker MG, Menikoff JA. Prophylaxis of endophthalmitis with topical povidone-iodine. *Ophthalmology.* 1991;98:1769-75.
11. Schaumberg DA, Sullivan DA, Buring JE, Dana MR. Prevalence of dry eye syndrome among U.S. women. *Am J Ophthalmol.* 2003;136:318-326.
12. Moss SE, Klein R, Klein BE. Incidence of dry eye in an older population. *Arch Ophthalmol.* 2004;122:369-373.

13. Kumar P, Elston R, Black D, Gilhotra S, DeGuzman N, Cambre K. Allergic rhinoconjunctivitis and contact lens intolerance. *CLAO J.* 1991;17(1):31-34.
14. Boorstein SM, Henk HJ, Elner VM. Atopy: A patient-specific risk factor for diffuse lamellar keratitis. *Ophthalmology.* 2003;110:1:131-137.
15. Yang HY, Fujishima H, Toda I, et al. Allergic conjunctivitis as a risk factor for regression and haze after photorefractive keratectomy. *Am J Ophthalmol.* 1998;125:1:54-58.
16. [No authors listed]. The definition and classification of dry eye disease: report of the Definition and Classification Subcommittee of the International Dry Eye WorkShop (2007). *Ocul Surf.* 2007;5(2):75-92.
17. [No authors listed]. The epidemiology of dry eye disease: report of the Epidemiology Subcommittee of the International Dry EyeWorkShop (2007). *Ocul Surf.* 2007;5(2):93-107.
18. [No authors listed]. Methodologies to diagnose and monitor dry eye disease: report of the Diagnostic Methodology Subcommittee of the International Dry Eye WorkShop (2007). *Ocul Surf.* 2007;5(2):108-152.
19. Luchs JI, Buznego C, Trattler W. Incidence of Blepharitis in patients scheduled for phacoemulsification. Poster presented at: American Society of Cataract and Refractive Surgery Annual Meeting; April 9-14, 2010; Boston, MA.
20. Trattler WB, Reilly CD, Goldberg DF, et al. Cataract and dry eye: prospective health assessment of cataract patients ocular surface study. Presented at American Society of Cataract and Refractive Surgery Annual Meeting; 2011. San Diego, CA.
21. Schiffman RM, Christianson MD, Jacobsen G, et al. Reliability and validity of the Ocular Surface Disease Index. *Arch Ophthalmol.* 2000;118(5):615-621.
22. Ngo W, Situ P, Keir N, Korb D, Blackie C, Simpson T. Psychometric properties and validation of the Standard Patient Evaluation of Eye Dryness Questionnaire. *Cornea.* 2013;32(9):1204-1210.
23. Tomlinson A, Khanal S, Ramaesh K, et al. Tear film osmolarity: determination of a referent for dry eye diagnosis. *Invest Ophthalmol Vis Sci.* 2006;47:4309-4315.
24. Bron AJ, Tomlinson A, Foulks GN, et al. Rethinking dry eye disease: a perspective on clinical implications. *Ocul Surf.* 2014;12(2 Suppl):S1-31.
25. American Academy of Ophthalmology. Preferred practice patterns: dry eye syndrome. www.aao.org/preferred-practice-pattern/dry-eye-syndrome-ppp--2013. Published October 2013. Accessed January 4, 2017.
26. Chotikavanich S, de Paiva CS, Li de Q, Chen JJ, et al. Production and activity of matrix metalloproteinase-9 on the ocular surface increase in dysfunctional tear syndrome. *Invest Ophthalmol Vis Sci.* 2009;50(7):3203-3209.
27. Sambursky R, Davitt WF III, Latkany R, et al. Sensitivity and specificity of a point-of-care matrix metalloproteinase 9 immunoassay for diagnosing inflammation related to dry eye. *JAMA Ophthalmol.* 2013;131(1):24-28.
28. Ohashi Y, Ishida R, Kojima T, Goto E, et al. Abnormal protein profiles in tears with dry eye syndrome. *Am J Ophthalmol.* 2003;136(2):291-299.
29. Zhou L, Beuerman RW, Chan CM, et al. Identification of tear fluid biomarkers in dry eye syndrome using iTRAQ quantitative proteomics. *J Proteome Res.* 2009;8(11):4889-4905.
30. Goren MB, Goren SB. Diagnostic tests in patients with symptoms of keratoconjunctivitis sicca. *Am J Ophthalmol.* 1988;106(5):570-574.
31. King-Smith PE, Kimball SH, Nichols JJ. Tear film interferometry and corneal surface roughness. *Invest Ophthalmol Vis Sci.* 2014;55(4):2614-2618.
32. Leonardi A, Motterle L, Bortolotti M. Allergy and the Eye. *Clin Exp Immunol.* 2008;153(Suppl 1):17-21.
33. Nomura K, Takamura E. Tear IgE concentrations in allergic conjunctivitis. *Eye (Lond).* 1998;12(Pt 2):296-298.
34. Savini G, Prabhawasat P, Kojima T, et al. The challenge of dry eye diagnosis. *Clin Ophthalmol.* 2008;2(1):31-55.
35. Rabinowitz YS. Keratoconus. *Surv Ophthalmol.* 1998;42(4):297-319.
36. Werblin TP, Hirst LW, Stark WJ, Maumenee IH. Prevalence of map-dot-fingerprint changes in the cornea. *Br J Ophthalmol.* 1981;65:401-409.
37. Laibson PR. Microcystic corneal dystrophy. *Trans Am Ophthalmol Soc.* 1976;74:488-531.

Chapter 5

Preoperative Testing for Refractive Cataract Surgery

Kevin Jwo, MD; William F. Wiley, MD; Ji Won Kwon, MD, PhD; and Jimmy Lee, MD

The promise of premium intraocular lenses (IOL) is as heady as it is bold; spectacle independence at all distances, something that is a distant memory for many cataract patients. Premium IOL options are categorized by the type of additional vision correction they provide: toric IOLs treat astigmatism, whereas multifocal (either diffractive or refractive) and accommodating IOLs address presbyopia. Given their downsides and risks, these options must be appropriately chosen and evaluated based on the lifestyle and personality traits of the patient. A comprehensive preoperative history, examination, and testing are essential for successful outcomes. Discussion of patient expectations and motivations should be one of the first goals, as they need to understand the benefits, limitations, and risks of premium IOLs. Unrealistic hopes among patients should be addressed. A thorough social, medical, and ocular history; manifest and cycloplegic refractions; a complete ophthalmic evaluation including pupillary exam, motility, slit-lamp, and fundus examinations; and testing of ocular dominance to discuss possible monovision correction may all be important elements of the preoperative evaluation.

Toric Lens

Assessing the type and degree of corneal astigmatism is important when considering toric IOL implants. Most studies that have shown superior postsurgical visual acuities following toric IOLs (compared with spherical IOLs) have been performed on patients with corneal astigmatism of at least 1.0 to 1.5 diopters (D), using IOL models with cylinder power of 1.5 D.[1-4] As such, it has been suggested that a minimum of 1.25 D of corneal astigmatism be present when considering a toric IOL.[5] Although patients with

Hovanesian JA.
Refractive Cataract Surgery: Best Practices and Advanced Technology, Second Edition (pp 41-60).

the classic "bowtie" astigmatism are ideal candidates, those with irregular astigmatism secondary to keratoconus,[6] pellucid marginal degeneration,[7] and post-keratoplasty[8] have also shown to benefit from toric IOLs. As these implants require precise centration and alignment for efficacy, the surgeon needs to screen for trauma, pseudoexfoliation, or even less common systemic conditions such as Marfan syndrome, homocysteinuria, ectopia lentis, and Weill-Marchesani syndrome, situations where weak zonules can compromise the centration of the IOL-capsule apparatus.

Multifocal Lens

Multifocal IOLs project multiple focal planes on the retina, from which the brain selects to process the clearest image. One tradeoff is that these lenses can create optical aberrations such as halos, especially under low-light conditions. Additionally, contrast sensitivity may be compromised. Therefore, it is paramount to gauge the patients' personality. Patients with moderate to high hyperopic refractive errors tend to be the best candidates, as they are unaccustomed to having excellent uncorrected near vision. Patients who are hypercritical with type A personalities, obsessive about crisp distance vision, or whose occupation relies on intermediate or night vision, are less than ideal candidates.[9]

Studies have shown that residual postoperative astigmatism after multifocal IOL implantation leads to worse visual outcomes and greater halo effects.[10] However, regular astigmatism can be addressed concurrently with manual or laser limbal relaxing incisions. Recently, multifocal toric platforms have been released outside the United States to address both astigmatism and presbyopia.

Irregular astigmatism remains a challenge, and significant amounts can be a relative contraindication. Ocular surface diseases such as dry eye syndrome and meibomian gland dysfunction can affect visual outcomes and should be aggressively treated preoperatively. Corneal scarring and dystrophies can also affect outcomes. For example, in Fuchs endothelial dystrophy, corneal edema and the light scattering effect of guttata can exacerbate glare and cause poor contrast sensitivity with multifocal IOLs.

Satisfaction with multifocal IOLs depends on proper implantation, centration, and pupil function. Patients with large, abnormal pupils or iris defects can have increased glare and photosensitivity. Iris colobomas and eccentric pupils can also lead to dissatisfaction. As with toric IOLs, conditions associated with zonular weakness, most commonly pseudoexfoliation, can lead to decentration and tilting, which causes increased aberrations, decreased contrast sensitivity, and poor visual acuity.[11] It is also important to assess angle kappa between the center of the pupil and the first Purkinje image on the cornea (corneal light reflex), as it has been shown that patients with a larger angle kappa have worse outcomes with diffractive multifocal lens.[12] As the multifocal IOL centers in the capsular bag, asymmetrically converging light rays of a patient with a large angle kappa may strike diffractive edges of the IOL at angles that cause light scatter and unwanted aberrations. Recently, Chang and Waring have described a new measure of centration to replace angle kappa and other indices, which are used inconsistently but thought to lack precision and specificity: the subject-fixed coaxially sighted corneal light reflex. This measurement relies on chord mu rather than angles: the 2-dimensional displacement

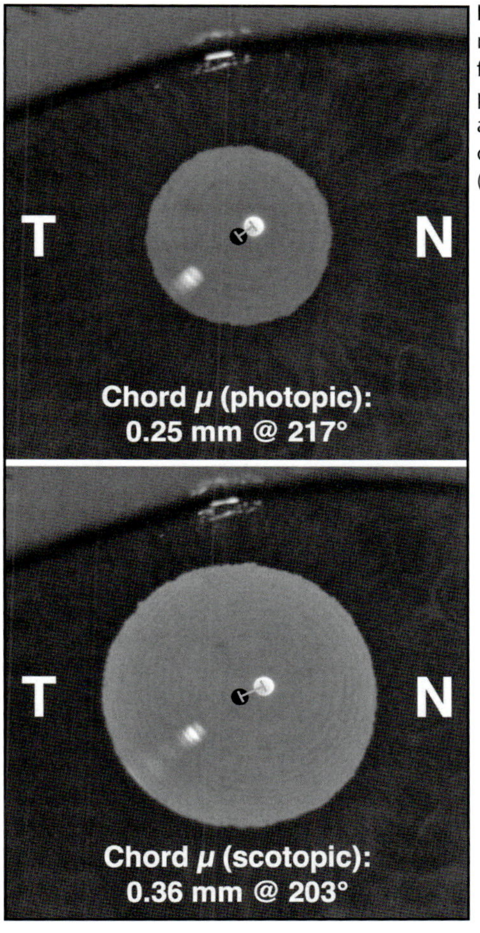

Figure 5-1. Chord mu is the 2-dimensional displacement of the entrance pupil center from the subject-fixated coaxially sighted corneal light reflex. Since the pupil center can shift with miosis and mydriasis, ideally chord mu should include a description of the state of the pupil. Chord mu as measured under photopic (top) and scotopic (bottom) light conditions.

of the entrance pupil center from the subject-fixed coaxially sighted corneal reflex[13] (Figure 5-1). Although it has yet to be incorporated into biometric devices, its appeal and utility lies in standardizing centration measurements.

Finally, it is important to screen for any pathology that limits visual potential, such as maculopathies (macular degeneration, diabetic retinopathy), optic nerve dysfunction, glaucoma, uveitis, or amblyopia, before deciding to implant a multifocal IOL. The decreased contrast sensitivity from multifocal IOLs can be compounded by underlying ocular pathology that threatens contrast sensitivity, visual acuity, color perception, or field of vision. Moreover, another consideration for patients with retinal diseases is that multifocal IOLs have been shown to hamper intraoperative visualization during vitrectomy.[14]

Preoperative Evaluation

Biometry for cataract surgery focuses primarily on three variables: axial length, corneal power, and estimated lens position (ELP).

Axial Length

Axial length traditionally has been measured by the A-scan ultrasound, in which a crystal oscillates to generate a high-frequency sound wave. There are 2 types of A-scan ultrasound biometry currently in use. The first is contact applanation biometry, in which an ultrasound probe is manually placed on the central cornea. Although this method is convenient and expedient, the operator may compress and indent the cornea. This can lead to a falsely low axial length, which can lead to an overestimation of IOL power. As the degree of compression is highly variable, this cannot be factored into a constant. The second method of A-scan ultrasound biometry is immersion A-scan biometry, in which a saline-filled scleral shell is placed between the probe and the eye, which avoids compression of the anterior chamber. Several studies have shown increased accuracy of immersion A-scan compared with contact A-scan, with an average of 0.25 to 0.33 mm shortening induced by contact.[15] The main disadvantage of immersion A-scan biometry is that it is more involved and time-consuming.

In a development that has significantly changed eye biometry, Carl Zeiss in 1999 introduced a noncontact partial coherence laser interferometer (IOLMaster 500, Carl Zeiss Meditec). This was followed in 2008 by the introduction of the Lenstar LS 900 (Haag-Streit), which uses optical low-coherence reflectometry. Optical biometry in general measures the delay and intensity of infrared light reflected back from a diode to determine the axial length of the eye. Beyond being fast and easy to use, it has several major advantages over A-scan biometry. First, optical biometry measures from the cornea to the retinal pigment epithelium, whereas ultrasound biometry measures the distance from the anterior cornea to the inner limiting membrane. Second, ultrasound measures the longest axis to the posterior pole, whereas optical biometry measures to the fovea. In eyes that are highly myopic, or have staphylomas, ultrasound biometry can overestimate the axial length. Finally, optical biometry is superior to ultrasound in the measurement of pseudophakic and silicone oil-filled eyes. Ultrasound measurements are performed with an assumed average velocity of 1555 meters/second for the sound wave as it travels through the cornea, aqueous, vitreous, and lens. Due to differing indices of refraction for various media, the velocity of sound through each of those media is different, which can confound measurements for very long or short eyes. Although optical biometers also average indices of refraction across different media, the correction factor is smaller in comparison, with less error. In long eyes, however, it's been shown that even optical biometry will overestimate axial length due to this assumption and lead to an overestimation of lens power.[16]

The main disadvantage of optical biometry relates to its need for a clear path for the infrared laser to travel from cornea to fovea. Opacities along the visual axis can block the infrared laser and interfere with proper measurement. Eyes with tear film abnormalities, corneal pathology, hypermature and posterior subcapsular cataracts, vitreous opacities, maculopathy, or retinal detachment are more difficult to measure. In addition, the patient must be able to maintain fixation. One group found that the Lenstar, IOLMaster, and immersion A-scan platforms are comparable in accuracy.[17]

Corneal Power

For most cataract patients, corneal power (K) is measured reliably with either manual or automated keratometry, which is available as independent units or as part of biometry devices such as the IOLMaster or Lenstar. Manual and automated keratometry platforms share an underlying principle: a well-lit target is placed in front of the cornea, which acts as a convex mirror and produces a virtual image of the target, and the radius of curvature is calculated via a simple vergence formula by the size of the reflected image. Corneal power is then derived from the radius of corneal curvature. Manual keratometers read either 2 or 4 points, whereas the autorefractor in the IOLMaster uses 6 reference points in a hexagonal pattern. In contrast, the Lenstar calculates Ks by analyzing the anterior corneal curvature at 32 reference points oriented in 2 circles.

Placido corneal topographers also measure corneal power: reflected images of multiple concentric circles are digitally captured, and the curvature of the cornea is calculated based on the distance between adjacent mires. These topographers measure more than 5000 points over the entire cornea and more than 1000 points within the central 3.0, yielding a simulated keratometry (sim K) value that is comparable to K values obtained from a manual keratometer or autorefractor. Recently, a novel corneal topographer, the Cassini corneal shape analyzer (i-Optics), has been introduced. This device uses 700 red, green, and yellow light-emitting diodes, each positioned in a unique relationship to 4 of its neighbors, to project light onto the cornea. The multiple colors and the asymmetric positioning prevent errors if reflections are smeared or overlapped to obtain more accurate Ks for irregular corneas.[18]

In comparison to keratometry and Placido topographers, corneal tomography can obtain actual true net corneal power by measuring both the anterior and posterior surfaces of the cornea. The Pentacam (Oculus), Galilei Dual Scheimpflug Analyzer (Ziemer Ophthalmic Systems), and Orbscan (Bausch & Lomb) calculate the total corneal power and astigmatism based on direct measurements of anterior and posterior cornea. These devices measure the topography of both anterior and posterior corneal surfaces and corneal thickness through direct measure of elevation, allowing 3-dimensional reconstruction of the cornea from 2-dimensional cross sections.[19] The Orbscan was the first developed; light is projected through vertical slits, 20 from the right and 20 from the left, at a fixed angle of 45 degrees, and a digital video camera analyzes the anterior and posterior edges of the slits to obtain true anterior and posterior elevation, corneal thickness, iris, and anterior capsule surface. Oculus' Pentacam utilizes a rotating Scheimpflug camera along with a static camera. The rotating camera sweeps across the surface of the cornea along with a monochromatic slit-light source to obtain slit images and anterior and posterior topography from height data. The Galilei combines 2 Scheimpflug cameras, which are able to capture slit images from opposite sides, along with Placido disc topography. Anterior chamber ocular coherence tomography (OCT) devices use low coherence interferometry to provide detailed 2-dimensional, cross-sectional images of the anterior chamber and can also be used to calculate true corneal power.[20] A listing of currently available biometric devices can be found in Table 5-1 (optical biometers) and Table 5-2 (corneal topographers).

Table 5-1
Optical Biometers

Device name	Lenstar LS 900	IOLMaster 500	IOLMaster 700	Aladdin	Galilei G6	OA-2000	AL-Scan
Company	Haag-Streit	Zeiss	Zeiss	Topcon	Ziemer	Tomey	Nidek
Axial length interferometry	x	x	x	x	x	x	x
Pachymetry	x		x	x	x	x	x
Anterior chamber depth	x	x	x	x	x	x	x
Lens thickness	x		x	x	x	x	
Pupillometry	x			x	x	x	x
Keratometry	x	x	x	x	True*	x	
Topography	Optional T-cone Placido add-on			Placido	Dual Scheimpflug/ Placido	Placido	
Toric calculator	Optional		x	x	x		x
OCT			x				

*True keratometry: evaluates both anterior and posterior corneal surfaces and provides a net corneal power.

Table 5-2

Corneal Topographers and Tomographers

Device Name	*Company*	*Category*	*Pupillometry*	*Keratometry*	*Autorefraction*	*Angle Kappa*	*Lens Thickness*	*Topography*
Atlas 9000	Zeiss	Topographer	x	x				Placido
OPD Scan III	Marco	Topographer	x	x	x	x		Placido
Kerato-graph 5M	Oculus	Topographer	x	x				Placido
Kerato-graph 4	Oculus	Topographer	x	x				Placido
Easygraph	Oculus	Topographer		x				Placido
CA-200F	Topcon	Topographer	x	x				Placido
CA-800	Topcon	Topographer	x	x				Placido
TMS-4	Tomey	Topographer		x				Placido
KR-1W	Topcon	Topographer	x	x	x			Placido
iTrace	Tracey Technologies	Topographer	x	x	x	x		Placido
Cassini	i-Optics	Topographer		x				Multicolor LED
Orbscan	Bausch & Lomb	Tomographer	x	True				Scanning slit
TMS-5	Tomey	Topographer		True			x	Scheimpflug/Placido

(continued)

Table 5-2 (continued)

Corneal Topographers and Tomographers

Device Name	*Company*	*Category*	*Pupillometry*	*Keratometry*	*Autore-fraction*	*Angle Kappa*	*Lens Thick-ness*	*Topography*
Pentacam	Oculus	Tomographer		True			x	Scheimp-flug
Pentacam HR	Oculus	Tomographer		True			x	Scheimp-flug
Galilei G4	Ziemer	Tomographer	x	True			x	Dual Scheimp-flug/ Placido
Galilei G2	Ziemer	Tomographer	x	True			x	Dual Scheimp-flug/ Placido

Abbreviation: LED, light-emitting diode

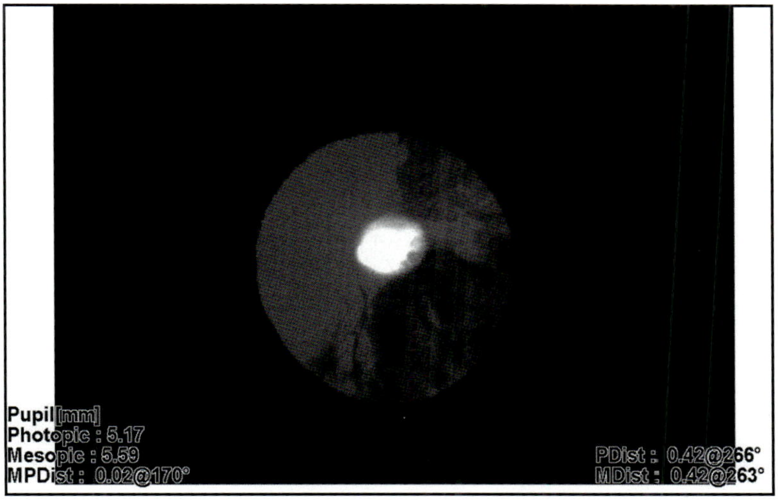

Figure 5-2. OPD-III retroillumination image highlighting the degree of cataract preoperatively.

Multifunctional devices such as OPD-III (Marco) and iTrace (Tracey Technologies) combine corneal topography, autorefraction, wavefront aberrometry, modulation transfer function, and pupillometry, all of which are important to consider when implanting premium IOLs. For example, for patients with high angle kappa, or chord mu, a multifocal implant may induce more aberration, glare, and halo; thus, an accommodative IOL may be a better solution for presbyopia. Some multifocal IOLs are more pupil-dependent than others. After measuring corneal spherical aberration, the proper IOL to reduce or neutralize the spherical aberration can be selected.

The OPD-III also offers features that can help in patient education as well as assisting the surgeon. Preoperatively, a retroillumination image shows the patient the degree of the cataract (Figure 5-2), and the toric summary uses lenticular landmarks and corresponding topographic overlay to verify the steep axis (Figure 5-3).

Estimated Lens Position and the Evolution of IOL Calculation Formulas

The evolution of IOL calculation formulas has largely revolved around progressive refinement of the ELP, which cannot be measured or chosen. In the 1980s, the first IOL calculation formulas created were regression formulas, which were empiric formulas generated by averaging large numbers of postoperative clinical results. These documented IOL implantations were plotted with respect to the corneal power, axial length, and IOL power and then a best-fit equation was determined by statistical regression analysis. The SRK I formula, developed by Sanders, Retzlaff, and Kraff in the 1980s, is the prototypical formula:

$P = A - (2.5L) - 0.9K$

P = lens implant power for target refraction (usually emmetropia) in diopters

L = axial length (mm)

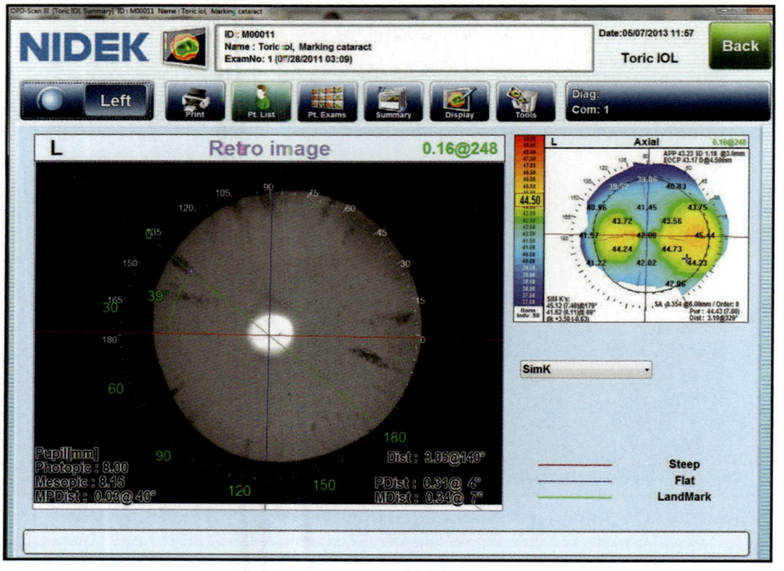

Figure 5-3. OPD-III toric summary display showing lenticular landmark and the corresponding topographic overlay to verify the steep axis.

K = average keratometric reading (diopters)

A = constant specific to lens implant

These regression formulas had the advantage of not being dependent on any theoretical assumptions regarding the eye. The A constant is a unit-less value that factors in the vagaries of the eye, measuring devices, and particular properties of the specific lens, such as its positioning tendencies, and are provided by each lens manufacturer. In these early formulas, the ELP was first termed *anterior chamber depth* (ACD), as most lenses were anterior-chamber IOLs. The ACD was a factor that was assumed to be a constant value (usually 2.8 or 3.5 mm) and was factored into the A constant. Since the 1990s, regression formulas have been largely replaced by newer theoretical formulas for IOL power calculations, and ELP replaced ACD as the term to describe the location of the IOL in the eye. Underlying all of the successive generations of theoretical formulas is the same basic formula generated by geometric optics holding the eye as a 2-element optical system, first mentioned earlier in this chapter.

$P = (n_V / AL - C) - K / (1 - K x (C / n_A)$

P = power of target IOL (diopters)

n_V = index of refraction of vitreous

AL = axial length

C = ELP

K = corneal power (diopters)

n_A = index of refraction of aqueous

In first-generation theoretical formulas, the ELP used was a constant of 4 mm for every lens, which sufficed, as most IOLs were of iris clip fixation type. Binkhorst improved the ELP prediction in 1981 by using a single variable: axial length, to scale for

ELP, which defined the second generation of theoretical formulas. Then in 1988, third-generation formulas were introduced, and keratometry was added to axial length as a second variable for predicting ELP, which was shown to significantly improve accuracy.[21] These formulas include the Holladay 1, SRK/T, and Hoffer Q. The Haigis-L is another 2-variable formula, which improves ELP determination by using 3 IOL- and surgeon-specific constants (a0, a1, and a2) and a measured ACD and is included in the IOLMaster's standard software package. Moreover, corneal power measurements are not required, which, as will be discussed later, benefits IOL calculations in post–refractive surgery eyes. The main limitation of the Haigis-L formula is that it requires the surgeon to generate a large number of cases (n > 50) over a wide range of axial lengths, as the constants are derived via regression analysis. In the fourth generation of theoretical formulas, Olsen introduced in 1995[22] a 4-variable predictor that added preoperative ACD and lens thickness. A year later, Holladay[23] introduced a 7-variable formula that uses axial length, corneal power, horizontal corneal diameter, ACD, lens thickness, preoperative refraction, and age. There is currently no formula that has been proven to be suitable for all eyes.[24] The largest study to date was conducted by Aristodemou et al, which showed that in 8108 eyes, the Hoffer Q was more accurate for eyes shorter than 24.5 mm, Holladay 1 for eyes ranging from 24.5 to 26.0 mm, and the SRK/T for eyes longer than 26.0 mm.[25] The Haigis-L, Olsen's formula, and the Holladay 2 formula are considered accurate for a broad range of axial lengths. However, there is lack of robust data to prove superiority of one particular formula.

The ACD required by the fourth-generation theoretical formulas can be measured in different ways, including A-scan ultrasonography, partial coherence interferometry (AC-Master [Carl Zeiss Meditec]), slit-scanning videokeratography, Scheimpflug imaging, and anterior segment optical coherence tomography (Visante OCT [Carl Zeiss Meditec]). The IOLMaster uses a slit-beam photographic technique to measure ACD. The anterior segment OCT provides high-resolution cross-sectional images of the anterior segment using infrared light. See Table 5-3 for a listing of commonly used modern formulas.

Recently, a novel software, tied in with the Lenstar LS 900, has been introduced, providing a probability distribution curve of possible expected final refraction outcomes based on the lens power chosen, using intensive computational analysis and the Monte Carlo Markov Chain statistical theory. This software aids in IOL power calculation by optimizing for future surgeries based on past results, using all of the current variables that are measured by modern formulas (corneal power, ACD, axial length, lens thickness, preoperative refraction, age) as well as 2 other variables: sulcus-to-sulcus widths and sulcus-to-sulcus perpendicular depth, which is the distance from the anterior cornea to the sulcus-to-sulcus line. The main advantage of this software is that it aids surgeons in automatically refining their A-constant for IOL calculations, although the effectiveness of this system has yet to be rigorously tested.

Table 5-3
Selected List of Formulas

Formula Name	*Generation of Theoretical Formula*	*Variables for ELP Prediction*	*Best Range of Use*
SRK I	Regression-based	n/a	22.0 to 24.5 mm
SRK II	Regression-based	n/a	Improved slightly from longer and shorter eyes compared with SRK I
Binkhorst	2nd	AL	Better for average-length eyes
SRK/T	3rd (combo regression with theoretical model)	AL, K	>26.0 mm
Hoffer Q	3rd	AL, K	<24.0 mm
Holladay I	3rd	AL, K	24.5 to 26.0 mm
Haigis-L	3rd	AL, ACD	Broad
Olsen	4th	AL, K, ACD, LT	Broad
Holladay II	4th	AL, K, ACD, WTW, LT, age, preoperative refraction	Broad
Barrett Universal Formula II	4th	AL, K, ACD, LT, WTW, preoperative refraction	Broad

Abbreviations: AL, axial length; K, keratometry; LT, lens thickness; WTW, white-to-white.

Special Occasions

IOL Calculation for Post–Refractive Surgery Eyes

Sources of Error

Often, patients who have had corneal refractive surgery are those most interested in refractive or multifocal IOLs, which makes accuracy of intraocular lens power calculation all the more important. There are 3 main challenges in calculating IOL power in post–refractive surgery eyes: index of refraction error, instrument error, and formula error.

Keratometry and keratoscopy estimate cornea power based on assumptions that the cornea is a spherocylinder, a thin lens, and has a fixed anterior-to-posterior corneal curvature. However, for corneas subjected to photorefractive keratectomy or LASIK, these assumptions are violated. The anterior surface of the cornea contributes roughly +49 D of power, whereas the posterior surface contributes on average -6 D of power, such that the overall net power averages to +43 D. As keratometers and topographers are only able to measure the anterior corneal curvature, they assume that the radius of curvature of the posterior surface is consistently 1.2 mm less than the anterior curvature. These platforms also use 1.3375 as the index of refraction for the cornea instead of the actual corneal refractive index of 1.376 to compensate for the negative power of the posterior surface.[26] Corneal refractive surgery alters the anterior curvature of the cornea, and thus the assumed relationship between anterior and posterior curvatures is no longer valid, resulting in the index of refraction error. The index of refraction of 1.3375 results in an overestimation of the true corneal power in myopic LASIK; for every 7.0 D of surgical correction, the cornea is overestimated by 1.0 D.

Unadulterated corneas are actually aspheric with a prolate shape: an effective optical zone with a central spherical zone of 1 to 2 mm and a paracentral 3 to 4 mm donut of progressive flattening. The aforementioned platforms measure the cornea at differing diameters. Manual keratometry measures a 3.2 mm ring, the IOLMaster measures a 2.5 mm ring, the Lenstar averages a 2.35 mm and a 1.64 mm ring, and simulated keratometry values from Placido topographers focus on the central 3.0 mm zone. Theoretically, the closer to the center of the visual axis the measurement, the more accurate it would be. However, none of the current platforms measure at the true center. LASIK and photorefractive keratectomy treatments tend to affect the center of the treated zone, resulting in instrument measurement error. For example, in myopic LASIK, the cornea is flattened in the center relative to the periphery. Current devices miss this central flattened zone of effective cornea power, overestimating actual corneal power, resulting in hyperopic refractive errors postoperatively. Conversely, in hyperopic LASIK, the postoperative cornea is steeper in the center, such that a myopic postoperative surprise occurs.

Finally, the third error arises from the fact that most third-generation IOL power formulas (Hoffer Q, Holladay 1 and 2, SRK/T) use axial length and corneal power to predict ELP. These formulas assume a certain proportionality to the anterior chamber, such that the steeper the cornea, the further away the ELP. In myopic laser refractive surgery, for example, postoperative flattening of the cornea calls for a more forward ELP, resulting in an underestimation of required IOL power.[27]

Solutions

The solutions for post–refractive cataract surgery IOL calculations historically focused on estimating post-refractive corneal power using historical data but now have shifted to focusing on directly measuring corneal power.

Traditionally, the clinical history method estimated post-refractive cornea power by simply subtracting the known change in spherical equivalent refraction from the prior preoperative keratometric power. There are a variety of formulas in current use that have been developed, such as the Double-K method by Aramberri, the Feiz-Mannis, and Masket methods, which all require preoperative data for estimation of corneal power. These formulas also separate the corneal power measurement from calculation of ELP. The main disadvantage of these formulas is that historical keratometry and refraction data are often unavailable.

Contact lens over-refraction was devised to circumvent missing historical data. The difference in manifest refraction, before and after applying a plano hard contact lens, is added to the known base curve power of the contact lens to derive the post-refractive K.

However, patients need a minimum of 20/80 vision, and this method has been critiqued as unreliable.[28]

Additional formulas that do not depend on historical data have been developed. The Haigis-L avoids measuring K altogether and is based entirely on surgeon-accumulated regression data, whereas Shammas and Shammas have a method which uses an average"K to calculate ELP.[29] These 2 formulas have shown promise.[30] Wang uses topography-measured corneal power for his formulas (the modified Maloney method).[31] Geggel described a novel method using a ratio of central to peripheral corneal thickness as measured by pachymetry to estimate the net change in corneal tissue removed by refractive surgery.[32] Most recently, the utility of true corneal power measurements derived from corneal tomography[33] and anterior segment OCT has been promising.[26] Potvin has shown with Pentacam that true net corneal power over the 4.0 mm zone, centered over the apex, produces accurate results for post–refractive surgery IOL calculations.[34]

As there are many different methods (Table 5-4), which rely on different combinations of devices and patient data, it has been standard practice for surgeons to use multiple methods. There are now online calculators that aggregate formulas and provide average post-refractive IOL calculations based on data provided. The American Society of Cataract and Refractive Surgery calculator (http://iolcalc.ascrs.org) and the Ocular MD calculator (http://iol.ocularmd.com/) are 2 popular online tools. Surgeons are able to compare the results from multiple different formulas and select the best option.

An alternative option for bypassing IOL calculations is intraoperative aberrometry. Intraoperative refractive biometry with wavefront aberrometry is performed after crystalline lens extraction to determine the aphakic spherical equivalent, which is then used to derive the emmetropic IOL power. The Optiwave Refractive Analysis (ORA) System (WaveTec Vision, Inc) was the first such device introduced[35] and has been shown to select IOLs that are comparable in accuracy to Pentacam and anterior OCT dependent formulas in post–refractive surgery eyes.[36] Intraoperative aberrometry is the only way to measure postsurgical astigmatism, because it takes the measurement after the main incision is made. Another intraoperative aberrometer with a new sequentially shifting wavefront device (HOLOS IntraOp, Clarity Medical Systems) and the newest ORA VerifEye offer real-time information regarding the refractive status of the eye during surgery.

IOL Calculations for Toric IOLs

The same instruments used to measure corneal power mentioned above are also used to measure corneal astigmatism: manual keratometers, automated keratometers, partial coherence interferometry, optical low-coherence reflectometry, Placido topographers, and scanning-slit and Scheimpflug tomographers. Studies to date have yet to determine which platforms measure astigmatism with the highest repeatability and reproducibility.[37] However, recent studies have shown that the posterior surface of the cornea indeed has an important contribution to total corneal astigmatism. In most eyes, the posterior corneal surface is steep vertically and exerts a negative refractive power vertically, resulting in net plus refractive power along the horizontal meridian. Although anterior corneal astigmatism changes with age, the posterior steep meridian has been shown to be constant throughout life. Thus, measuring true corneal power with tomographers should

Table 5-4
Selected List of Solutions to Post-Refractive Surgery IOL Calculations

Formula/ Method Name	*Historical Data Required*	*Special Measurements/ Equipment Required*	*Notes**
Clinical history method	Yes	None	Even if historical data available, 2 major disadvantages: 1) it can be difficult to determine if postoperative refraction is accurate/stable, 2) there is often a myopic shift secondary to development of cataract
Double-K by Aramberri	Yes	None	Bypasses the ELP prediction error by using preoperative K reading to calculate the ELP, whereas IOL power is calculated using postoperative K reading: hence double K
Feiz-Mannis	Yes	None	
Masket	Yes	None	
Contact lens over-refraction	No	Rigid contact lens	Vision needs to be at least 20/80 for this method to be accurate; also, the patient's refraction in the presence of a cataract needs to be reliable.
Maloney	No	Corneal topography	
Wang	No	Corneal topography	
Shammas and Shammas average K	No	None	Does not have ELP calculation vary with corneal curvature. There is an arbitrary average corneal power used to calculate the ELP
Haigis-L	No	None	Uses empirical linear regression analysis of postoperative surgery results to optimize the estimate of corneal power from standard keratometry

(continued)

Table 5-4 (continued)
Selected List of Solutions to Post-Refractive Surgery IOL Calculations

Formula/ Method Name	*Historical Data Required*	*Special Measurements/ Equipment Required*	*Notes**
Geggel	No	Corneal pachymetry	Uses a ratio of central and peripheral corneal thickness measured post–refractive surgery to estimate surgical change in spherical equivalence induced by the refractive surgery
Povkin	No	Corneal tomography (Pentacam)	Given that tomography measures both anterior and posterior K, a true net K can be measured.

* Preoperative = pre–refractive surgery; postoperative = post–refractive surgery.

give the most precise measurement of corneal astigmatism. Based on studies that have verified the influence of the posterior corneal curvature on total astigmatism, Koch et al have suggested that 0.5 D should be subtracted in with-the-rule astigmatism and 0.3 D should be added for against-the-rule astigmatism when astigmatism is calculated with anterior corneal measurements.[27]

Currently, most studies reviewing toric IOL implantation are done with the *3-step* marking procedure, in which the patient's eye is physically marked pre- and intraoperatively. This process has been shown to have, on average, 5 degrees of error, with as high as 10 degrees in individual patients.[38] Several new intraoperative techniques for aligning toric IOLs have been introduced. First, in 2010 Osher described a technique in which a preoperative image of the eye was taken with a high-resolution camera, printed, and brought to the surgical suite to align the toric IOL based on iris morphology. Second, the aforementioned intraoperative wavefront aberrometer can also be used to help align toric IOLs. The surgeon can measure intraoperatively residual astigmatism and adjust appropriately. Finally, several systems have been introduced that track the eye intraoperatively to help surgeons optimize incision placement and toric IOL alignment. Prior to surgery, a high-resolution image of the eye, which details blood vessel and iris morphology, is captured and matched to keratometry to determine the steep and flat corneal meridians. Intraoperatively, an overlay showing the alignment axis is visible through the oculars of the operating microscope and aids in aligning the toric IOL. The TrueGuide Computer-Guided Surgery system (TrueVision), which has been integrated with the Cassini topographer, and Callisto Eye System (Carl Zeiss Meditec) are similar systems that have recently been developed. Alcon also has an intraoperative system that combines the intraoperative aberrometry with real-time eye tracking based

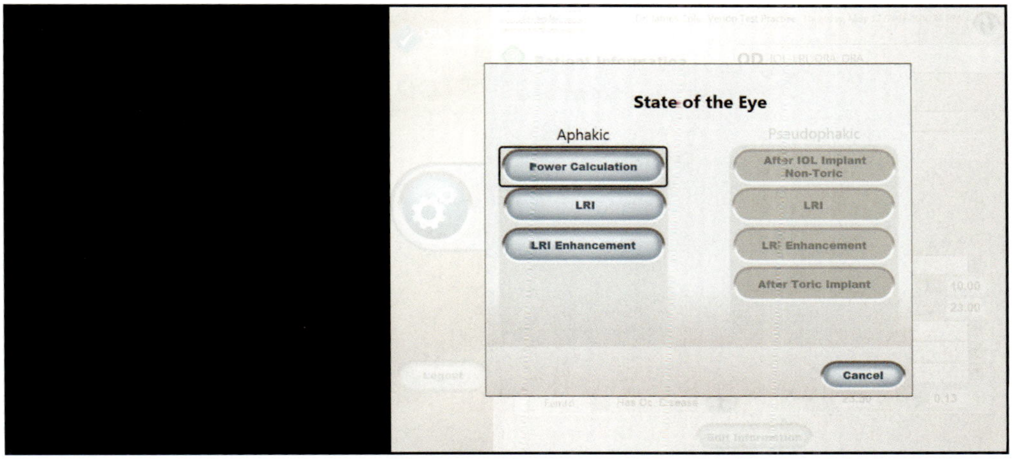

Figure 5-4. ORA display screen enabling selection of lens status of eye. Measurements can be taken in a variety of situations: for power calculation cataract removal, after IOL implantation for verification of power, for limbal relaxing incisions, and confirming toric IOL implant alignment.

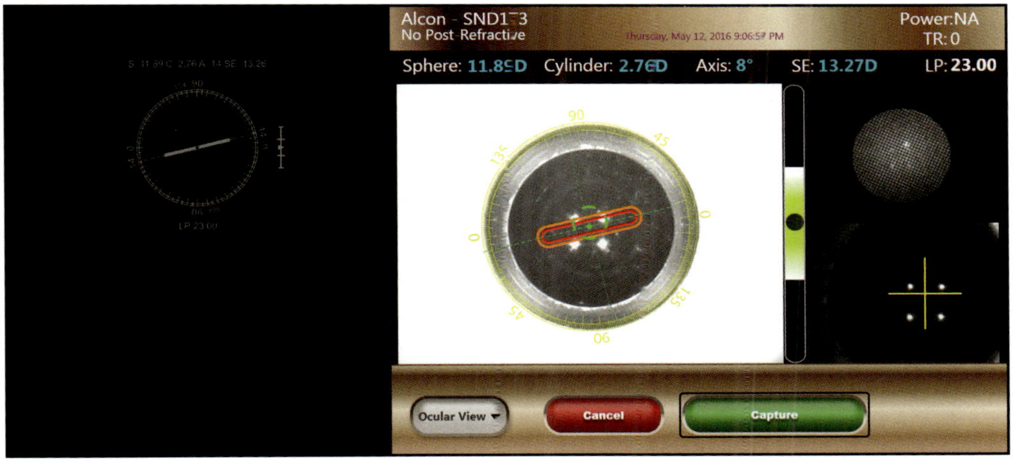

Figure 5-5. View of ORA display during orientation and alignment of targeting reticule to enable accurate aberrometry readings.

on iris and blood-vessel characteristics (Verion Image Guided System and ORA System with VerifEye+ Technology, Alcon). After the cataract is extracted and aphakic status is selected (Figure 5-4), the eye is scanned (Figure 5-5), implant selected (Figure 5-6), and pseudophakic scans are performed until the measured residual refractive error is minimal or in the case of toric IOL implants, no rotation is recommended (Figure 5-7).

Light-Adjustable Intraocular Lenses

The landscape of premium intraocular lenses is exciting, as it is constantly in flux. Preoperative diagnostics may become more or less crucial as technology advances. One example of this is the introduction of light-adjustable IOLs. Light-adjustable IOLs are

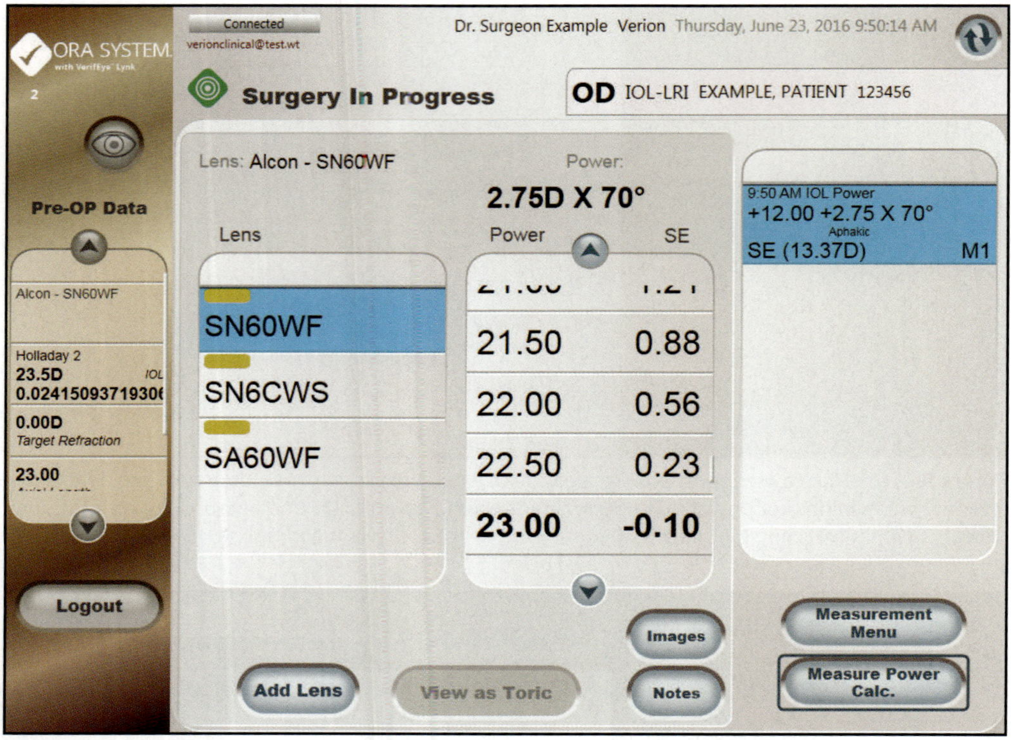

Figure 5-6. Screenshot of ORA display for toric IOL selection

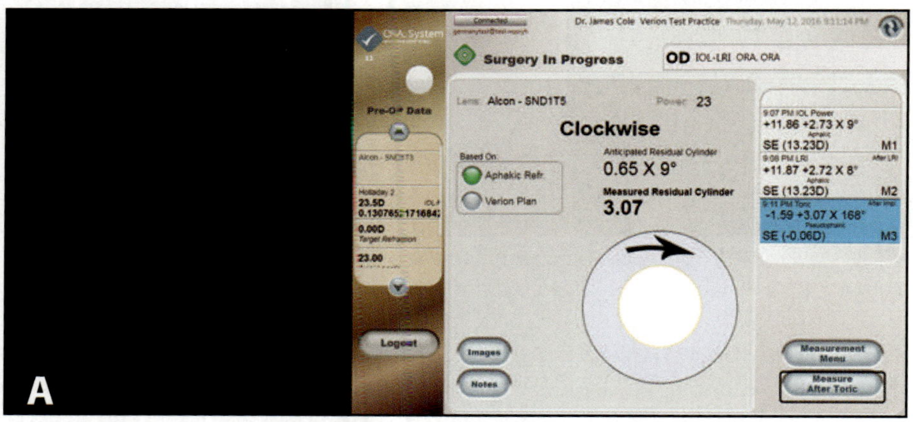

Figure 5-7. View of ORA display (A) showing the suggested degree of rotation after a toric IOL has been inserted. *(continued)*

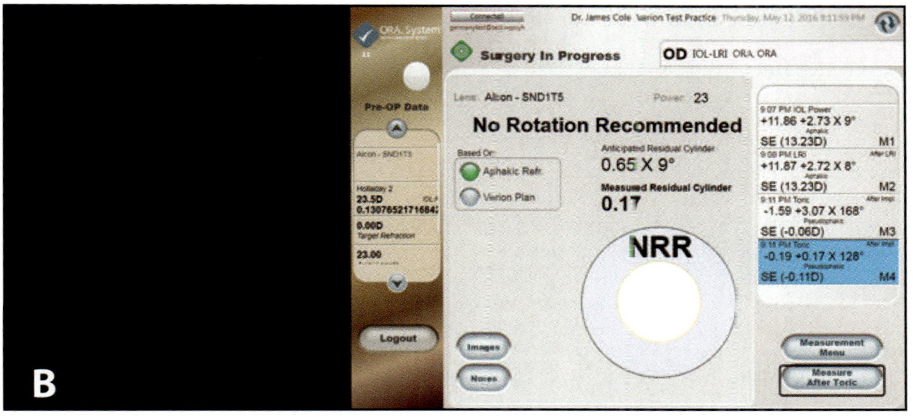

Figure 5-7 (continued). The lens is rotated (B) until no further rotation is recommended.

silicone lenses that can be irradiated with ultraviolet light after implantation to induce a change in the shape and power of the IOL. Myopic, hyperopic, and even astigmatic shifts are possible. This technology is still under development and not approved by the Food and Drug Administration. However, if successful, it may in fact make biometry less relevant in the future.

References

1. Ahmed II, Rocha G, Slomovic AR, et al. Visual function and patient experience after bilateral implantation of toric intraocular lenses. *J Cataract Refract Surg.* 2010;36(4):609-616.
2. Ernest P, Potvin R. Effects of preoperative corneal astigmatism orientation on results with a low-cylinder-power toric intraocular lens. *J Cataract Refract Surg.* 2011;37(4):727-732.
3. Bauer NJ, de Vries NE, Webers CA, Hendrikse F, Nuijts RM. Astigmatism management in cataract surgery with the AcrySof toric intraocular lens. *J Cataract Refract Surg.* 2008;34(9):1483-1488.
4. Holland E, Lane S, Horn JD, Ernest P, Arleo R, Miller KM. The AcrySof Toric intraocular lens in subjects with cataracts and corneal astigmatism: a randomized, subject-masked, parallel-group, 1-year study. *Ophthalmology.* 2010;117(11):2104-2111.
5. Visser N, Bauer NJ, Nuijts RM. Toric intraocular lenses: historical overview, patient selection, IOL calculation, surgical techniques, clinical outcomes, and complications. *J Cataract Refract Surg.* 2013;39(4):624-637.
6. Visser N, Gast ST, Bauer NJ, Nuijts RM. Cataract surgery with toric intraocular lens implantation in keratoconus: a case report. *Cornea.* 2011;30(6):720-723.
7. Luck J. Customized ultra-high-power toric intraocular lens implantation for pellucid marginal degeneration and cataract. *J Cataract Refract Surg.* 2010;36(7):1235-1238.
8. Kersey JP, O'Donnell A, Illingworth CD. Cataract surgery with toric intraocular lenses can optimize uncorrected postoperative visual acuity in patients with marked corneal astigmatism. *Cornea.* 2007;26(2):133-135.
9. Braga-Mele R, Chang D, Dewey S, et al. Multifocal intraocular lenses: relative indications and contraindications for implantation. *J Cataract Refract Surg.* 2014;40(2):313-322.
10. Hayashi K, Manabe S, Yoshida M, Hayashi H. Effect of astigmatism on visual acuity in eyes with a diffractive multifocal intraocular lens. *J Cataract Refract Surg.* 2010;36(3):1323-1329.
11. Montes-Mico R, Lopez-Gil N, Perez-Vives C, Bonaque S, Ferrer-Blasco T. In vitro optical performance of nonrotational symmetric and refractive-diffractive aspheric multifocal intraocular lenses: impact of tilt and decentration. *J Cataract Refract Surg.* 2012;38(9):1657-1663.
12. Prakash G, Prakash DR, Agarwal A, Kumar DA, Agarwal A, Jacob S. Predictive factor and kappa angle analysis for visual satisfactions in patients with multifocal IOL implantation. *Eye.* 2011;25(9):1187-1193.

13. Chang DH, Waring GO IV. The subject-fixated coaxially sighted corneal light reflex: a clinical marker for centration of refractive treatments and devices. *Am J Ophthalmol.* 2014;158(5):863-874.
14. Yoshino M, Inoue M, Kitamura N, Bissen-Miyajima H. Diffractive multifocal intraocular lens interferes with intraoperative view. *Clin Ophthalmol.* 2010;4:467-469.
15. Shammas HJ. A comparison of immersion and contact techniques for axial length measurement. *J Am Intraocul Implant Soc.* 1984;10(4):444-447.
16. Wang L, Shirayama M, Ma XJ, Kohnen T, Koch DD. Optimizing intraocular lens power calculations in eyes with axial lengths above 25.0 mm. *J Cataract Refract Surg.* 2011;37(11):2018-2027.
17. Montes-Mico R, Carones F, Buttacchio A, Ferrer-Blasco T, Madrid-Costa D. Comparison of immersion ultrasound, partial coherence interferometry, and low coherence reflectometry for ocular biometry in cataract patients. *J Refract Surg.* 2011;27(9):665-671.
18. Kent C. Making the Most of high-tech biometry. *Review of Ophthalmology.* www.truevisionsys.com/pdf/2014-04ReviewofOphthalmology_Making.pdf. Published April 2, 2014. Accessed January 4, 2017.
19. Oliveira CM, Ribeiro C, Franco S. Corneal imaging with slit-scanning and Scheimpflug imaging techniques. *Clin Exp Optom.* 2011;94(1):33-42.
20. Tang M, Wang L, Koch DD, Li Y, Huang D. Intraocular lens power calculation after previous myopic laser vision correction based on corneal power measured by Fourier-domain optical coherence tomography. *J Cataract Refract Surg.* 2012;38(4):589-594.
21. Holladay JT, Prager TC, Chandler TY, Musgrove KH, Lewis JW, Ruiz RS. A three-part system for refining intraocular lens power calculations. *J Cataract Refract Surg.* 1988;14(1):17-24.
22. Olsen T, Corydon L, Gimbel H. Intraocular lens power calculation with an improved anterior chamber depth prediction algorithm. *J Cataract Refract Surg.* 1995;21(3):313-319.
23. Holladay JT, Gills JP, Leidlein J, Cherchio M. Achieving emmetropia in extremely short eyes with two piggyback posterior chamber intraocular lenses. *Ophthalmology.* 1996;103(7):1118-1123.
24. Lee AC, Qazi MA, Pepose JS. Biometry and intraocular lens power calculation. *Curr Opin Ophthalmol.* 2008;19(1):13-17.
25. Aristodemou P, Knox Cartwright NE, Sparrow JM, Johnston RL. Formula choice: Hoffer Q, Holladay 1, or SRK/T and refractive outcomes in 8108 eyes after cataract surgery with biometry by partial coherence interferometry. *J Cataract Refract Surg.* 2011;37(1):63-71.
26. Tang M, Li Y, Avila M, Huang D. Measuring total corneal power before and after laser in situ keratomileusis with high-speed optical coherence tomography. *J Cataract Refract Surg.* 2006;32(11):1843-1850.
27. Koch DD, Wang L. Calculating IOL power in eyes that have had refractive surgery. *J Cataract Refract Surg.* 2003;29(11):2039-2042.
28. Haigis W. Corneal power after refractive surgery for myopia: contact lens method. *J Cataract Refract Surg.* 2003;29(7):1397-1411.
29. Shammas HJ, Shammas MC. No-history method of intraocular lens power calculation for cataract surgery after myopic laser in situ keratomileusis. *J Cataract Refract Surg.* 2007;33(1):31-36.
30. McCarthy M, Gavanski GM, Paton KE, Holland SP. Intraocular lens power calculations after myopic laser refractive surgery: a comparison of methods in 173 eyes. *Ophthalmology.* 2011;118(5):940-944.
31. Wang L, Booth MA, Koch DD. Comparison of intraocular lens power calculation methods in eyes that have undergone laser-assisted in-situ keratomileusis. *Trans Am Ophthalmol Soc.* 2004;102:189-196; discussion 196-187.
32. Geggel HS. Pachymetric ratio no-history method for intraocular lens power adjustment after excimer laser refractive surgery. *Ophthalmology.* 2009;116(6):1057-1066.
33. Savini G, Calossi A, Camellin M, Carones F, Fantozzi M, Hoffer KJ. Corneal ray tracing versus simulated keratometry for estimating corneal power changes after excimer laser surgery. *J Cataract Refract Surg.* 2014;40(7):1109-1115.
34. Potvin R, Hill W. New algorithm for intraocular lens power calculations after myopic laser in situ keratomileusis based on rotating Scheimpflug camera data. *J Cataract Refract Surg.* 2015;41(2):339-347.
35. Ianchulev T, Hoffer KJ, Yoo SH, et al. Intraoperative refractive biometry for predicting intraocular lens power calculation after prior myopic refractive surgery. *Ophthalmology.* 2014;121(1):56-60.
36. Fram NR, Masket S, Wang L. Comparison of intraoperative aberrometry, oct-based iol formula, haigis-l, and masket formulae for IOL power calculation after laser vision correction. *Ophthalmology.* 2015;122(6):1096-1101.
37. Lee H, Kim TI, Kim EK. Corneal astigmatism analysis for toric intraocular lens implantation: precise measurements for perfect correction. *Curr Opin Ophthalmol.* 2015;26(1):34-38.
38. Visser N, Berendschot TT, Bauer NJ, Jurich J, Kersting O, Nuijts RM. Accuracy of toric intraocular lens implantation in cataract and refractive surgery. *J Cataract Refract Surg.* 2011;37(8):1394-1402.

Chapter 6

Practice Management Considerations of Refractive Cataract Surgery

Kevin J. Corcoran, COE, CPC, CPMA, FNAO

The goal of cataract surgery is to improve vision by removing the lenticular opacity that scatters light. Coincidentally, with precise biometry and sophisticated intraocular lens (IOL) calculations, pre-existing myopia or hyperopia can be reduced or eliminated. As the surgical technique and planning has improved, patients and surgeons have established 2 concurrent goals: remediate cataract and simultaneously minimize residual refractive errors after cataract surgery, and obtain the best possible uncorrected visual acuity or the desired ametropia as planned for in pseudophakic monovision. This approach has been termed *refractive cataract surgery,* recognizing the twin objectives.

Refractive Cataract Surgery

From the perspective of the Medicare program as well as other third-party payers, the improved refractive outcomes have been taken for granted as a byproduct of the evolution of the cataract procedure. Better results have not generated higher payment rates to surgeons. Instead, better results have led to higher volumes of procedures, which, in turn, reduce payment per procedure but increase total revenue for busier surgeons.

Refractive cataract surgery gained momentum and recognition from the understanding that astigmatism and presbyopia are not so easily dealt with in IOL calculations, but that ancillary diagnostic testing, corneal refractive procedures, and/or premium IOLs were needed to ameliorate them.[1] These additional items and services are not required in cataract surgery—they are optional. Indeed, Medicare established in 1990 that beneficiaries are entitled to "one pair of conventional eyeglasses or contact lenses furnished subsequent to each cataract surgery with insertion of an intraocular lens,"[2] which addresses

Hovanesian JA.
Refractive Cataract Surgery: Best Practices and Advanced Technology, Second Edition (pp 61-73). © 2017 SLACK Incorporated.

all postoperative refractive errors other than egregious IOL miscalculations. Under a number of Medicare rules,[3,4] sometimes imitated by other third-party payers, patients desiring a greater degree of spectacle independence may elect these additional items and services and pay for them out of pocket, because they are performed solely for refractive purposes and "are not reasonable and necessary for the diagnosis or treatment of illness or injury or to improve the functioning of a malformed body member."[5]

Femtosecond Lasers

Many patients ask, "Do you perform cataract surgery using a laser?" Surgeons carefully explain the difference between primary cataracts and secondary cataracts, the myths about cataract, and the surgical procedures involved. While lasers have been used for posterior capsulotomy to soften cataracts and speed up emulsification,[6] phacoemulsification remains the favored technique in the developed world. Several femtosecond lasers have been developed for use in refractive cataract surgery (eg, Catalys [Abbott Medical Optics], LenSx [Alcon], VICTUS [Bausch & Lomb]), with the goal of improving surgical precision and patient outcomes.[7] Like phacoemulsification before it, the femtosecond laser represents another technological advancement, but one with a high price tag; a kind of golden scalpel. Femtosecond lasers have 4 capabilities: 1) create a self-sealing, stepped corneal incision for the insertion of surgical instruments into the anterior chamber, 2) perform precise capsulorrhexis, 3) fragment the crystalline lens to facilitate removal, and 4) make corneal relaxing incisions to ameliorate clinically significant regular astigmatism. Of these capabilities, only the last one can be separately charged to the beneficiary as a noncovered procedure, while the others are part of the covered cataract surgery.[8,9]

Covered Versus Noncovered

In the context of practice management, covered services are subject to strict limitations on balance billing, while noncovered services are the beneficiary's financial responsibility (Table 6-1). Balance billing is the practice of asking a beneficiary to pay the difference between the actual charge and the assigned benefit amount for covered services that the provider has contractually accepted as payment in full.[10] It does not refer to the collection of copayments and deductibles. At the very least, the provider who balance-bills patients may breach his or her pre-existing agreement with the payer, which could result in termination of his or her provider agreement and/or other contractual remedies, such as monetary penalties. Some state insurance laws or consumer protection laws also might be implicated. Despite the prohibitions against balance billing, third-party payers generally agree that enrollees may be billed for noncovered services. Consequently, it is necessary to clearly define and separate covered from noncovered services and to obtain the patient's voluntary acceptance of financial responsibility for the latter (Table 6-2).

Table 6-1
Reimbursement Grid

	Facility	*Physician*
Covered	Cataract surgery	Cataract surgery
Not covered	Astigmatism-correcting or presbyopia-correcting IOL, refractive keratoplasty	Screening, preventive and refractive services

Table 6-2
Covered and Non-Covered Services

	Facility	*Surgeon*
Eye exam	—	Covered
Biometry[a]	—	Covered
Refractive testing[b]	—	Not covered
Corneal topography[c]	—	Rarely covered
Specular microscopy[d]	—	Covered
Screening[e]	—	Not covered
Laser capsulorrhexis[f]	Covered	Covered
Laser lens fragmentation[f]	Covered	Covered
Phacoemulsification	Covered	Covered
Postoperative care	—	Covered
Refractive surgery[g]	Not covered	Not covered

[a]NCD 10.1 A-scan or Optical Coherence Biometry (either one but not both).[11]
[b]Testing for refractive errors including refraction (sphere, cylinder, add, prism) are noncovered services in Medicare. Beneficiaries with supplemental insurance that includes a vision benefit may have separate coverage.[12]
[c]Regular astigmatism is not a covered indication for Medicare; irregular astigmatism is a covered indication, as may occur after corneal trauma. Corneal pathology, such as keratoconus, may be covered.[13]
[d]NCD 80.8 states: "When a presurgical examination for cataract surgery is performed and the conditions of this section are met, if the only visual problem is cataracts, endothelial cell photography is covered as part of the presurgical comprehensive eye examination or combination brief/intermediate examination provided prior to cataract surgery, and not in addition to it."[14]
[e]Prophylactic testing (eg, screening with scanning computerized ophthalmic diagnostic imaging) is not a Medicare benefit, unless specifically authorized by Congress.
[f]Laser capsulorrhexis and lens fragmentation are an integral part of cataract surgery, so there is no merit for a separate charge.
[g]NCD 80.7 states: "The use of radial keratotomy and/or keratoplasty for the purpose of refractive error compensation is considered a substitute or alternative to eyeglasses or contact lenses, which are specifically excluded by §1862(a)(7) of the Act (except in certain cases in connection with cataract surgery). In addition, many in the medical community consider such procedures cosmetic surgery, which is excluded by section §1862(a)(10) of the Act. Therefore, radial keratotomy and keratoplasty to treat refractive defects are not covered."[15]

Deluxe Items

One very helpful concept that has been well established in other aspects of reimbursement is the notion of a *deluxe item*, which incorporates both covered and noncovered elements (eg, wheelchairs, hearing aids). Within ophthalmology, the classic example is eyeglass frames. The payer establishes a preset covered amount for eyeglass frames and permits the optician to accept payment from the beneficiary for any additional amount to upgrade the frame. It is important to note that this billing method is not balance billing, and that the mechanism for claim submission includes 2 distinct lines on the claim form to discriminate between the covered and noncovered elements.

For example, your pseudophakic patient orders a $300 frame. Medicare allows $60 for a standard frame (Healthcare Common Procedure Coding System [HCPCS] V2020). The beneficiary agrees to pay $240 for a deluxe frame (HCPCS V2025)—the difference between $300 and $60. As with eyeglasses, Medicare and some third-party payers have applied the deluxe concept to specifically designated IOLs, permitting providers (ie, hospitals and ambulatory surgery centers [ASCs]) to collect an extra fee from beneficiaries for the noncovered aspect of an otherwise covered IOL. To assist with bookkeeping, the Centers for Medicare and Medicaid Services (CMS) created 2 HCPCS codes to identify the noncovered or deluxe portion of a presbyopia-correcting IOL and an astigmatism-correcting IOL. Respectively, they are V2788 and V2787. Hospitals and ASCs use them on claim forms to identify the noncovered part of the premium IOL. Commonly, these premium IOLs cost significantly more than conventional IOLs. Since reimbursement for a conventional IOL is included in the facility fee for the hospital outpatient department (HOPD) or ASC, we must estimate its value. As a useful point of reference, the January 2016 CMS Durable Medical Equipment, Prosthetics, Orthotics, and Supplies fee schedule allows $113.04 for a posterior chamber IOL (HCPCS V2632).[16] Alternately, the average purchase price of a conventional IOL in the HOPD or ASC is a reasonable value. For example, if the premium IOL is valued at $950, including shipping, handling, and applicable taxes, and a conventional IOL is valued at $113, then the noncovered portion payable by the beneficiary is $837.

The purchaser of the premium IOL is almost always the HOPD or ASC, because it is supplied in the facility, and the conventional portion of the IOL is billed and paid to the facility. The exception is in-office cataract surgery.

Financial Waivers

An Advance Beneficiary Notice of Noncoverage (ABN; form CMS-R-131) is a written notice a health care provider gives to a Part B Medicare beneficiary when the provider believes that Medicare will not pay for items or services. An ABN cannot be used for a Part C Medicare beneficiary; follow the Medicare Advantage Organization's instructions for predetermination of benefits.[17] By signing an ABN, the Medicare beneficiary acknowledges that he or she has been advised that Medicare will not pay and agrees to be responsible for payment, either personally or through another insurance plan. For an ABN to have any utility, it must be signed before providing the item or service.

An ABN is voluntary for items or services that are statutorily excluded from coverage or fails to meet a technical benefit requirement by Medicare.[18,19,20]

The format of an ABN cannot be modified to any significant degree. You must add your name, address, and telephone number to the header. You may add your logo and other information if you wish. The "Items or Services," "Reason Medicare May Not Pay," and "Estimated Cost" boxes are customizable so you can add preprinted lists of common items and services or denial reasons. Anything you add in the boxes must be high-contrast ink on a pale background. Blue or black ink on white paper is preferred. You may not make any other alterations to the form. It must be one page, single-sided.

You must complete your portion of the form before asking the beneficiary to sign. Fill in the beneficiary's name and identification number (but not the health insurance claim number) at the top of the form. Complete the "Items or Services" box, describing what you propose to provide. Use simple language the beneficiary can understand. You may add current procedural terminology or HCPCS codes, but codes alone are not sufficient without a description. Complete the "Reason Medicare May Not Pay" box with the reason(s) you expect a denial. The reason(s) must be specific to the particular patient; general statements such as "medically unnecessary" are not acceptable. The "Estimated Cost" field is required.

The beneficiary must personally choose from Option 1, 2, or 3. The patient must sign and date the form; an unsigned or undated form is not valid. Once the patient has signed the completed form, he or she must receive a legible copy. The same guidelines apply to the copy as to the original—blue or black ink on white paper is preferred; a photocopy is fine. You keep the original in your files.

If the beneficiary chooses Option 1, you must file a claim and append an appropriate modifier to the reported item(s) or service(s). In CMS Transmittal R1921CP, effective April 1, 2010, 2 modifiers were updated to distinguish between voluntary and required use of liability notices. This change addresses the fact that most beneficiaries will elect Option 1 in the hope that Medicare might pay, despite your assurances to the contrary.

Modifier GA was redefined as "Waiver of Liability Statement Issued as Required by Payer Policy." For example, screening for potential disease, such as macular degeneration or epiretinal membrane, using scanning computerized ophthalmic diagnostic imaging of the retina is not covered because prophylactic testing is not a Medicare benefit unless specifically authorized by Congress. In contrast, testing patients with a history of macular degeneration or other retinal pathology is a covered service. When coverage is uncertain, you ask the patient to sign an ABN and submit your claim with modifier GA, allowing the payer to decide if the test is covered.

Modifier GX is defined as "Notice of Liability Issued, Voluntary Under Payer Policy." For example, in conjunction with covered cataract surgery, the patient elects a refractive procedure such as limbal relaxing incisions to correct pre-existing astigmatism. If the patient selects Option 1, append modifiers GX and GY to that claim, as those services are noncovered. Modifier GY is defined as "Item or Service Statutorily Excluded or Does Not Meet the Definition of Any Medicare Benefit."

Option 2 applies to situations in which Medicare is precluded from paying for the item or service and the beneficiary does not dispute the point. Do not file a claim; do post the item or service in your computer system with modifier GY.

Table 6-3
Hierarchy of Options

Problem	*Options*	*Noncovered Surgeon Charge*	*Noncovered Facility Charge*
Presbyopia, no astigmatism	Pseudophakic monovision	Small cost	None
Mild astigmatism (≤1 D)	Refractive corneal surgery	Moderate cost	Refractive corneal surgery
Significant astigmatism (>1 D)	A-C IOL	Moderate cost	A-C IOL
Presbyopia	P-C IOL	High cost	P-C IOL
Presbyopia + mild astigmatism	P-C IOL and refractive corneal surgery	High cost	P-C IOL and refractive corneal surgery
Presbyopia + significant astigmatism	P-C/A-C IOL	High cost	Dual purpose P-C/A-C IOL

Abbreviations: A-C, astigmatism-correcting; P-C, presbyopia-correcting.

The preceding discussion applies to the surgeon as well as the facility. Two separate ABNs are needed; one for each provider.

For non-Medicare beneficiaries, some of the previously outlined principles are just as applicable. While the concept of waiver of liability may not be present, or at least not as vigorously, it is still prudent to ensure that patients appreciate the distinction between covered and noncovered services and accept financial responsibility for the latter.

Developing Your Professional Charge

Refractive cataract surgery has many options (Table 6-3). There is no one-size-fits-all solution. Each option has a different charge for the noncovered portion based on the elements involved. As a practical matter, the more treatment options presented to patients, the more confused they become, and the more likely that indecision will result. In the interest of simplicity and patient acceptance, a fixed global charge is preferred to variable a la carte charges. To derive a fee for an option, consider the following approach.

1. Develop a comprehensive list of all noncovered services, such as the following:
   - ▲ Refraction to determine refractive error
   - ▲ Contact lens trial fitting to assess refractive error
   - ▲ Wavefront aberrometry to assess higher-order optical aberrations
   - ▲ Corneal topography to assess regular astigmatism; no corneal disease
   - ▲ Corneal pachymetry to plan refractive surgery
   - ▲ Pupillometry to assess pupil size under photopic, mesopic, and scotopic conditions

- ▲ Screening for dry eye disease with tear osmolarity testing
- ▲ Prophylactic testing with scanning computerized ophthalmic diagnostic imaging to rule out potential retinal problems that could affect the desired outcome; no prior history of retinal disease or disorder
- ▲ Refractive keratoplasty for the purpose of reducing dependence on eyeglasses or contact lenses (eg, limbal relaxing incisions, corneal relaxing incisions, photorefractive keratectomy, LASIK, enhancements)
- ▲ IOL exchange necessitated by inaccurate biometry or patient dissatisfaction with the refractive outcome
- ▲ Early yttrium-aluminum-garnet capsulotomy in-office for trace posterior capsule fog reducing near vision
- ▲ Additional postoperative care office visits after 90 days for routine eye care (eg, to cope with refractive error)
- ▲ Exclude the purchase of an IOL; this is the responsibility of the hospital or ASC.

2. Assign your usual and customary charge to each service. Include any fees that you might have to pay to others (eg, facility fee for IOL exchange or enhancements).
3. Determine the frequency with which each service is likely to occur within the population of patients who elect a premium IOL, refractive surgery, or pseudophakic monovision. As you develop experience, use retrospective chart review to reassess your frequency estimates.
4. Multiply the frequency times the usual and customary fee to arrive at a weighted average fee.
5. Total the weighted average fees to establish the charge for the noncovered portion of refractive cataract surgery.

This approach is analogous to CMS's methodology for establishing relative value units for a procedure using estimates of the time and resources involved. Tables 6-4, 6-5, and 6-6 illustrate the process; charges and frequencies are hypothetical.

At the same time that you are developing your professional charge, work with the facility where you perform cataract surgery to identify its charge for items and services that are noncovered. These include the facility fee for the femtosecond laser used for corneal relaxing incisions and the portion of a premium IOL for the correction of astigmatism and/or presbyopia. Then, when the time comes, you can explain to the beneficiary what to expect. Do not assume that you have to handle the financial transaction for the HOPD or ASC. From a legal perspective, it would be best not to handle other providers' money.

Co-Management

Some parts of the postoperative care following refractive cataract surgery may be provided by someone other than the surgeon under a co-management arrangement. The Office of Inspector General (OIG) of the Department of Health and Human Services published a tightly worded favorable opinion on this topic.[21] While OIG Advisory Opinions have strict limitations, the co-management of refractive cataract surgery using the following practice management policies does not involve prohibited remuneration under the federal anti-kickback statute.

Table 6-4
Creating a Charge for Pseudophakic Monovision Without Concurrent Astigmatism Correction

Item Or Service	*Surgeon's Charge*	*Frequency*	*Weighted Charge*	*Facility Fee*
Refraction OU	$40	200%	$80	$0
Screening corneal topography OU	$75	100%	$75	$0
Screening SCODI retina OU	$125	100%	$125	$0
Total charge (first eye)			$280	$0
Total charge (second eye)‡			$0	$0

Abbreviations: OU, both eyes; SCODI, scanning computerized ophthalmic diagnostic imaging.
All fees are only for illustration purposes.
‡ Diagnostic testing is OU and does not need to be repeated on the second eye surgery. Alternately, to establish a fee for unilateral testing, reduce the charge 50%, and charge the same for each surgery.

Table 6-5
Creating a Charge for Astigmatism-Correcting IOL

Item Or Service	*Surgeon's Charge*	*Frequency*	*Weighted Charge*	*Facility Fee*
Refraction OU	$40	300%	$120	$0
Screening corneal topography OU	$75	100%	$75	$0
Screening SCODI retina OU	$125	100%	$125	$0
Measure/position toric IOL on axis	$200	100%	$200	$0
Astigmatism-correcting IOL				$450
Enhancement (global*)	$1250	15%	$188	TBD*

(continued)

Table 6-5 (continued)

Creating a Charge for Astigmatism-Correcting IOL

Item Or Service	*Surgeon's Charge*	*Frequency*	*Weighted Charge*	*Facility Fee*
IOL exchange (global*)	$3000	2%	$60	TBD*
Total charge (first eye)			$768	$450
Total charge (second eye)‡			$448	$450

Abbreviations: TBD, to be determined

All fees are only for illustration purposes.

* Global fee includes professional fee and facility fee. Surgeon contracts with HOPD or ASC to pay the facility fee (TBD) instead of the patient at a mutually agreeable amount, likely similar to Medicare allowed amount.

‡ Diagnostic testing is OU and does not need to be repeated on the second eye surgery. Alternately, to establish a fee for unilateral testing, reduce the charge 50% and charge the same for each surgery.

Table 6-6

Creating a Charge for Presbyopia-Correcting IOL and Corneal Relaxing Incision

Item Or Service	*Surgeon's Charge*	*Frequency*	*Weighted Charge*	*Facility Fee*
Refraction OU	$40	300%	$120	$0
Screening corneal topography OU	$75	100%	$75	$0
Screening SCODI retina OU	$125	100%	$125	$0
Pachymetry OU to plan CRI	$30	100%	$30	$0
Screening tear osmolarity test OU	$35	100%	$35	$0
Femtosecond laser corneal relaxing incisions	$500	100%	$500	$700
Presbyopia-correcting IOL				$837
Early YAG capsulotomy (global*)	$750	20%	$150	TBD*
Enhancement (global*)	$1,250	15%	$188	TBD*

(continued)

Table 6-6 (continued)
Creating a Charge for Presbyopia-Correcting IOL and Corneal Relaxing Incision

Item Or Service	*Surgeon's Charge*	*Frequency*	*Weighted Charge*	*Facility Fee*
IOL exchange (global*)	$3000	2%	$60	TBD*
Extended postoperative care (1 year)	$225	100%	$225	$0
Total charge (first eye)			$1,508	$1,537
Total charge (second eye)‡			$1,123	$1,537

Abbreviations: CRI, corneal relaxing incision; YAG, yttrium-aluminum-garnet.
All fees are only for illustration purposes.
*Global fee includes professional fee and facility fee. Surgeon contracts with HOPD or ASC to pay the facility fee (TBD) instead of the patient at a mutually agreeable amount, likely similar to Medicare allowed amount.
‡ Diagnostic testing is OU and does not need to be repeated on the second eye surgery. Alternately, to establish a fee for unilateral testing, reduce the charge 50% and charge the same for each surgery.

- ▲ The surgeon would have no written or unwritten agreements to co-manage patients with optometrists. Instead, the surgeon would explain to all patients that they may receive their postsurgical care from the surgeon or from their referring optometrist, following a determination of clinical appropriateness—an option that the referring optometrist may have already presented to the patient.
- ▲ The surgeon would inform patients receiving premium IOLs that, if they choose to return to their optometrist for postoperative care, the optometrist may charge them for any services related to the premium IOL that the optometrist may deem necessary.
- ▲ Co-management of postoperative care for a beneficiary receiving a premium IOL does not increase costs to the Medicare program.
- ▲ The surgeon would transfer a patient back to his or her optometrist only upon the patient's request.

A number of key points can be gleaned from the OIG's Advisory Opinion that amount to best practices.

- ▲ Both the surgeon and the co-managing doctor exhibit the proper motivation consistent with professionalism.
- ▲ The surgeon determines suitability for surgery.
- ▲ The surgeon and patient discuss postoperative care options prior to surgery.
- ▲ Co-management depends on what's best for the patient.
- ▲ Document the patient's choice.
- ▲ Adhere to Medicare and other payers' billing instructions where applicable.

- Ensure professional charges represent fair market value for services performed.
- Use transparent billing so the patient knows the amount paid to each physician.

Subsequently, the American Academy of Ophthalmology and American Society of Cataract and Refractive Surgery issued joint guidance on co-management in general.[22] The updated position paper:

- Acknowledges that sharing postoperative management can serve legitimate patient interests and can be done appropriately.
- Improves and updates key definitions, such as *co-management* and *transfer*, and distinguishes between them.
- Emphasizes mutually agreed standards for postoperative care.
- Identifies circumstances that justify co-management: barriers to patient travel, unavailability of operating ophthalmologist, and patient prerogatives.
- Identifies several acceptable arrangements.
- Recommends written consent but allows verbal consent with documentation.

Avoiding Problems

Experience with refractive cataract surgery has shown that the worst problems arise from poor communication with patients. This may occur due to the following:

- Promising outcomes that cannot be achieved
- Inadequate or incomplete explanation of patient financial responsibility
- Failure to obtain financial waivers (ie, ABN)
- Lack of communication with other providers impacted by refractive cataract surgery (eg, HOPD, ASC)
- Ignorance of coverage and payment policies outside the Medicare system
- Not educating staff about this topic

Like with LASIK surgery, there are a different mindset and orientation for refractive cataract surgery from those of conventional cataract surgery, and they place added responsibilities on the physician and his or her staff. In fact, the patients most likely to opt for a premium IOL will have much in common with refractive surgery patients. This means that the patients will likely have high expectations and a lower tolerance for less-than-ideal outcomes.

Conclusion

Refractive cataract surgery is a combination of covered cataract surgery and noncovered refractive services. Medicare providers can only bill beneficiaries for noncovered services, and then only if the beneficiary understands and accepts financial responsibility in advance, usually by signing an ABN. Balance billing Medicare beneficiaries for covered services is prohibited under the assignment agreement or restricted under the nonparticipation rules. Other third-party payers have a similar attitude, although they are not obliged to follow Medicare precepts.

From a bookkeeping perspective, the office staff should make the same distinction between covered and noncovered services when posting charges and payments. Good

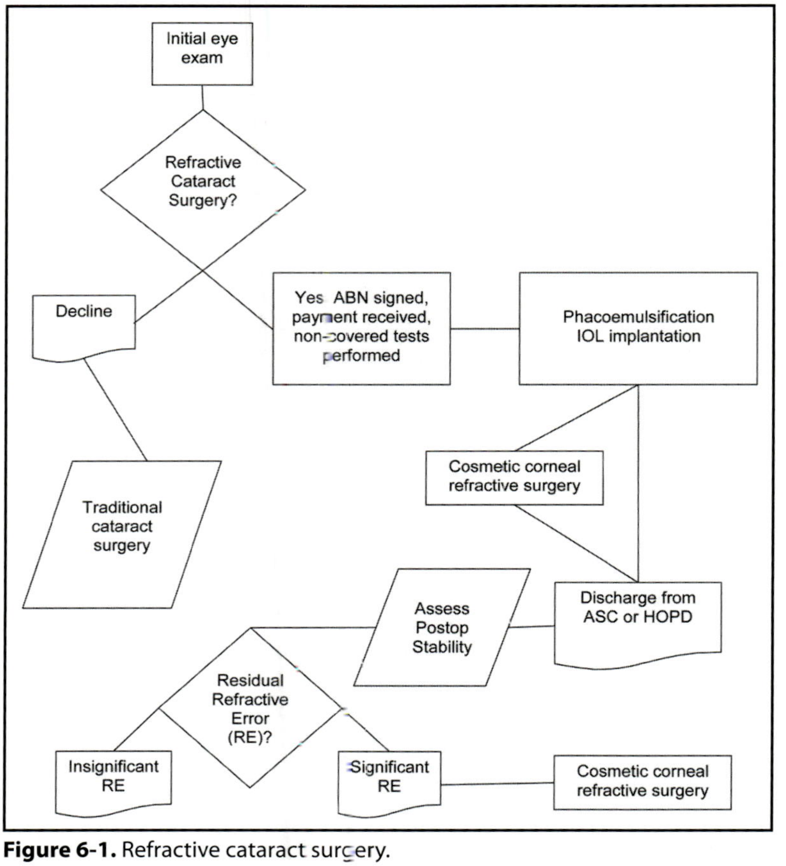

Figure 6-1. Refractive cataract surgery.

record keeping is essential—it entails maintaining a comprehensive paper trail of patient consents, complete and clear operative notes for each procedure, financial waivers and disclosures, and also all communication with payers and patients.

Figure 6-1 diagrammatically represents all of the concepts discussed. The reader is encouraged to use it as a mechanism for sorting out all the varied intersecting issues.

Management Tips

- ▲ The surgeon may not charge extra for "better" cataract surgery, only for refractive items and services.
- ▲ A presbyopia-correcting or astigmatism-correcting IOL can be thought of as 2 IOLs: 1 for cataract (covered) and 1 for refractive error (not covered).
- ▲ Medicare beneficiaries may not be compelled to pay for elective services as a precondition for obtaining covered services.
- ▲ Treatment of most complications of cataract surgery is a covered service. For example, treatment of infection or inflammation after surgery is covered.
- ▲ Enhancements to correct unplanned or unintended ametropias are not covered.

- With appropriate patient consent and a signed ABN, the beneficiary is responsible for all noncovered professional services to address refractive errors.
- Don't commingle funds that belong to separate organizations. For example, a surgeon's practice is usually distinct from an ASC or HOPD, so the surgeon's professional fees are payable to the practice, while the facility fees are payable to the ASC or HOPD. Don't mix them.
- Do not assume that all third-party payers follow Medicare precepts.

References

1. Corcoran, KJ. Macroeconomic landscape of refractive surgery in the United States. *Curr Opin Ophthalmol.* 2015;26(4):249-254.
2. Omnibus Budget Reconciliation Act of 1990, HR 5835, 101st Cong (1990)
3. CMS Ruling 05-01. Presbyopia-correcting intraocular lens. May 2005.
4. CMS Transmittal 1536-R. Astigmatism-correcting intraocular lens. September 2007.
5. Social Security Act §1862(a)(1)(A).
6. Hughes EH, Mellington FE, Whitefield LA. Aqualase for cataract extraction. *Eye.* 2007;21:191-194.
7. Donaldson KE, Braga-Mele R, Cabot F, et al. Femtosecond laser-assisted cataract surgery. *J Cataract Refract Surg.* 2013;39:1753-1763.
8. CMS Guidance, Laser-Assisted Cataract Surgery, and CMS Rulings 05-01 and 1536-R. November 16, 2012.
9. AAO/ASCRS guidelines for billing medicare beneficiaries when using the femtosecond laser. http://ascrs.org/sites/default/files/resources/12-04-2012%20FS%20Laser%20Guidelines%20Document%20(2)_0.pdf. Revised November 2012. Accessed January 4, 2017.
10. Health Insurance Glossary. Definition of balance billing. www.healthinsurance.org/glossary/balance-billing/.
11. CMS DMEPOS Fee Schedule. CY2016.
12. 42 CFR §§ 422.568 and 422.572, CMS instructions to Medicare Advantage contractors on improper use of advance notices of non-coverage. May 5, 2014.
13. CMS Medicare Learning Network. MM6136 Revised. Revised Form CMS-R-131 Advance Beneficiary Notice of Noncoverage. Effective March 3, 2008.
14. CMS Transmittal R1921CP. Billing for services related to voluntary uses of advance beneficiary notices of noncoverage (ABNs). Effective April 1, 2010.
15. DHHS OIG Advisory Opinion 11-14. Issued September 30, 2011.
16. Ophthalmic Postoperative Care. A joint position paper of the American Academy of Ophthalmology and the American Society of Cataract and Refractive Surgery. September, 2015.
17. NCD 10.1. Use of visual tests prior to and general anesthesia during cataract surgery. www.cms.gov/medicare-coverage-database/details/ncd-details.aspx?NCDId=60&ncdver=1&bc=AAAAgAAAAAAA&. Effective date August 31, 1992. Accessed January 4, 2017.
18. Medicare Benefits Policy Manual. Chapter 16 §90.
19. Corcoran Consulting Group. FAQ on Medicare reimbursement for corneal topography. www.corcoranccg.com/products/faqs/medicare-reimbursement-for-corneal-topography/. Published 2015. Accessed January 4, 2017.
20. CMS Medicare Learning Network, MM6563 Revised, Billing for Services Related to Voluntary Uses of Advance Beneficiary Notices of Noncoverage (ABNs), Effective April 1, 2010
21. NCD 80.8. Endothelial cell photography. www.cms.gov/medicare-coverage-database/details/ncd-details.aspx?NCDId=213&ncdver=1&MCDId=10&McdName=Factors+CMS+Considers+in+Referring+Topics+to+the+Medicare+Evidence+Development+%26+Coverage+Advisory+Committee&bc=BAAAgAAAAAAA&. Effective August 31, 1992. Accessed January 4, 2017.
22. NCD 80.7. Refractive keratoplasty. www.cms.gov/medicare-coverage-database/details/ncd-details.aspx?NCDId=72&ncdver=1&bc=BAAAgAAAAAAA&. Effective May 1, 1997. Accessed January 4, 2017.

Chapter 7

Advertising and Public Relations for Premium Cataract Surgery

Paul Stubenbordt, BS

Nothing Ventured, Nothing Gained

My friend and colleague Mike Malley with Centre for Refractive Marketing once had quite an interesting marketing experience. Mike was hired by a practice in Florida to do marketing for LASIK. After the LASIK campaign proved a success, Mike asked his client about doing a campaign for laser cataract surgery. The client turned the idea down; he said that he had other partners, and at the moment they were not interested in pursuing a marketing campaign for cataracts.

Several months went by, and one day Mike's client called and said they were ready start a marketing campaign for cataracts. Mike asked what happened, and the client explained:

"Mike, I just had one of my longtime patients come in for a visit, and I noticed that they had had cataract surgery. I asked, 'Where did your cataracts go?' The patient said that they had the surgery across the street. I asked why they didn't come to me for surgery, and the patient replied that they wanted laser cataract surgery, and we 'didn't offer it.'

"I was dumbfounded! I told the patient that we do indeed offer this technology, and I wished they would have come to us for their cataract removal. The patient said they heard an ad on the radio about laser cataract surgery and met with the doctor. The doctor (who happened to be a friend of mine) told the patient that we were friends, we played golf together, etc, and he could remove the cataract and send them back to me for postoperative care.

"Mike, can you believe that I'm co-managing my own patient's cataract case? We need to get the word out now!"

Hovanesian JA.
Refractive Cataract Surgery: Best Practices and Advanced Technology, Second Edition (pp 75-86). © 2017 SLACK Incorporated.

Moral of the story: If you don't advertise what you do, someone else can take your market share.

"Doing business without advertising is like winking at a girl in the dark. You know what you are doing, but nobody else does."

—Steuart Henderson Britt

Why Market Your Practice?

Marketing your practice is crucial for many reasons. The most basic reason for marketing is, of course, to grow your practice. Other benefits from marketing and advertising that lead up to practice growth include the following:

- ▲ Generating new patients
- ▲ Positioning your practice as an innovative leader in cataract surgery
- ▲ Increasing credibility with patients and referring doctors
- ▲ Retaining existing patients
- ▲ Creating buzz

Advertising does not have to be an arduous undertaking. It all starts with a plan.

Start With Internal Marketing

The most cost-effective way to market to cataract patients is by establishing a strong internal marketing program that educates your existing patients. This should include posters throughout the office, an education DVD loop in the waiting room, a customized on-hold message, quarterly patient newsletters, and expanded staff education. Beyond external advertising, internal marketing also gives your practice a solid professional veneer. With the right internal marketing efforts, the ophthalmologist in Mike's story would not have lost his patient.

Your Marketing Plan—Your Budget, Your Message, Your Placement

Although a marketing plan can be quite extensive, any marketing plan consists of a budget, your message (what you want to say), and your placement (where you are going to say it).

A good rule of thumb for your budget is to spend 3% to 6% of your total revenue on marketing. If your practice generates $1.5 million/year in cataract revenue, then plan to spend $45,000 to $90,000/year promoting that segment of your practice. It is important to select a marketing budget you will be comfortable with. Remember, it is an investment, not an expense.

Next, you need to decide on a message. What are you going to say? The simplest message is, "Here is what I have, and here is what it can do for you." Any number of variations on how you want to say that can help your campaign.

Most patients who are interested in premium intraocular lenses (IOL) want to eliminate the need for glasses, particularly reading glasses. In our society, wearing reading glasses is one of the first signs of getting old, right up there with graying hair and nocturia. Today's baby boomers want visual freedom, they want independence, they want the best, and they are willing to pay for it.

Key Items Every Ad Should Have

Honesty

Seniors are turned off by ads that look too much like you are trying to sell something. They like educational ads that are toned down, honest, and authentic.

Value

Seniors spend time researching major purchases and look for value in everything they purchase. Show the benefits of a premium IOL to demonstrate value.

Emotions

Seniors are attracted to ads that use story-telling and emotions to drive their purchase decisions.

Reinform

Older patients may remember their parents' cataract surgery, which might scare them. Reiterate that modern procedures are fast and effective, with little to no down time.

Contact Information

Make it easy for seniors to find your phone number, website, and physical address.

Figure 7-1 is an advertisement for cataract removal and implants. I like this example for many reasons, but mainly because it appeals to that "restoration of youth" psychology that most people can relate to. Also, this ad is succinct. Long-winded messages are not memorable.

Where to Advertise

Media placement can be tricky. Just like eyes, no 2 practices or markets are alike. For example, you might be a huge practice willing to spend 12% of your revenue toward marketing, which could open up broadcast television, radio, print, and other options. Alternatively, you could be a solo practitioner who has never marketed and wants to keep marketing efforts on the conservative side. Whatever your situation, a little media knowledge can guide your decisions.

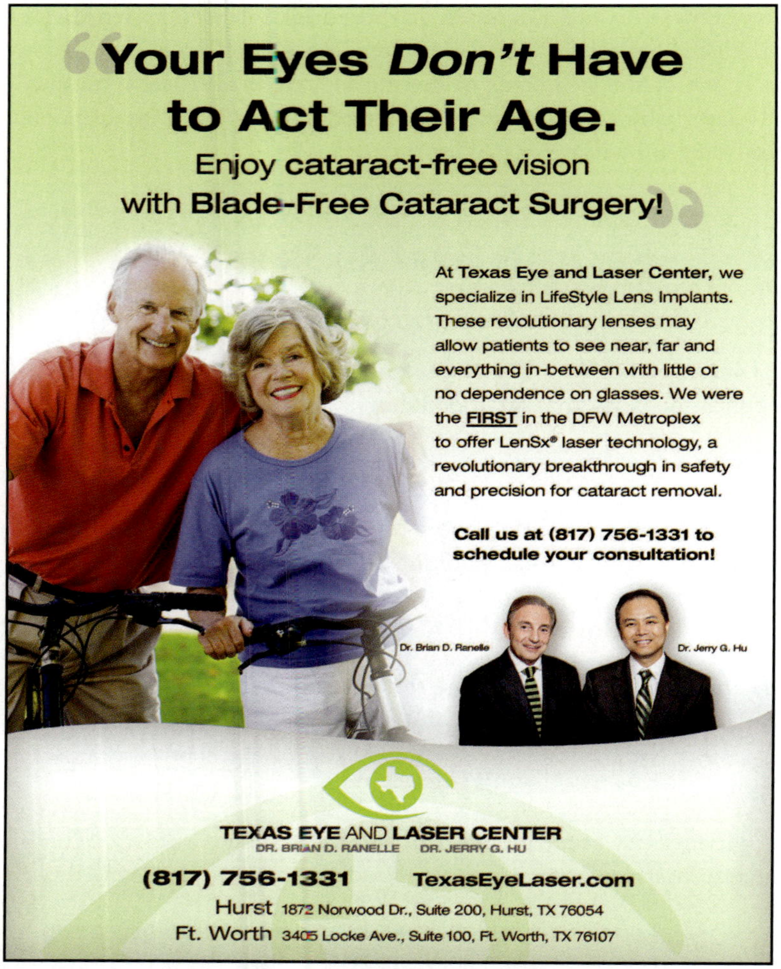

Figure 7-1. Sample of a premium IOL magazine advertisement.

Radio

Talk radio can work really well for branding a premium IOL practice. I tend to run ads during drive times, which are from 6 AM through 9 AM and 3 PM through 7 PM. I do this because that is when the majority of people listen. Ideally, your radio representative will give you additional fill spots for free if you spend a decent amount with a station. To get the most bang for your buck, also consider a hybrid message, with the first 30 seconds focusing on another service your practice offers, such as LASIK, and the final 30 seconds discussing cataract surgery and premium IOLs.

Television

"As Seen on TV" is a marketing gimmick that has been used to sell products through supermarkets and retailers for years. What "As Seen on TV" does is add credibility. The idea is the same when marketing your practice. Television also has the benefit of reaching the viewer through sight and sound, which is even more memorable. With TV, you can actually visually demonstrate cataract symptoms and the visual results after cataract surgery.

Broadcast TV (eg, CBS, NBC, FOX, and ABC) reaches a lot of viewers, especially during primetime, but also tends to be very expensive. The good news is our target cataract market of 55+ tends to watch a lot of daytime TV, which is much lower in cost then prime or evening television.

A great alternative to broadcast TV is cable. You can target specific geographic zones, and you can bombard consumers with tremendous frequency. Cable is great for practices with a smaller budget.

Newsprint

Although newspapers may be a dying medium, they tend to do very well for practices promoting cataract surgery and premium IOLs. For print ads, develop a compelling headline and include text and photos that will draw reader attention. I also like using color as opposed to black and white ads. If your practice has a distinct color scheme, readers will have instant recognition just by seeing your practice colors. Try to keep your ads in sections of the paper that are most read by seniors. From my experience, this includes the weather, lifestyle, and obituary sections. I also recommend using smaller ad sizes with more frequency rather than expensive larger ads with less frequency.

Some research shows readers equate large ads with large businesses and small ads with small businesses. Don't be tempted to use a large ad to make people believe you're a large business. They'll be disappointed when they arrive at your door—and you'll discover your ploy was all for naught.

Social Media

Who says social media is only for the young? Not only are people 65 years of age and older jumping on the Internet in greater numbers, the Pew Research Center social media update for 2014 shows more than half of all online adults age 65 and older (56%) use the social networking site Facebook, representing 31% of all seniors.[1] Overall, 71% of Internet users are on Facebook, and 70% of Facebook users engage with the site on a daily basis. Now, are patients going to like their eye doctor's Facebook page and follow your post? Probably not; however, Facebook offers some innovative ways to market to seniors. One of the biggest advantages to advertising on Facebook is the ability to target specific groups of highly engaged people based on their unique interest. You can get as targeted as having your ads appear to only those who live within 10 miles, are between 65 and 80 years old, enjoy crocheting, and are followers of Dave Ramsey. At this time, Facebook is the only social media I see valuable for reaching out to seniors.

Hire a Professional Agency

Most of us believe we can do anything, but for advertising, it is best to use an advertising agency. If this seems out of reach, use your local media sales representative for placement assistance. One of my favorite quotes is from Red Adair: "If you think it's expensive to hire a professional to do the job, wait until you hire an amateur."[2]

The Patient Experience

Seth Godin, one of the country's leading marketing experts, says, "Our job is to connect to people, to interact with them in a way that leaves them better than we found them, more able to get where they'd like to go."[3] This connection needs to take place at every point your practice comes into contact with your patients or potential patients. Everything from your website, to how the phones are answered, to what kind of information patients received prior to their appointment, to the visit, to the discussion with the doctor, to the surgery, to the outcome, to how you treat them after they are 1-year postoperative patients—it all matters. When details are missed, patients become frustrated, and they invariably share their frustration with their friends, family members—and yes, even the co-managing optometrist who sent the patient over in the first place.

A good place to start looking at the details is by stepping outside of your own practice. Try to look at it from an outsider's perspective. Visit your website, mystery telephone shop your own practice; step out into the waiting room and have a seat. Do you like what you see and hear? Next, have a counselor explain the difference between basic cataract surgery and premium IOL surgery using laser technology. Does it make sense? Are you pleased? From my experience, most practices think they are doing well. From a consultant's perspective, most practices seem to struggle in certain areas. You can improve the patient experience even further by offering free Internet access, snacks, coffee, and even bottled water.

Hire the Right Staff

Four- and five-star hotels never hire for experience; they hire for personality. They put their staff "on show" every single day. They know that indifference is the ultimate enemy to customer satisfaction and they combat this enemy by treating everyone like family.

The following are some tips you can learn from them:

- Greet patients by name when they arrive.
- Hold the patient's hand during surgery.
- Arrange courtesy transportation.
- Hire for personality, not experience.
- Look at your practice from an outsider's viewpoint to nail the details.
- Offer free Wi-Fi, gourmet coffee, and snacks in your lobby.
- Treat everyone like family.

Taking it one step further, I have even seen a practice provide food for their patient's entire family the day of surgery, reducing the family's number of concerns for the evening. This practice has a certain buzz about everything they do for the patient and the patient's family.

Finally, it is a good idea to send out a survey to patients once a year. You can do this on your own by choosing 100 or so patients to send the survey to, or you can use a service to take care of it for you. Once the surveys are returned, the surgeon or administrator can use the data provided to make improvements.

Telephones—The Front Line

For many premium cataract surgeons, the most common first experience a patient will have of your practice is the initial phone call. This is when you will really want to make a great first impression, and it is up to your staff to do so.

Start by having a friendly voice, and listen to what the patient is asking. What are his or her concerns? Is he or she a co-managed patient? How did he or she hear about your practice? For most practices, even those who are fairly successful, the telephone tends to be an area of weakness.

Improve the quality of your phone calls by doing the following:

- ▲ Use a friendly voice.
- ▲ Answer within 3 rings.
- ▲ Never put the patient on hold for more than 30 seconds.
- ▲ Have empathy.
- ▲ Use the patient's first name or something like "Mrs. Jones" to make the call more personal.
- ▲ Build rapport.

Scripting and Role Playing

Practices should focus on preparing staff members by creating phone scripts. Phone scripts help employees with the flow of how a call should be handled, keep the message consistent, and will prevent employees from making guesses during various scenarios. It is recommended to use these scripts as guides until employees become more comfortable with the flow of conversation.

The best way for a staff member to become effective on the telephone is by role playing. Role playing will make the scripts sound more natural and less forced. During role-play sessions, it is good to focus on various situations, such as, "What if the patient is co-managed?" or "If he or she had LASIK, is he or she still a good candidate for a premium IOL?" The goal is to have your staff discuss cataract surgery and premium IOL options with potential patients just as if they were family members.

Do Not Educate Over the Phone; Just Get Them In

The goal on the telephone is simple: get the patient in for an exam, create rapport and trust, and prepare the patient for what to expect. It is important to listen to the patient's concerns and address them accordingly, but do not go over all of the premium lens options, cost, and other details on the telephone. Save the details for the exam, because you will find answering questions in the office to be much more rewarding.

One way to educate patients prior to their appointment is by directing them to your website or by sending them an informative brochure on cataracts and their options. You can also send them a questionnaire, which helps them consider their needs and concerns prior to their appointment while providing the surgical counselor with important information. This way, you might be able to avoid the "deer-in-headlights" look when discussing premium IOLs and the associated costs during the office visit.

Scheduling Time for Discussions With Patients

In general, people are afraid of what they do not understand. Most patients are already under stress because they have been told they need cataract surgery. Can you imagine what they go through when we throw premium IOLs at them?

Using a questionnaire prior to the patient's meeting with the doctor will help. The questionnaire or survey is a series of questions that the patient will answer prior to his or her appointment, thus helping the surgeon determine if the patient would be better suited for a multifocal, accommodative, or standard IOL.

I have heard complaints from patients ranging from, "I didn't know it would cost more," to "I was told I would be able to see like I was 25 again," to "No one told me I would have to pay thousands of dollars just to wear glasses when I read." That is why time spent with patients improves overall satisfaction. Teach your staff to set reasonable expectations and not to make promises that can backfire.

Taking the time to explain the benefits of a premium IOL is absolutely crucial. If the patient senses the slightest amount of hesitation or urgency in the surgeon's or staff member's voice, he or she will begin to put his or her guard up. On the other hand, if the doctor (or staff) takes the time to explain the benefits and drawbacks and to answer any questions the patient might have, you will find a much higher satisfaction rate among your premium lens patients.

Evaluating Every Cataract Patient

Several years ago, I was visiting a practice that had a very unhappy cataract patient. Did she have a bad result? No. Did she experience some type of abnormal pain? No. Did we put the wrong lens in her eye? No. "So…what's the problem?" I asked.

The doctor answered, "She was mad because my practice never informed her that she could reduce her dependency on glasses with a premium IOL." I asked what set her off, only to find out that her neighbor had had surgery just weeks after our upset patient did and was offered a premium IOL. The patient was angry that the option was offered to her friend but not to her. The patient had normal cataracts, normal corneas, and was indeed a good candidate for a premium IOL. When I asked the doctor why she was not asked, he replied, "We don't evaluate every patient for a premium IOL."

There is an important lesson to be learned here. Although lens selection can be challenging, deciding whether or not patients should be offered the option should never be the issue.

Lifestyle Questionnaire

Name: ______________________________ Date: ________________

We would like to know how you use your eyes on a daily basis. Along with your eye exam, this information will assist us in recommending the best options for your eyes and your lifestyle.

- Do you currently wear glasses? ☐ Yes – All the time ☐ Yes – sometimes ☐ No
- Would you like to be able to read or use the computer without glasses? ☐ Yes ☐ Don't mind wearing glasses
- How many hours a day do you.............. Read?______ Use a computer? ______
- Would it be okay if you had to wear glasses once in a while? ☐ Yes ☐ No
- Does the thought of **NOT** having to wear glasses all of the time appeal to you? ☐ Yes ☐ No
- Do you drive at night? ☐ No If Yes: ☐ Occasionally ☐ Night ☐ As a profession

****** Please check any of the following activities that you do on a regular basis: ******

☐ Read Newspaper / Books	☐ Musician / Choir	☐ Drive Daytime
☐ Needlepoint	☐ Shop	☐ Drive Nighttime
☐ Paperwork	☐ Play Cards / Dominos	☐ Hunt / Fish
☐ Read Medicine Bottles	☐ Dine out / Cook	☐ Bicycle
☐ Use Computer / PDA	☐ Paint / Artist	☐ Golf / Tennis
☐ Photography	☐ Theatre	☐ Spectator Sports

****** Circle the above activities you would like to do without glasses if possible. ******

- What occupational, recreational or other activities are you currently engaged in that are not listed? ________________________
- Please place an "X" on the following personality scale to best describe your personality and adaptability.

Easy going, I take things in stride. ←――――――――――――→ Perfectionist, I have to have things "just so."

Patient's Signature ________________________ **Doctor's Initials:** ______

Figure 7-2. Premium IOL and LRI wavier form.

How to Evaluate Every Patient

Have each and every cataract patient complete a patient survey prior to his or her appointment. This will not only help determine if he or she is interested in reducing or eliminating his or her need for glasses, but it will also help determine which lens would be best suited for his or her needs.

Review each patient surgery, review the cataract exam, determine candidacy, and discuss options with the patient.

Finally, have each patient sign a premium IOL waiver (Figure 7-2). This is a basic form that explains that you have discussed his or her candidacy for premium IOLs and other options such as limbal relaxing incisions (LRIs), and that he or she chooses to waive the option to upgrade.

Offering Astigmatism Surgery for Those Who Do Not Choose Presbyopia-Correcting Intraocular Lenses

One of the biggest misconceptions I have seen staff members and even some surgeons say to patients is that standard IOLs will allow them to see in the distance just fine, but

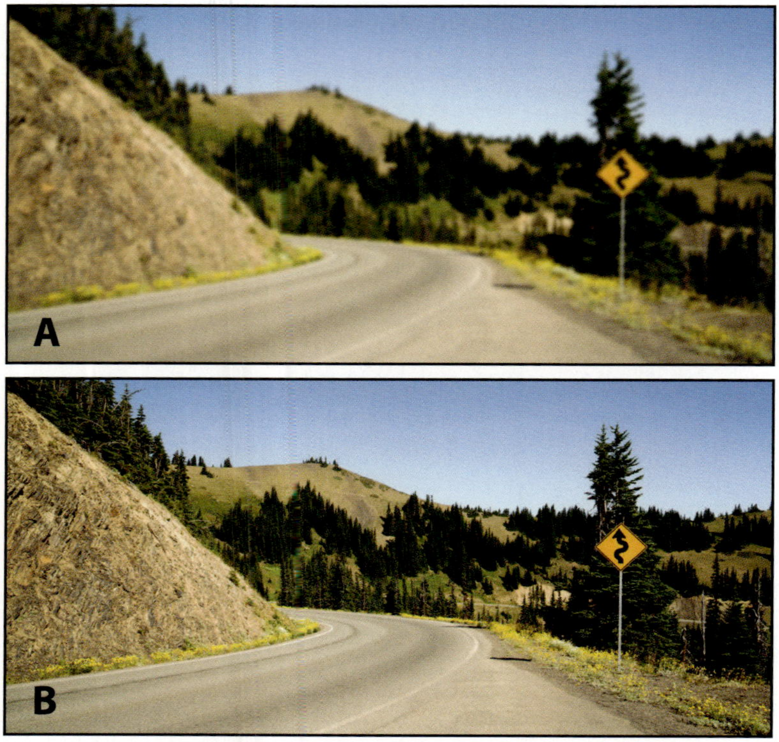

Figure 7-3. Simulation of (A) residual and (B) corrected corneal astigmatism after cataract surgery

they will need glasses for seeing objects at intermediate and reading distances. Of course, they are forgetting about corneal astigmatism.

Astigmatism correction with an LRI is a very simple procedure that can make your standard implant cataract patients much happier. Even correcting a small amount of astigmatism can add a great deal of satisfaction to the results (Figure 7-3).

Another solution for correcting astigmatism simultaneously with cataract surgery is toric lenses. Toric IOLs seem to be a good option for cataract surgeons who want to start offering premium IOLs. In most practices I see, doctors will elect to use LRI for low amounts of astigmatism and toric IOLs for patients with a higher amount of astigmatism.

If a cataract patient has astigmatism, do not be reluctant to suggest correcting it during cataract surgery. It is worth it for them, and it is worth it for you. Reiterate to your staff that just because a patient does not elect to have a premium IOL, this does not mean we should not help them reduce corneal astigmatism.

Laser-Assisted Cataract Surgery

Cataract removal using femtosecond technology is slowly becoming incorporated into most premium practices. Patients should be aware that this technology can allow the surgeon to perform many of the cataract surgery's key steps, which have traditionally been performed manually, with the precision of a laser. When a patient is undergoing cataract removal with the use of a premium IOL, laser-assisted, patients should be aware that this technology is more precise and predictable when compared with manual cataract surgery and may produce a better visual outcome. I recommend having your femtosecond technology bundled into your premium pricing tiers. If a patient balks at the price, I recommend telling him or her that if he or she had to choose between a multifocal IOL or femtosecond technology, a multifocal IOL is more beneficial, as he or she will benefit from this technology for the rest of his or her life.

Preparing Counselors and Staff

Educating and preparing your staff is paramount, because one weak link can ruin the chain. You must educate everyone involved in the process about what to say (and what not to say) when discussing premium IOLs. A good way to start is by handing out a list of frequently asked questions and having the staff study it. They should not only memorize the answers, but also know why they are the right answers. Remember to keep a consistent message throughout the office.

Your surgical counselor is usually the key person in charge of discussing and converting premium IOLs with patients. He or she will be responsible for properly educating and setting realistic expectations for the patient, so it is essential you hire someone suited to the job. Using a lifestyle questionnaire can help the surgical counselor know where to start, but he or she also must be ready to listen to the patient and avoid common selling techniques. Instead, focus on the benefits to the patient and his or her real needs and real desires. Remind the patient that this is something he or she will use every waking moment for the rest of his or her life. By the time the patient reaches the surgeon, he or she should be well educated about his or her options.

Lastly, try to do quarterly training with your staff. We teach Caring, Sharing, Information. For the first part of the meeting, *caring*, we discuss personal topics that the practice could help individual employees with, both personal and business. Second, for *sharing*, the staff shares ideas with the practice on what they think the practice can do to improve. Finally, for *information*, the doctors or administrator will update staff on new technologies, protocols, or any other type of improvements to the premium IOL/cataract practice. Having staff meetings like this instead of individual meetings will help keep a consistent message throughout the office.

Summary

- ▲ Educate everyone about the process of premium IOLs.
- ▲ Have the staff memorize and understand FAQs.
- ▲ Keep a consistent message throughout the office.
- ▲ Have only one person in charge of the program, if possible; usually, the surgical counselor.
- ▲ Educate patients so that when they reach the surgeon, they are fully aware of their options.
- ▲ Implement monthly or quarterly staff training.

Conclusion

Although seniors have many competing health care choices, such as cosmetics and hearing, their vision is extremely important to them, and they are willing to pay a premium price for premium technology. Although today's technology may not be perfect, it is very good and can help many patients correct their vision so that they may reduce or eliminate their dependency on reading glasses or bifocals. There are also very few things that we will purchase that we will use every waking moment for the rest of our lives, but cataract surgery using a multifocal, accommodative, or toric IOL is one of those things. Explain this rationale to your patients, and they will make the investment in their vision.

References

1. Duggan M, Ellison NB, Lampe C, Lenhart A, Madden M. Social media update 2014. *Pew Research Center*. www.pewinternet.org/2015/01/09/social-media-update-2014/. Published January 9, 2015. Accessed January 4, 2017.
2. BrainyQuote. www.brainyquote.com/quotes/quotes/r/redadair195665.html. Accessed November 30, 2011.
3. Lazzaroni, D. 75 Quotes to inspire marketing greatness. *LinkedIn Marketing Solutions Blog*. http://marketing.linkedin.com/blog/75-quotes-to-inspire-marketing-greatness/. Published June 9, 2014. Accessed July 30, 2015.

Chapter 8

Educating Patients About Refractive Cataract Surgery

John A. Hovanesian, MD, FACS

Presbyopia-correcting lens implants and femtosecond laser cataract surgery are becoming the standard of care among practices that have learned to conquer the technical and psychological aspects of setting up expectations and then delivering them. Delivering spectacle freedom to patients has a snowball effect in which happy patients refer their friends and family specifically for these premium lenses. It is not unusual for 60% to 70% of cataract patients to choose elective refractive options in practices that are experienced in delivering these results.

In my own private practice, Harvard Eye Associates in southern California, we have seen similar enthusiastic acceptance of these technologies by patients, yet we don't believe this is just the result of the greater awareness of lifestyle in California. Like colleagues from more rural states who have had similar success, we believe that the value of spectacle freedom is universally appealing. However his or her lifestyle is compromised by age or illness, every patient can benefit from spectacle freedom and deserves to fully understand the options before undergoing cataract surgery. Furthermore, observing 10 simple principles will lead every practice to success in educating patients about the best technologies.

Principle 1: Believe in the Technology

It takes a certain leap of faith for the surgeon who is new to refractive cataract surgery to educate patients enthusiastically about it. As surgeons, we should always have our patients' best interests in mind. We understand that our ethics and our reputation depend on delivering the same treatment to our patients that we would to family

Hovanesian JA.
Refractive Cataract Surgery: Best Practices and Advanced Technology, Second Edition (pp 87-92).

members. We also understand that refractive surgical options entail significant added cost for patients and a much higher expectation of what will be delivered. Gaining confidence that this greater expectation can be met takes both knowledge and experience. It is the hope of the authors of this book that readers will gain the knowledge necessary to deliver results. Confidence takes some time to develop. With experience and many happy patients, this excitement develops naturally, not just in the surgeon but also in staff members. Meanwhile, remind your staff members that we always remember a patient who is unhappy, but we easily forget the vast majority who love their results and refer their friends.

Principle 2: Understand the Importance of the Discussion, and Include Family Members

What takes a few minutes for us or our staff to discuss has a lifelong impact on a patient. For most of our patients, the costs involved in refractive cataract surgery can be daunting. Be sure to take adequate time for this discussion. Rushing the process will leave questions unanswered and create angst for the patient. If asked, many will say, "I don't mind wearing glasses. I've done it all my life." That automatic response usually comes out because the patient has never seriously considered the alternative. Yet once these same patients understand that no (or minimal) additional surgery will be needed to greatly reduce spectacle dependence, their latent need for refractive cataract surgery may become manifest.[1] For this reason, we do not begin our discussion by asking whether the patient is interested in refractive options. Instead, we take the time to explain the benefits of these options in understandable terms to every single patient. We schedule extra time for this discussion for patients who we expect may be ready for cataract surgery. We also recommend that a family member be present for this cataract consent process. This truly enhances our older patients' retention, and having a loved one present allows the patient to make a decision (and remember it) with confidence.

Principle 3: Match the Technology to the Patient

Before meeting the doctor, we ask each patient to fill out a questionnaire that rates his or her visual disability and determines his or her needs for distance, intermediate, and near vision. Derived from the survey developed by Steven Dell, MD,[2] this questionnaire (Figure 8-1), which can be downloaded at www.bettereyesurgery.com, helps us understand the patient's needs. But it doesn't substitute for asking directly what activities the patient enjoys. We then describe the implant's benefits in the context of these activities. Retailers tell us that most big-ticket purchases are driven more by emotional motivation than exhaustive analysis. Showing the individualized lifestyle benefit of each surgical choice helps patients understand its advantages on a very personal and emotional level.

HARVARD EYE ASSOCIATES History Update

Please update **ANY CHANGES** to the following since you last visit:	
Home address/phone	
Email address	
Medical insurance	
Medicine or allergies	
New surgeries	
New medical conditions	

Are you interested in learning more about procedures like LASIK that can reduce your need for glasses/contacts? (circle) YES NO

How many years old are your current glasses?

Primary Pair:________ Sunglasses:______ Reading Glasses: ________
Computer Glasses:______ Sports Glasses:______ Occupational Glasses: _________

How much of a vision problem do you have with…	**None←→Severe**
Glare from sunlight while driving	N/A 0 1 2 3 4
Glare around headlights in a car after dark	N/A 0 1 2 3 4
Difficulty reading street signs far away	N/A 0 1 2 3 4
Difficulty reading for long periods of time	N/A 0 1 2 3 4
Difficulty reading with your glasses in dim light	N/A 0 1 2 3 4
Difficulty with vision for sports (following golf ball, tennis ball)	N/A 0 1 2 3 4
Difficulty with hobbies requiring fine vision (sewing, carpentry)	N/A 0 1 2 3 4
Difficulty playing games like cards, bingo, etc.	N/A 0 1 2 3 4
Difficulty seeing small captions on the TV	N/A 0 1 2 3 4
Reading fine print (medicine bottles, telephone book, food labels)	N/A 0 1 2 3 4

Do you drive after dark? (circle)	OFTEN	SOMETIMES	RARELY/NEVER
Do you use a computer? (circle)	OFTEN	SOMETIMES	RARELY/NEVER
Do you do a lot of close detail work, like sewing or building models? (circle)	OFTEN	SOMETIMES	RARELY/NEVER

Have you ever tried mono-vision contact lenses (one eye near, one eye distance)? YES NO

If you **had** to wear glasses after surgery for one activity, for which activity would you be **most willing** to wear glasses? ____**Reading fine print** ____**Computer** ____**Driving**

Please place an "X" on the following scale to **describe your personality** as best you can:
[---|---]
Easy Going Perfectionist

Patient Signature Date

Dr. Initial

v2007_04_13

Figure 8-1. Patient questionnaire available for download at www.bettereyesurgery.com/download.

Principle 4: Let the Doctor Do the Educating

We use a number of educational tools: brochures, our website (www.harvardeye.com), videos, consent forms, and patient testimonials on the walls of our waiting room to make patients aware of refractive options before their cataract consultation. Direct-to-consumer advertising provided by some implant manufacturers also enhances awareness of these technologies.[3] The first verbal discussion about choices, though, is with the doctor. This ensures reasonable expectations and reduces the chance that a staff member will over-sell the technology. It allows customizing the education process to the patient's needs. It allows information to come from the most trusted source: the surgeon. The discussion need not require significant time of the surgeon, yet the importance of the patient hearing a recommendation from the surgeon cannot be overestimated.

Principle 5: Keep It Simple

Rather than presenting brand names of products and their relative benefits to patients, generally it is best to make a recommendation of 1 or 2 sets of options. Again, most of our patients do not want to analyze the unique features of every available choice. They want to know what will be the best choice for their own situation, and most feel it's the doctor's duty to make this choice. In your discussion and in your paperwork, be careful about using the word *standard* to refer to traditional phaco with a monofocal implant. Also avoid the term *premium* to refer to elective refractive surgical options. While some patients are drawn to products labeled as premium, others have an aversion to any kind of upgrade option. Try to focus on how vision will be affected by various options, and use familiar references to help the patient understand. For example, instead of referring to *intermediate vision*, instead mention "seeing the computer screen, dashboard, or a music stand at arm's length." Instead of *distance vision*, talk about "passing a driver's test without glasses, recognizing faces across the room, and being able to use nonprescription sunglasses to drive." These examples help patients visualize value points they might not otherwise consider and help them make a decision from a more personal perspective.

Principle 6: Offer More Than One Type of Implant

With the online availability of information about various implants, patients often ask us for a specific lens, whether or not it is the same choice the surgeon would have made. When patients make this request, we are happy to comply if we feel it to be an appropriate choice. If not, we can explain from experience why their preference might fall short of their expectations. Either way, the fact that we have experience with all available implants allows us to speak credibly about the patient's best interests rather than our one-size-fits-all personal preference.

Principle 7: Be Clear and Unapologetic About Limitations

I frequently tell patients, "Don't expect perfect. Let's face it, your body is out of warranty." This bluntness almost always provokes a laugh and helps the patient understand the role an aging eye plays in limiting vision, even with a high-tech lens implant. It's useful to explain, "Ninety percent of people can pass a driver's test without glasses, but you may need glasses to feel comfortable reading road signs at night. Ninety percent can read a newspaper, but expect to need glasses for some things, like prolonged, fine-print, or dim light reading." Again, giving these specific examples of activities that may require glasses is much more memorable than just saying "sometimes," and patients very much appreciate the honesty.

Principle 8: Be Clear and Unapologetic About Extra Costs

Most patients have no frame of reference for the cost of a premium implant, and any 4-digit price is likely to be met with some shock. There are 3 helpful strategies to soften this. First, though it is an uncomfortable topic for some, it is best for the surgeon—the most trusted individual—to explain price to the patient. Second, present the implant costs in the context of the overall cost of cataract surgery, including anesthesia, surgery center fees, and the surgical fee itself. Compared to this larger cost of all elements (surgeon's fee, facility fee, anesthesia fee), the patient understands that upgrading to a refractive surgical option is an incremental cost.[4] Third, let the patient know that financing is available to allow patients to spread the cost of refractive options over time.

Principle 9: Tell What You Would Do for Your Sister

If you would honestly recommend a refractive cataract surgery option to a loved one, end this discussion on this point. There is no way to more genuinely express your belief that better technology will lead the patient to a better life. Again, your ability to make this statement credibly depends on your experience and heartfelt feelings.

Principle 10: Follow Up and Follow Through

With refractive cataract surgery, there are 2 critical follow-up efforts after the consultation. At the end of your consultation, make a notation in the chart as to how likely you believe the patient is to choose a refractive surgery option. Because most patients give some verbal or nonverbal feedback as to their feelings, this is easy enough information to obtain. If you learn later that the same patient who you thought was likely to want a presbyopia-correcting option or a toric implant has instead changed his or her mind and chosen a monofocal implant, pick up the phone and make sure he or she hasn't based his or her decision on misinformation. This occurs all too often when patients talk with friends. For example, a patient with significant corneal astigmatism is told by a friend that he should expect perfect uncorrected distance vision with a "no-cost" implant. A patient with preoperative myopia in both eyes might assume that she will be able to read without glasses after surgery with a monofocal implant and a plano result simply because she has taken for granted her fantastic uncorrected near acuity since birth. Sometimes we have to explain things again. If we don't, patients may expect more than they will get, however unrealistic this may be. If they are disappointed, they will naturally blame their surgeon rather than their choice of implant.

The second and most important time to follow through is a month or so after the final surgery is performed. Some patients may already develop posterior capsule opacity, and some may have mild residual refractive error that is interfering with spectacle independence. These marginally happy people may not be bothered enough to initiate a visit to your office, but they will tell their friends how disappointed they are with their expensive implants. This can be very damaging to your reputation. In our practice, we don't wait for patients to complain. We routinely survey all postoperative cataract surgery patients using an automated follow-up care system called MDbackline

(MDbackline, LLC, www.mdbackline.com). If patients report even mild disappointment with their results, we get in touch with them to schedule a follow-up visit to undertake whatever treatment is appropriate. Our mantra is "You deserve to be happy." Patients love us for this extra effort, and they tell their friends.

Conclusion

Organize your discussion with patients about premium implants, take extra time, say what you believe, and believe what you say. Your practice will be rewarded with higher patient adoption of and satisfaction with these exciting technologies.

References

1. Bosworth MT. *Solution Selling: Creating Buyers in Difficult Selling Markets.* Columbus, OH: McGraw-Hill; 1994.
2. Chang DF. *Mastering Refractive IOLs: The Art and Science.* Thorofare, NJ: SLACK Incorporated; 2008:870.
3. Bausch & Lomb Inc. Crystalens website. www.crystalens.com.
4. Lane SD. Distinguishing cataract surgery from refractive correction. Eye World. www.eyeworld.org/article---65279-distinguishing-cataract-surgery-from-refractive-correction. Published June 2014. Accessed February 7, 2017.

Section II

Surgical Technique and Implants

Chapter 9

Femtosecond Laser-Assisted Cataract Surgery

Kendall E. Donaldson, MD, MS

The Origin of Femtosecond Laser–Assisted Cataract Surgery

Femtosecond laser–assisted cataract surgery (FLACS) has recently become part of our armamentarium as cataract surgeons. It has given us another option to upgrade our patients with hopes of achieving the most advanced, safest, customized option in cataract surgery. The primary potential goals of FLACS are to achieve better refractive outcomes and safer surgery relative to traditional cataract surgery.

There has been great debate over the proper terminology used to describe this technology. Acronyms include ReLACS (refractive laser–assisted cataract surgery), FALCS (femtosecond-assisted laser cataract surgery), and T-LACS (therapeutic laser–assisted cataract surgery). Finally, the most widely used acronym has become FLACS.

The availability of FLACS and its increasing usage by cataract surgeons has come at a time of a refractive revolution in cataract surgery. Its development has occurred alongside the continued development of presbyopic intraocular lenses. The past decade has seen a dramatic improvement in this technology, allowing us to feel more confident while offering our patients these expanded options for vision correction. Fifty years ago, cataract surgery was performed with one goal in mind: removal of the cloudy lens and replacement with aphakic spectacles. However, by today's standards, this result would be considered a travesty by both the surgeon and the patient. Our surgery then evolved to include the replacement of the cloudy lens with a spherical distance lens, which was very effective in many patients but left them wearing glasses for astigmatism correction and for near vision. Now, cataract surgery has 2 primary goals: removal of the cloudy lens and replacement with a lens that either gives the best possible distance, near, or both, while

Hovanesian JA.
Refractive Cataract Surgery: Best Practices and Advanced Technology, Second Edition (pp 95-113).

correcting astigmatism to give patients high-quality vision at a broader range of distances while providing more freedom from glasses. FLACS has become a tool toward achieving this goal, while giving us a mechanism to achieve better outcomes and improving the safety of the procedure.

How Does a Femtosecond Laser Work?

Femtosecond lasers work through the process of photodisruption, which is characterized by the coalescence of expansive gas bubbles that unite to form a cleavage plane through a solid tissue. Essentially, the gas bubbles are placed in a line, and then the dots are connected to form the intended, preprogrammed incision. Femtosecond lasers are extremely fast, functioning at subpicosecond pulse durations in the near infrared range.

Femtosecond lasers were initially used to create corneal flaps in LASIK with the approval of the IntraLase femtosecond laser (Abbott Medical Optics) by the United States Food and Drug Administration in 2000.[1] Laser application to the cornea, however, was much simpler, as the cornea was applanated, essentially flattening it so that the laser could be applied in a plane parallel to the surface at a preset distance beneath the applanating interface. The laser had to pass through and cut only one structure, the cornea, and there were no other interfering or surrounding structures that could potentially be damaged by inadvertent laser application. Additionally, with LASIK surgery, patients are generally much younger and healthier, allowing them the flexibility to be positioned as needed and to tolerate the high levels of vacuum required during their laser treatment.

For FLACS, we now need to be able to use these lasers to cut corneal tissue as well as capsular tissue and lens material, while avoiding collateral damage to surrounding structures such as the iris or posterior capsule. Thus, imaging capabilities have been enhanced so that the laser can accurately detect and avoid these surrounding structures to ensure the safety of the procedure.

Currently Available Laser Platforms

There are currently 5 laser platforms available in the United States: 1) LenSx (Alcon), 2) VICTUS (Bausch & Lomb), 3) Catalys (Abbott Medical Optics), 4) LensAR, and 5) the LDV Z8 femtosecond laser (Ziemer), which was CE marked in Europe and recently cleared by the US Food and Drug Administration for use in cataract surgery (corneal incisions, capsulotomy, and lens fragmentation). Each laser is unique on several levels. Four of them can be compared based on the essential features illustrated in Table 9-1 and Figure 9-1.

The Patient Interface

The patient interface is a key differentiating factor among the laser platforms. Both the LenSx and the VICTUS platforms are derived from LASIK-based applanation platforms, whereas the Catalys and LensAR platforms evolved de novo for cataract surgery. In addition, due to the minimal rise in intraocular pressure (10 to 16 mm Hg), the Catalys and the LenSx lasers have been approved for usage in glaucoma patients.[2,3]

Table 9-1
Four of the Five Femtosecond Lasers Available for Cataract Surgery in the United States‡

Laser	LenSx (Alcon)	VICTUS (Bausch & Lomb)	Catalys (Abbott)	LensAR (LensAR, LLC)
Pulse Frequency (Khz)	50	Up to 160	120	80
Patient Interface Design	SoftFit, curved lens, applanating, 1-piece	Dual modality curved lens, applanating, 2-piece, spherical, solid + liquid, vacuum	Liquid optics, nonapplanating, liquid interface, 2-piece design, vacuum	Robocone nonapplanating, fluid interface, 2-piece vacuum docking
Patient Interface Dimensions	Inner diameter: 12.5 mm; outer diameter: 19.8 mm	Curved, > 12 mm; inner diameter suction clip: 15.5 mm; outer diameter suction clip: 21 mm	2 Options: 1) Inner diameter: 12.7 mm; outer diameter: 24.0 mm 2) Small: 12 mm inner diameter	Inner diameter: > 12.7 mm; outer diameter: 24.0 mm
Docking	Curved applanation	Soft docking for capsulotomy and lens frag: hard docking for corneal incisions	No applanation; liquid	No applanation; liquid
Imaging	3D Spectral domain OCT	3D Spectral domain OCT	3D Spectral domain OCT	3D RayTracing CSI*
Integrated Bed	No	Yes	Yes	No
Dimensions	1.524 m x 1.828 m	2.075 m x 0.825 m (without bed)	0.68 m x 0.37 m (on floor without bed)	1.65 m x 1.97 m

Abbreviations: CSI, confocal structural illumination; OCT, optical coherence tomography.
‡ This does not include the LDV Z8 femtosecond laser.
* 3D-CSI uses a super diode to create the infrared light that illuminates the eye. The illumination beam scans the eye, and a video camera records the images. The Scheimpflug principle is used to maintain focus throughout.

Since the inception of laser-assisted cataract surgery, Alcon has modified the patient interface from a standard applanating interface to the SoftFit modified applanating interface, with a customized soft contact lens within the applanating cone. This allows the applanating surface to conform to the surface of the eye more accurately. This

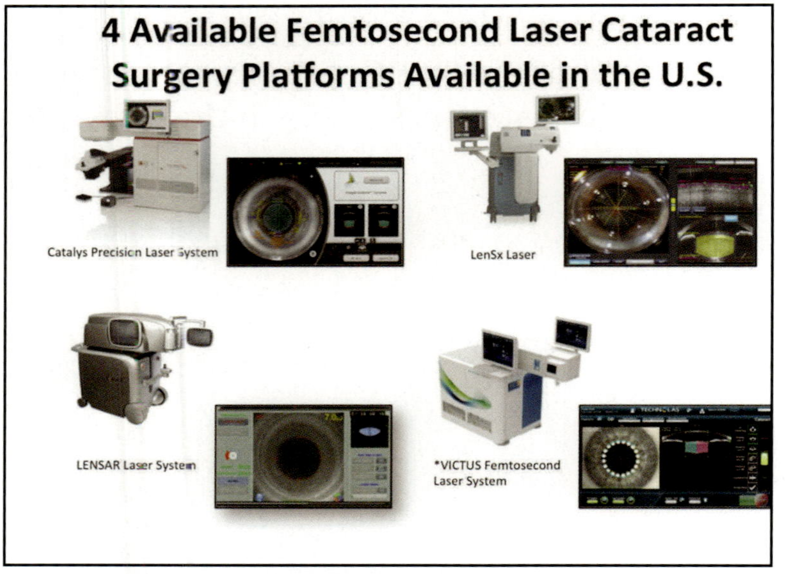

Figure 9-1. Four of the 5 femtosecond lasers available for use in cataract surgery in the United States. This does not include the LDV Z8 femtosecond laser.

interface modification significantly decreased the incidence of capsular discontinuities, as it reduced the applanation-induced corneal deformation, or folding, that can occur when pressure is applied to the ocular surface. This modification occurred along with a decrease in the diameter of the patient interface, while also reducing the intraocular pressure elevation necessary to provide adequate vacuum. Corneal folds may introduce artifacts during imaging, ultimately resulting in areas devoid of laser application. These *skip lesions* result in capsular tags, which, if not identified and managed proactively, can result in anterior capsular tears and, in some cases, posterior capsular extension and potential vitreous loss.

The VICTUS laser is unique with its dual modality patient interface that uses a hard dock for the corneal portion of the procedure and a soft dock for the intraocular portion of the procedure. The VICTUS has a standard, solid, curved 2-piece applanating interface that serves to flatten the corneal surface to perform the corneal incisions. Then a lower pressure liquid docking system is used to complete the capsulotomy and lenticular fragmentation portion of the procedure.

The Catalys femtosecond laser uses a liquid optics interface with 2-piece vacuum docking. Imaging through liquid allows for high-resolution OCT imaging with no interference through other solid interfaces that may induce any deformation of the cornea. A very low intraocular pressure elevation of 10.2 mm Hg occurs during vacuum application.[3]

The LensAR laser also images through a liquid interface through a patented Robocone 3-piece applanating system. The liquid interface provides high-quality imaging without interference, which is similar to the Catalys laser.

The Zeimer laser also has a liquid optics interface designed to optimize lens fragmentation, while it still has corneal refractive procedure capabilities, including cataract incisions, LASIK flap creation, channels for corneal ring segments, and keratoplasty applications.

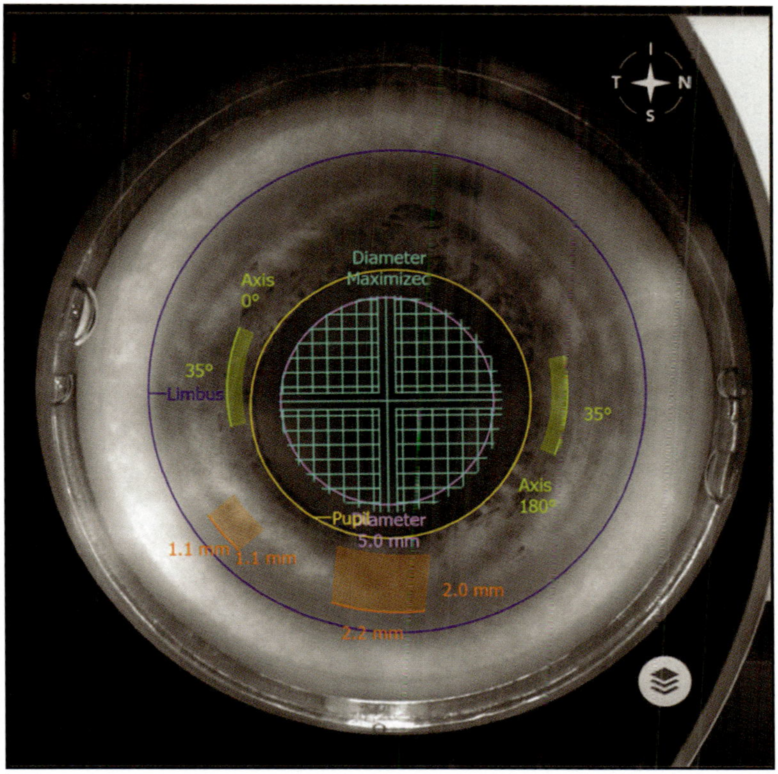

Figure 9-2. FLACS Treatment Plan including capsulotomy, lens fragmentation, and corneal incisions.

Imaging

All of the lasers require precise 3-dimensional imaging capabilities in order to accurately apply the intended laser treatment. Three of the lasers image the structures through spectral domain OCT. Through a series of OCT images taken in rapid succession, the images are merged to create a 3-dimensional reconstruction of the patient's eye. The programmed treatment is then illustrated in an overlay using the recreated image (Figure 9-2). The image must accurately determine position of the structures and account for any induced lens tilt in order to avoid inadvertent lasing of surrounding structures. Although safety zones are preset by the surgeon, strict imaging requirements are critical to avoid complications. In contrast to the other laser platforms, the LensAR femtosecond laser uses the Scheimpflug principle to align the camera lens, taking a series of 10 photographs with a rotating camera, which are then fused to create a high-resolution 3-dimensional model of the essential ocular structures. A scanning superluminescent diode with a variable scan rate creates the infrared light that illuminates the eye. It uses a lower scan rate on more highly reflective surfaces to avoid reflection (ie, for the iris) and a higher scan rate for lower reflective surfaces (ie, for the lens and posterior capsule). Through accurate reconstruction of the anterior segment structures, lens tilt is accounted for, and the treatment profile is applied accurately, avoiding surrounding structures.

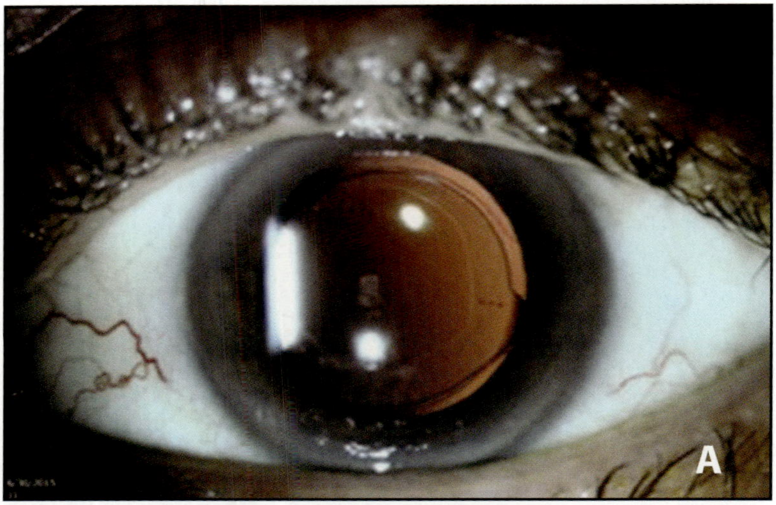

Figure 9-3. (A) Complete femtosecond capsulotomy: good centration, accurate size and shape. *(continued)*

The Procedure

Capsulotomy

The anterior capsulotomy is arguably the most important portion of laser application, with the lowest margin of error (requiring the most precision). Some may argue that the lens fragmentation is more critical; however, we generally program a significant safety zone for lens fragmentation, so capsular discontinuities, although rare, are much more common than inadvertent lasing of the posterior capsule. Fortunately, as the lasers have evolved over the past few years, the average laser time necessary to complete a capsulotomy has decreased from 13 to 15 seconds to 1 to 6 seconds for most laser platforms. This allows less time for patient movement, making the incidence of capsular discontinuities much more rare. An incomplete capsulotomy can be a very frustrating problem for the surgeon, taking a simple traditional case and turning it into a challenging FLACS case (Figure 9-3A). This may result from lens tilt, a corneal opacity (such as a scar or fold), an opacity within the anterior chamber (such as a bubble in viscoelastic after placement of a Malyugin ring), misalignment of the laser beam, or a suction break during laser application. Recovery after an incomplete capsulotomy may be challenging in some cases, as it may be difficult to visualize, particularly in those cases involving more complex lens fragmentation patterns that end near the capsulotomy edge. For this reason, many surgeons have advocated the *dimple down technique*, using a Utrata forceps (or similar tool) to slightly indent the central portion of the capsule, allowing the capsular edge to slightly retract centrally, revealing a 360-degree gutter ensuring a complete treatment pattern before the capsule is removed abruptly.

Since the capsulotomy is created by the coalescence of gas bubbles (through photodisruption, as previously discussed), we know that the capsule edge will not be quite as smooth as it would be in comparison to a manually torn capsulorrhexis. Electron microscopy studies have shown that the capsulotomy edge is irregular (and has been likened to

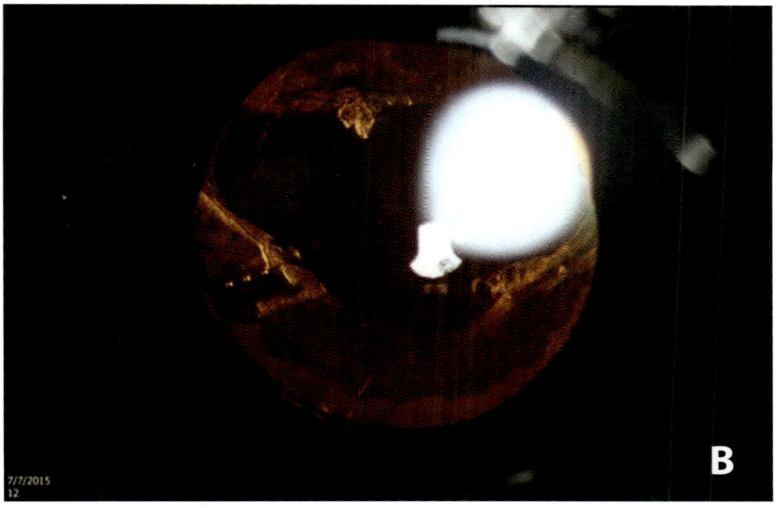

Figure 9-3 (continued). (B) Incomplete anterior capsulotomy resulting in anterior capsular tear without posterior extension. Toric intraocular lens within the capsular bag with proper orientation.

a postage stamp), even with a complete treatment pattern.[4] Fortunately, studies have also revealed that the strength of a femtosecond capsulotomy is similar to or stronger than a manual capsulotomy.[4-6] The speed of laser capsulotomy creation makes the laser a particularly useful tool with white cataracts in which the potential increased pressure from capsular distension and the friable nature of the capsule itself makes those cases prone to extension of a capsular tear (known as an *Argentinian Flag sign*).

The laser has an exceptional ability to create a capsulotomy of a preset size, shape, and centration[7-9] (Figure 9-3B). All of the laser platforms have shown extremely accurate reproducibility and accuracy. The capsulotomy may be centered on the pupil, limbus, scanned capsule, or by some other customized parameter as designated by the surgeon. An accurate centered capsulotomy may not be essential for every monofocal case with current intraocular lens technology; however, this degree of accuracy may be necessary for best results with accommodating lens technology, and particularly with some of the newer lens designs involving dual optics.

Lens Fragmentation

The ability of the laser to prefragment the lens has become a useful tool, particularly in denser cataracts and in eyes vulnerable to ultrasound-induced trauma (ie, Fuchs dystrophy). We currently have a variety of treatment patterns available on all of the laser platforms, allowing us to customize the lens treatment according to surgeon preference and lens density. The treatment patterns are generally divided into 3 categories: cuts, cylinders, and grids. Cuts can be used to divide the lens into 2, 4, 6, or 8 equal segments. Cylinders can be added to create circumferential ring segments and be increased to form a more complicated spider-web pattern, creating smaller segments to facilitate nuclear removal. A grid pattern creates small cubes of a preprogramed size (approximately 100 to 2000 microns), ultimately subdividing the lens into the smallest possible fragments.

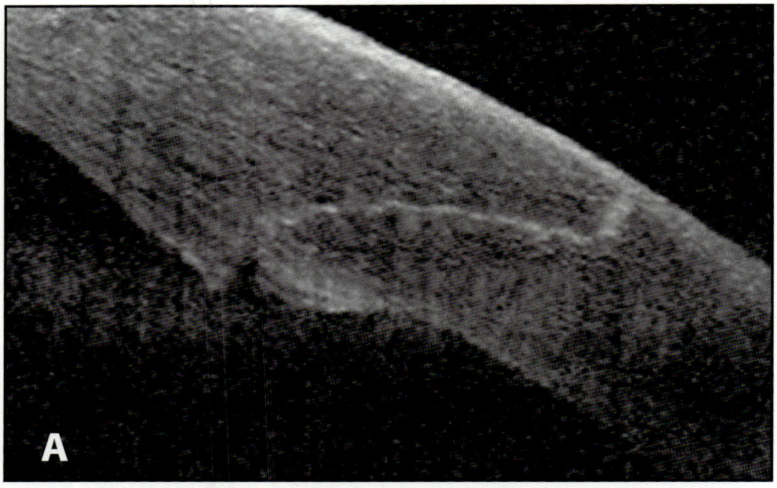

Figure 9-4. Primary wound architecture. (A) FLACS primary incision, OCT image. *(continued)*

These treatment patterns can be combined or used alone, according to the surgeon's preference for a particular case.

Corneal Incisions

Clear Corneal Incisions

The femtosecond laser is able to produce a customized, reproducible corneal incision. It can be programed to create a complicated triplanar beveled incision of differing inner and outer diameters, it can create a simple stab incision for a paracentesis, and it can create exceptionally accurate astigmatic incisions (Figure 9-4). The laser can only cut through transparent corneal tissue and not through the opaque limbal tissue. Thus, the laser is limited in its ability to create a truly limbal or scleral primary incision, as some surgeons tend to initiate their manual incision at the limbus. Improvements in imaging have allowed the laser to better identify the true limbus and have allowed us to bring our incisions out more peripherally with upgrades in both hardware and software over the past few years. If incisions are inadvertently made too centrally within the cornea, they may induce irregular astigmatism, corneal edema, and poor wound closure (see Figure 9-4).

Limbal Relaxing Incisions

The ability of the laser to customize limbal relaxing incisions (LRI) is unsurpassable. However, most of the evidence for increased accuracy of laser-based incisions is derived primarily from studies comparing manual with femtosecond laser incisions after penetrating keratoplasty.[10] We can create a particular arc length and apply it much more accurately than we ever could achieve with a manual LRI. Manual nomograms have been modified with the introduction of FLACS technology, with an average reduction of treatment plan (length of arc) of approximately 30% from the manual nomograms (personal communication with Skip Nichamin, April 25, 2014). However, surgeons are

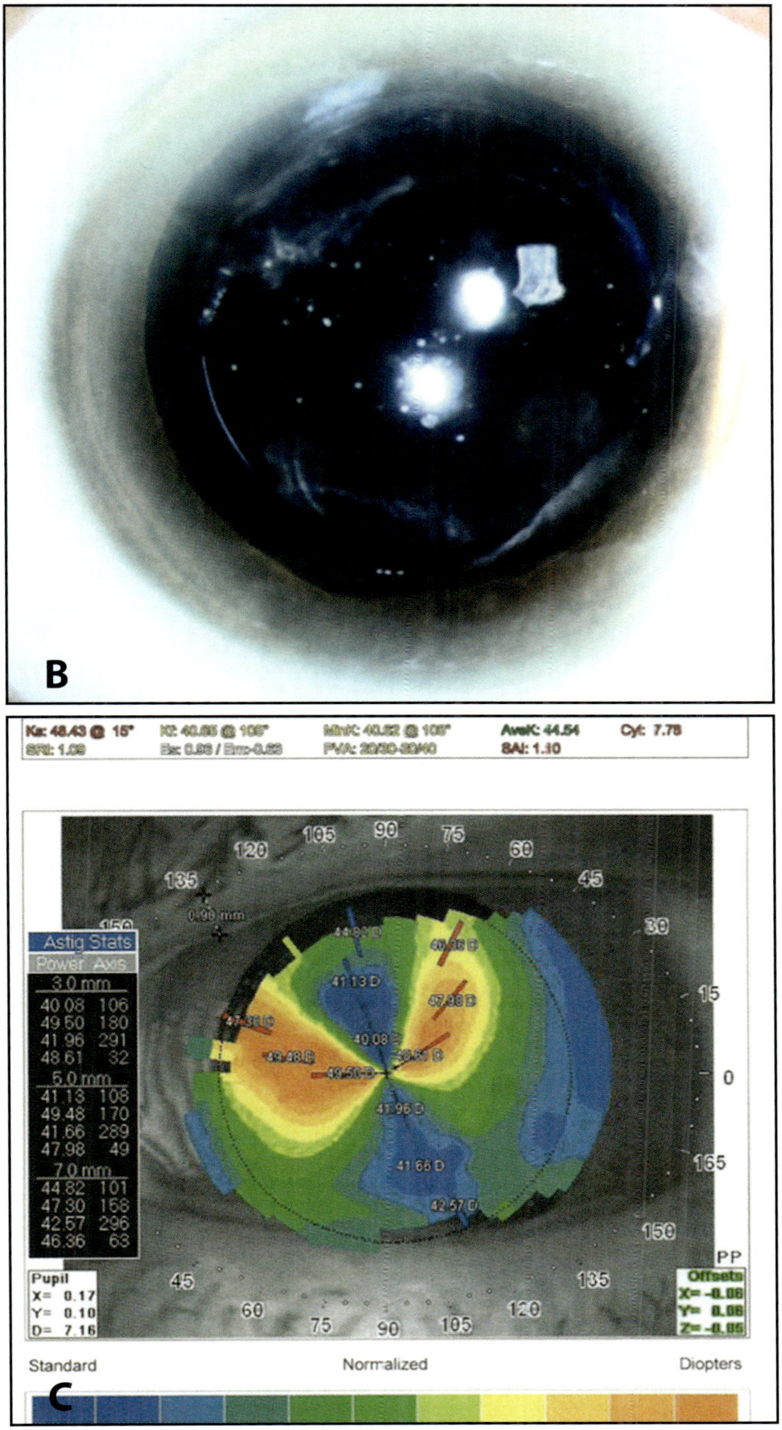

Figure 9-4 (continued). (B) FLACS wound inadvertently placed too central inducing astigmatism, slit-lamp photo; (C) central FLACS wound inducing astigmatism, Tomey topography.

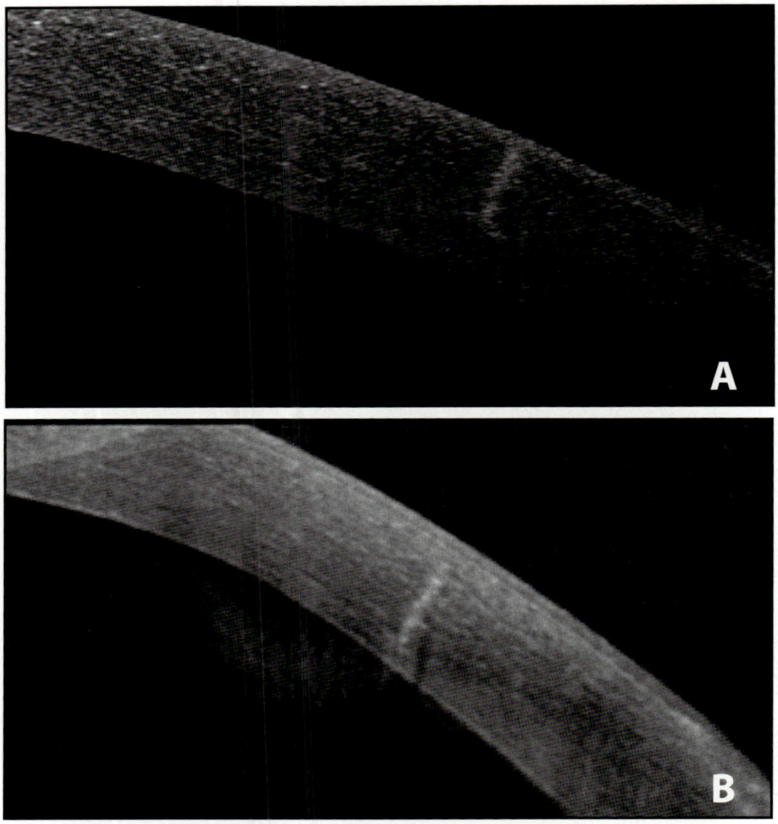

Figure 9-5. (A) Surface incisions; (B) intrastromal incisions.

modifying nomograms in a variety of ways, so much variability still exists among current treatment nomograms. Although most surgeons are not opening their LRIs, some surgeons are using intraoperative aberrometry to open incisions either partially or fully at the time of surgery. Other surgeons are opening incisions postoperatively with the guidance of corneal topography and refraction. Incisions can be opened many months postoperatively, as indicated by refractive error and topographic imaging. Although most surgeons are using surface LRIs, femtosecond lasers also have the ability to create intrastromal incisions (Figure 9-5). Intrastromal incisions are programmed to extend from one preset depth within the cornea to another (eg, sparing 20% anteriorly and 40% posteriorly). Intrastromal incisions exert less astigmatic effect; however, they may also induce less surface irritation with a decreased risk of infection. Many surgeons opt to use 10- to 15-degree intrastromal incisions to mark their steep corneal axis for toric intraocular lens alignment.

Logistics

As with the integration of any new technology into one's practice, femtosecond cataract surgery is associated with practice alterations in the operating room as well as in the clinic. The most direct change is in the operating room, as the cataract surgery now has 2 components (femto and phaco) instead of just 1 (phaco). The laser can be placed in the operating room or in a separate laser suite. Although pretreatment with a laser in a separate laser suite may decrease the time spent in the operating room, one must also account for the time spent in the laser suite. Studies have shown that when the laser is housed in the operating room, the cataract surgery takes longer than it would with traditional phacoemulsification.[11] Additional staffing may also be necessary in the operating room (to operate the laser), as well as in the office (for patient education).

New technology also brings with it a cost or investment for the practice. Each practice must assess its own ability to support this new technology, as the investment may be in excess of a half million dollars between the cost of the laser, the service contract, marketing costs, and the cost of any additional staffing. Internal and external marketing helps attract new patients to the practice or may serve to upgrade current patients, with additional revenue offsetting the added cost of the laser technology.

Given the costs to the practice as far as the initial investment and the compromised efficiency (particularly during the learning curve), the practice needs to be committed to making the investment successful. This starts with internal changes promoting the potential benefits for the patients. Marketing initiatives are often worthwhile investments when making the initial commitment. Teaching both patients and staff about the new technology also helps propagate understanding of the benefits of this technology to patients throughout the practice.

Outcomes

Safety and Complication Rates

Femtosecond cataract surgery has been well established as a safe procedure.[12-14] Several studies have compared the incidence of complications in FLACS cases to traditional cases and found no significant increase in complications.[12-14] Studies with residents in training have shown the safety of FLACS, even among residents with minimal prior experience with traditional phacoemulsification.[12,13]

As would be expected, during the learning curve, complications may occur more frequently.[15,16] However, the learning curve with FLACS is relatively quick compared with that of traditional cataract surgery or with some other ophthalmic procedures (such as Descemet membrane endothelial keratoplasty or deep anterior lamellar keratoplasty).[15,16]

Refractive Outcomes

FLACS outcomes have been compared with outcomes with traditional cataract surgery in only a few studies. Thus, we are still awaiting more conclusive results from larger randomized prospective trials. Some studies have shown refractive outcomes to be similar between FLACS and traditional cataract surgery, whereas other studies have shown improved accuracy of refractive outcomes with FLACS.[17,18] As we improve nomograms for astigmatism correction and maximize the ability to create the most accurate astigmatic incisions, our outcomes should continue to improve and exceed conventional surgery.

FLACS in Complicated Cases

1. Hypermature/white cataracts
2. Pseudoexfoliation syndrome
3. Small pupils
4. Loose zonules
5. Traumatic cataracts
6. Dense/mature cataracts
7. Fuchs dystrophy
8. Posterior polar cataracts

FLACS may serve as an extremely useful tool in complicated cataract cases. As previously mentioned, white cataracts, although soft and easily fragmented, can be associated with capsular distension and increased tension on the capsule during capsulorrhexis creation (Figure 9-6). The ability of the femtosecond laser to create a capsulotomy in 1 to 2 seconds prevents radial tearing and facilitates lens removal within the intact capsular bag.

FLACS serves as a tool in patients with pseudoexfoliation syndrome, as prefragmentation facilitates lens removal with less manipulation and less stress on the zonules. Some pseudoexfoliation patients may have small pupils, precluding the use of laser; however, most patients with adequate mydriasis are potential candidates for FLACS. If the laser is in the operating room, even patients who might otherwise be precluded from FLACS may be prepped and draped in the usual sterile fashion and have a Malyugin ring (or other pupillary expansion device) placed. The patient may then be rotated under the femtosecond laser to undergo capsulotomy and lens fragmentation (Figure 9-7). The patient can then be rotated back under the operating scope to complete the procedure. The laser portion of the procedure may be done through balanced salt solution or through viscoelastic. However, there must be no bubbles or balanced salt solution/viscoelastic interfaces in the anterior chamber, and the wound must be adequately sealed to tolerate the application of the patient interface to the corneal surface.

FLACS may also be useful for traumatic cataracts or in other cases with suspected zonular laxity. Lens prefragmentation is particularly useful in these patients, as it allows phacoemulsification to proceed with less manipulation and less energy expenditure in an eye with pre-existing compromised support.

Posterior polar cataracts may pose a challenge during FLACS.[19,20] The typical surgical technique needs to be modified in order to incorporate the entirety of the lens opacity into the posterior safety zone. Hydrodelineation is key to safe and effective removal of a posterior polar cataract; thus, the cleavage plane for fluid must be anterior to the lens opacity so that hydrodissection is not performed inadvertently. Abby Vasavada has promoted the "inside out" phaco technique, avoiding all nuclear rotation, for safe removal of posterior polar cataracts, reducing the risk of posterior capsular rupture[20] (Figure 9-8).

Dense cataracts generally require increased ultrasound power and longer phaco time for lens removal with traditional phacoemulsification. As surgery itself is a form of trauma and increased energy expenditure translates into increased intraocular trauma, this

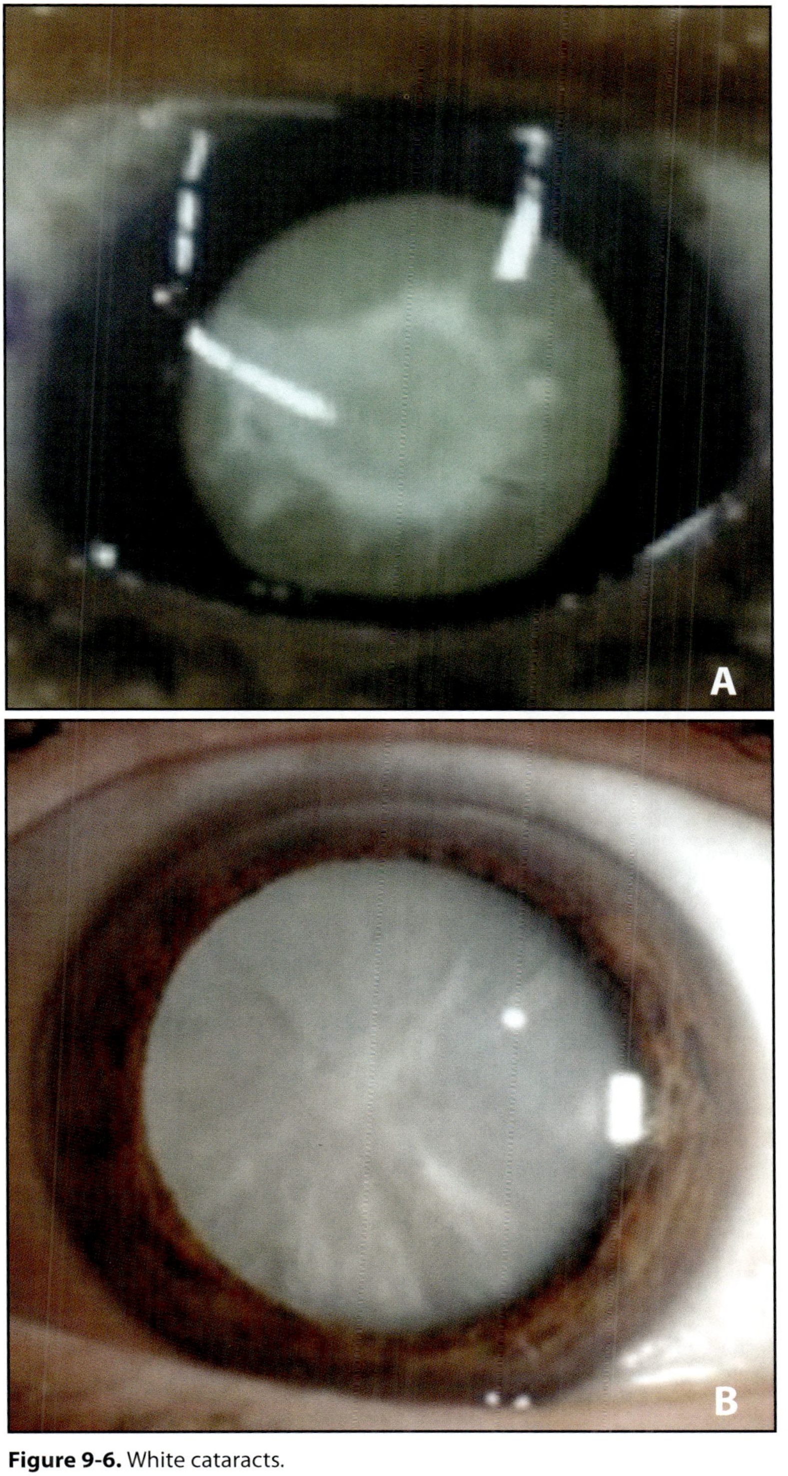

Figure 9-6. White cataracts.

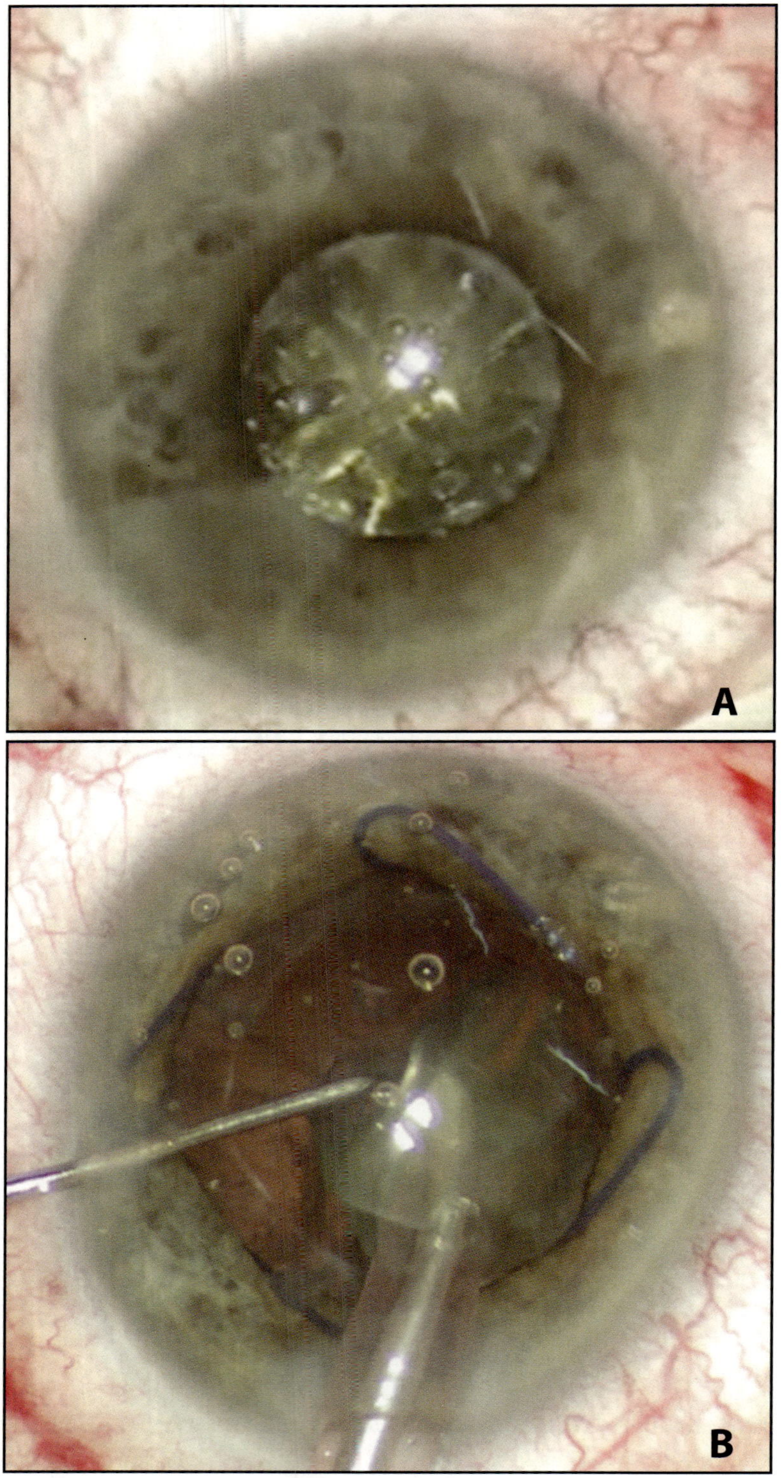

Figure 9-7. Small pupil case with Malyugin ring.

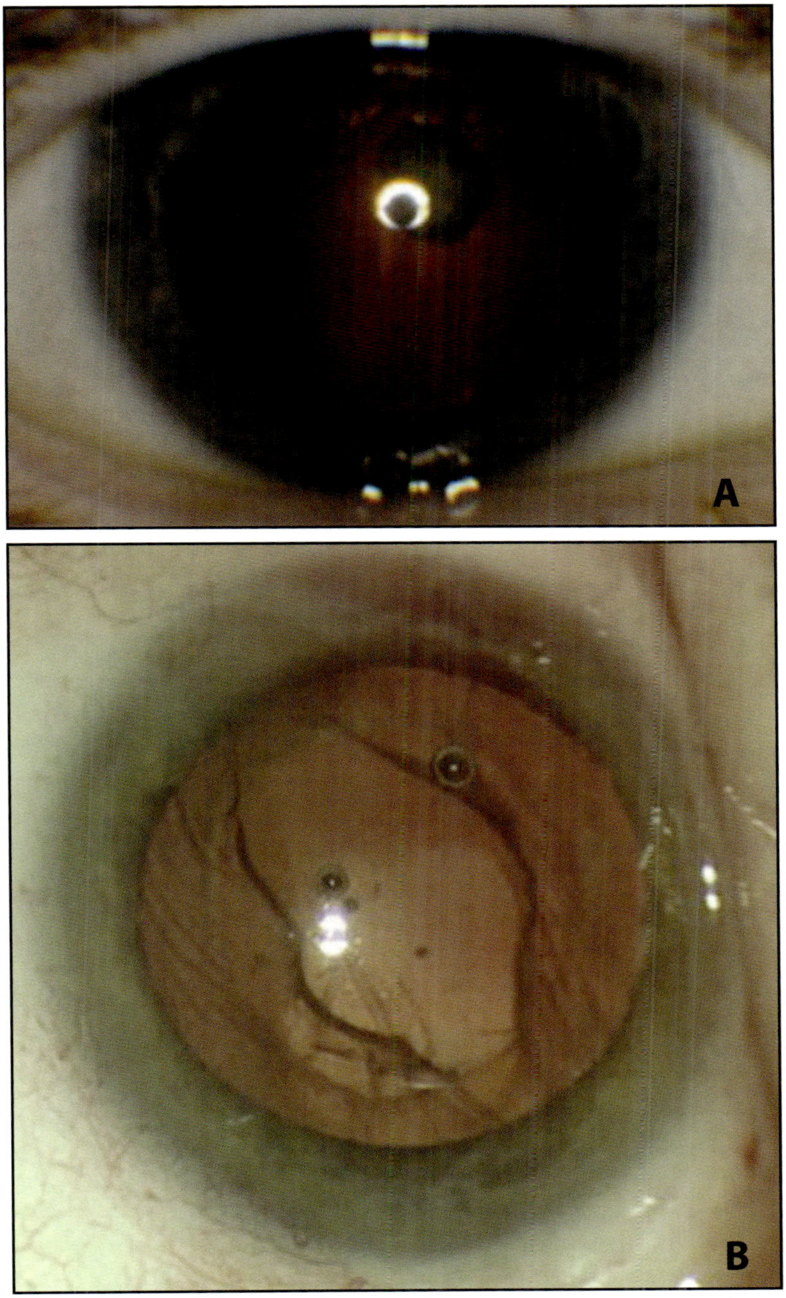

Figure 9-8. (A) Posterior polar cataract; (B) posterior capsular rupture during FLACS with posterior polar cataract.

trauma may be associated with increased damage to the corneal endothelial cells. Several studies have consistently shown that FLACS pretreatment reduces ultrasound power and phaco time in comparison with traditional cataract surgery.[21,22] Although, theoretically, a reduction in ultrasound energy should translate into preservation of endothelial cells, several studies have found endothelial cell loss to be similar between FLACS and traditional surgery.[23-25] Larger prospective randomized trials are still needed to establish this relationship.

FLACS-Induced Pupillary Miosis

Pupillary miosis is a known concern with FLACS.[26-28] It is well-established that the release of prostaglandins into the anterior chamber during laser application causes pupillary constriction. The various stages of laser application during surgery have been analyzed individually, and it has been determined that the greatest prostaglandin release occurs during the creation of the capsulotomy.[28]

In addition to prostaglandin release, miosis may be induced by corneal applanation, as miosis has been observed during repeat applanation or extended applanation without laser application.

In order to decrease the incidence and severity of pupillary miosis, all patients should be pretreated with a topical nonsteroidal agent in preparation for surgery. Preoperative regimens vary from 3 days prior to surgery to treatment on the day of surgery. In addition, compounded intracameral preservative-free dilating agents may be used to reverse any induced miosis associated with the laser treatment. This miosis is reversible in most cases once an intracameral mydriatic is instilled. Alternatively, the recently released ketorolac 0.3%/phenylephrine 1% solution (Omidria [Omeros Corp]) is now available to add to the irrigating solution during phacoemulsification to help maintain a dilated pupil throughout surgery. Given the reversibility of this phenomenon, no associated complications have been directly linked to the pupillary miosis induced by FLACS. However, it is well known that conventional phacoemulsification in cases with small pupils is associated with a higher rate of complications.[29]

Ethical Dilemmas and Controversies

The introduction of FLACS has brought with it ethical dilemmas, as is often the case with services not covered by third-party payers. There has been much discussion among surgeons and patients as the costs and benefits have been debated. As surgical options for patients increase, the differences among procedures and the potential benefits needs to be accurately and honestly discussed with the patient, with hopes of guiding them through the decision-making process. Unfortunately, as surgeons, we may not always have the luxury of spending adequate time reviewing this important decision with patients. Many surgeons work with the assistance of support staff, who can spend the necessary time for adequate patient education and to avoid patient confusion. With the concurrent expansion of presbyopic lens technology and options for astigmatism correction, patients have multiple decisions to make regarding their surgery; thus, counseling throughout this process is almost an imperative measure to avoid preoperative misunderstandings and dissatisfied postoperative patients.

Practice patterns are changing, and surgeons are becoming more aggressive with regard to astigmatism correction. Part of this evolution has stemmed from the increasing usage of presbyopic lens technology that requires minimal residual astigmatism to achieve a successful outcome. Additionally, toric lenses have become increasingly popular among surgeons. Finally, the ability of the femtosecond laser to create customized LRIs has increased surgeons' confidence with astigmatism correction as compared with manual incisions, which are known for their potential for variation and unpredictability.

Although FLACS may provide an added benefit for many of our patients, particularly those with astigmatism and denser lenses, some patients with smaller degrees of astigmatism and softer lenses may not appreciate a significant benefit for the added cost at this point in time.

Future Directions

Although cataract surgery is continuously evolving, over the past decade we have seen a dramatic transition from simple cataract removal to refractive cataract surgery, with increased patient expectations and improved outcomes. FLACS is just one tool that is helping us to achieve the next level with the potential for improved refractive outcomes and higher levels of safety.

The uses of the femtosecond laser are expanding into 2 areas: corneal procedures and presbyopia correction. In addition to the ability to perform LASIK surgery (the origin of the femtosecond laser), the femtosecond laser has the ability to create channels for corneal ring segments, intrastromal ablations for presbyopia correction (Intracor), flaps for corneal inlays, and the potential to perform various forms of lamellar keratoplasty. Additionally, the LensAR laser has been used to perform lens softening procedures for presbyopia correction. We will surely see the uses of the femtosecond laser expand during the upcoming years.

The future of cataract surgery will be dependent on the increasingly seamless integration of technology between the clinic and the operating room. We are in the early stages of integration, as we are beginning to use technology to help plan our surgeries in the clinic, and this plan is translated through the femtosecond laser and the operating microscope to be applied to the patient. Intraoperative aberrometry is being used to guide and adjust our treatment during surgery. And finally, our postoperative results are being used to adjust our nomograms and alter future treatments customized by both surgeon and patient. The future of cataract surgery is dependent upon increasing integration. The femtosecond laser is an integral tool that will help us move closer toward our quest for emmetropia.

References

1. US Food and Drug Administration. Ophthalmic devices panel meeting summary for November 8, 2000. www.fda.gov/advisorycommittees/committeesmeetingmaterials/medicaldevices/medicaldevicesadvisorycommittee/ophthalmicdevicespanel/ucm124831.htm. Updated July 31, 2013. Accessed January 4, 2017.
2. Kerr NM, Abell FG, Vote BJ, Toh T'. Intraocular pressure during femtosecond laser pretreatment of cataract. *J Cataract Refract Surg* 2013;39:339-342.
3. Schultz T, Conrad-Hengerer I, Hengerer FH, Dick HB. Intraocular pressure variation during femtosecond laser–assisted cataract surgery using a fluid-filled interface. *J Cataract Refract Surg*. 2013;39:22-27.
4. Bala C, Xia Y, Meades K. Laser capsulotomies are approaching the smoothness of the manual capsulorhexis. *J Cataract Refract Surg*. 2014;40(8):1382-1389.

5. Friedman NJ, Palanker DV, Schuele G, et al. Femtosecond laser capsulotomy. *J Cataract Refract Surg.* 2011;37(7):1189-1198.
6. Auffarth GU, Reddy KP, Ritter R, Holzer MP, Rabsilber TM. Comparison of the maximum applicable stretch force after femtosecond laser-assisted and manual anterior capsulotomy. *J Cataract Refract Surg.* 2013;39(1):105-109.
7. Palanker DV, Blumenkranz MS, Anderson D, et al. Femtosecond laser-assisted cataract surgery with integrated optical coherence tomography. *Sci Transl Med.* 2010;2(58):58ra85.
8. Reddy KP, Kandulla J, Auffarth GU. Effectiveness and safety of femtosecond laser-assisted lens fragmentation and anterior capsulotomy versus the manual technique in cataract surgery. *J Cataract Refract Surg.* 2013;39(9):1297-1306.
9. Nagy ZZ, Kranitz K, Takacs AI, Mihaltz K, Kovacs I, Knorz MC. Comparison of intraocular lens decentration parameters after femtosecond and manual capsulotomies. *J Refract Surg.* 2011;27(8):564-569.
10. Bahar I, Levinger E, Kaiserman I, Sansanayudh W, Rootman DS. IntraLase-enabled astigmatic keratotomy for postkeratoplasty astigmatism. *Am J Ophthalmol.* 2008;146(6):897-904.
11. Lubahn JG, Donaldson KE, Culbertson WW, Yoo SH. Operating times of experienced cataract surgeons beginning femtosecond laser–assisted cataract surgery. *J Cataract Refract Surg.* 2014;40(11):1773-1776.
12. Scott W, Tauber S, Ohly J, Owsiak R, Eck C, Gessler JA. Comparison of vitreous loss rates between manual phacoemulsification cataract surgery and femtosecond laser–assisted cataract surgery. Paper presented at: 7th World Cornea Congress; April 15-17, 2015; San Diego, CA.
13. Hou JH, Prickett AL, Cortina MS, Jain S, de la Cruz J. Safety of femtosecond laser-assisted cataract surgery performed by surgeons in training. *J Refract Surg.* 2015;31(1):69-70.
14. Abell RG, Darian-Smith E, Kan JB, Allen PL, Ewe SYP, Vote BJ. Femtosecond laser–assisted cataract surgery versus standard phacoemulsification cataract surgery: outcomes and safety in more than 4000 cases at a single center. *J Cataract Refract Surg.* 2015;41(1)47-52.
15. Bali SJ, Hodge C, Lawless M, Roberts TV, Sutton G. Early experience with the femtosecond laser for cataract surgery. *Ophthalmology.* 2012;119(5):891-899.
16. Roberts TV, Lawless M, Bail SJ, Hodge C, Sutton G. Surgical outcomes and safety of femtosecond laser cataract surgery: a prospective study of 1500 consecutive cases. *Ophthalmology.* 2013;120(2):227-233.
17. Lawless M, Bali SJ, Hodge C, Roberts TV, Chan C, Sutton G. Outcomes of femtosecond laser cataract surgery with a diffractive multifocal intraocular lens. *J Refract Surg.* 2012;28(1):859-864.
18. Filkorn T, Kovacs I, Takacs A, Horvath E, Knorz MC, Nagy ZZ. Comparison of IOL power calculation and refractive outcome after laser refractive cataract surgery with a femtosecond laser versus conventional phacoemulsification. *J Refract Surg.* 2012;28(8):540-544.
19. Alder BD, Donaldson KE. Comparison of 2 techniques for managing posterior polar cataracts: Traditional phacoemulsification versus femtosecond laser-assisted cataract surgery. *J Cataract Refract Surg.* 2014;40(12):2148-2151.
20. Vasavada AR, Vasavada V, Vasavada S, Srivastava S, Vasavada V, Raj S. Femtodelineation to enhance safety in posterior polar cataracts. *J Cataract Refract Surg.* 2015;41(4):702-707.
21. Conrad-Hengerer I, Hengerer FH, Schultz T, Dick HB. Effect of femtosecond laser fragmentation on effective phacoemulsification time in cataract surgery. *J Refract Surg.* 2012;28(12):879-883.
22. Daya SM, Nanavaty MA, Espinosa-Lagana MM. Translenticular hydrodissection, lens fragmentation, and influence on ultrasound power in femtosecond laser-assisted cataract surgery and refractive lens exchange. *J Cataract Refract Surg.* 2014;40(1):37-43.
23. Abell RG, Kerr NM, Howie AR, Mustaffa Kamal MA, Allen PL, Vote BJ. Effect of femtosecond laser-assisted cataract surgery on the corneal endothelium. *J Cataract Refract Surg.* 2014;40(11):1777-1783.
24. Krarup T, Holm LM, la Cour M, Kjaerbo H. Endothelial cell loss and refractive predictability in femtosecond laser-assisted cataract surgery compared with conventional cataract surgery. *Acta Ophthalmol.* 2014;92(7):617-622.
25. Takacs AI, Kovacs I, Mihaltz K, Filkorn T, Knorz MC, Nagy ZZ. Central corneal volume and endothelial cell count following femtosecond laser-assisted refractive cataract surgery compared to conventional phacoemulsification. *J Refract Surg.* 2012;28(6):387-391.
26. Jong HJ, Kyu YH, Sung DC, Choun-Ki J. Pupil-size alterations induced by photodisruption during femtosecond laser–assisted cataract surgery. *J Cataract Refract Surg.* 2015;41(2)278-285.
27. Nagy ZZ, Takacs AI, Filkorn T, et al. Complications of femtosecond laser-assisted cataract surgery. *J Cataract Refract Surg.* 2014;40(1):20-28.

28. Schultz T, Joachim SC, Stellbogen M, Dick B. Prostaglandin release during femtosecond laser-assisted cataract surgery: main inducer. *J Refract Surg.* 2015;31(2):78-81.
29. Hashemi H, Seyedian MA, Mohammadpour M. Small pupil and cataract surgery. *Curr Opin Ophthalmol.* 2015;26(1):3-9.

Chapter 10

Intraoperative Wavefront Aberrometry

Joel M. Solano, MD and John P. Berdahl, MD

Intraoperative wavefront aberrometry is a method of measuring the refractive error of an eye at the time of cataract surgery to aid in the determination of the best intraocular lens (IOL) for the desired refractive target. Currently, there are 3 devices that couple with the operating microscope to allow for such wavefront measurements: ORA (Alcon; Food and Drug Administration [FDA] approved), HOLOS (Clarity Medical Systems, Inc; FDA approval pending), and Aston (under development at Solihull Hospital and Aston University, Birmingham, United Kingdom). This chapter will discuss how wavefront aberrometry grows the ophthalmic surgeon's confidence in selecting an IOL compared with previously available methods and provide guidelines for optimization of data acquisition during surgery.

Intraocular Lens Power Calculations

The standard of care in ophthalmology is to use IOL power formulas when selecting an IOL at the time of cataract surgery. These formulas rely on measuring axial length, corneal power, and anterior chamber depth. They are known to have a high predictive value in eyes with normal, previously unoperated anatomy. However, even the newer generation formulas have suboptimal performance when predicting postoperative refractive outcomes for patients with extremes of refractive error or those with a history of refractive surgery. The challenges in IOL prediction for these patients include variability in effective lens position and difficulty with acquiring true corneal powers. Keratometers and topographers measure only the anterior corneal curvature and assume a standard relationship between the anterior and posterior curvatures. With refractive surgery,

Hovanesian JA.
Refractive Cataract Surgery: Best Practices and Advanced Technology, Second Edition (pp 115-122). © 2017 SLACK Incorporated.

the relationship between anterior and posterior corneal curvatures is altered, and thus the predicted corneal powers are inaccurate. When making a cornea more oblate, as is done with myopic refractive surgery, the estimated IOL power can lead to postoperative hyperopia and the unpleasant "refractive surprise." Several options are available to help combat the difficulty with post–refractive surgery IOL selection, including the contact lens method, historical method, nomogram method, targeting myopia method, and the widely accepted American Society of Cataract and Refractive surgery online post–keratorefractive IOL power calculator (http://iolcalc.org/). These are all viable options for the preoperative selection of the IOL power. Intraoperative aberrometry is the only method for IOL selection that can take place during surgery and will account for both the anterior and posterior curvatures as well as any surgically induced astigmatism.[1-6]

Astigmatism

Astigmatism can be managed at the time of cataract surgery with either incisional corneal surgery or toric IOL placement. The complete treatment of cylinder requires conceptualizing the astigmatism as a vector with power and direction. In the visual system, astigmatism can be induced at the anterior cornea, posterior cornea, or the lens. When removing the lens during cataract surgery, we are left with correcting the total corneal astigmatism, but it is important to remember that topography and keratometry are based on the anterior surface only. Koch et al have shown that the posterior cornea contributes to the total corneal power, and this must be accounted for when treating astigmatism at the time of cataract surgery.[7] They showed that the mean magnitude of astigmatism of the posterior cornea was -0.3 ± 0.15 diopter (D; range -0.01 to -1.10 D). Their data allows for the generalization that the posterior cornea adds against-the-rule astigmatism, but the range of data is such that some patients can have with-the-rule astigmatism on the posterior cornea. Thus, when trying to account for this when treating corneal astigmatism, many patients will be left with unexpected cylinder. One approach to better managing astigmatism is to actually measure both the anterior and posterior power contributions from the cornea. At this time, measuring the posterior curvature preoperatively has been difficult.

Surgically induced corneal astigmatism (SIA) also needs to be factored in when managing cylinder in the cataract patient. SIA can be measured and tracked over time for an individual surgeon, but the range of data can be such that using an average will lead to postoperative surprises.

Intraoperative Wavefront Aberrometry

Intraoperative wavefront aberrometry is a method of determining the refractive error of an aphakic or pseudophakic eye during cataract surgery. The aim of intraoperative aberrometry is to measure the optical system after the corneal incisions have been made so that the optics are as close to the postoperative state as possible while the measurements are acquired. Indeed, corneal wound healing and remodeling can change the power of the cornea; however, this approach remains as close to the final postoperative state as one can obtain before selecting and placing the IOL. The advantage of delaying the measurements for IOL power calculation until this point is that the total power of the cornea is included, as opposed to the preoperative method, in which just the anterior surface curvature is measured and the power calculated based on an assumption between the anterior and posterior surfaces. In addition, the measurements are captured after the corneal incisions have been created, which allows for a patient-specific account of SIA, thus obviating the need for the surgeon to calculate SIA. A search of the ophthalmology literature shows 3 aberrometers that are either available or in development: ORA (FDA approved), HOLOS (FDA approval is pending), and Aston (under development at Solihull Hospital and Aston University, Birmingham, United Kingdom).

ORA

ORA (formerly Wavetec's Optiwave Refractive Analysis system) is currently the only intraoperative wavefront aberrometer commercially available in the United States. The device attaches to the cataract surgeon's operating microscope and is capable of capturing phakic, aphakic, and pseudophakic refractions.

After phacoemulsification and removal of the lens cortex, the capsular bag and anterior chamber are filled with a cohesive viscoelastic and the images are captured. There is an art to quick and accurate image capture, and it is up to the surgeon to decide which values are most reproducible. On occasion, the data at the time of image acquisition are substantially different from the expected values calculated preoperatively. Several repetitions of image capture are then performed, and the surgeon will decide which measurements have the most similar spherical equivalents to guide the surgeon's selection. Additionally, the surgeon may compare preoperative and intraoperative measures of magnitude and direction of the cylinder for guidance.

HOLOS

HOLOS is an intraoperative wavefront aberrometer that is currently being developed by Clarity Medical Systems, Inc. HOLOS is not yet commercially available and is pending FDA approval.

The instrument uses a sequentially shifting wavefront device to rapidly sample the wavefront and acquires data in real time. All data is acquired real-time, and therefore there is no need to pause and have the surgical assistant push a data capture button.[8]

ORA: Image Capture

Many surgeons use ORA almost exclusively in the aphakic or pseudophakic state, but the device is able to capture data during the phakic state as well. In the phakic state of the eye, the measurements can be taken before incision or at the time of limbal relaxing incision or enhancement. When capturing data during the aphakic state, the user must ensure a clear path for the wavefront for IOL selection. Once all of the cataract is removed, the surgeon should make sure the posterior capsule is clean and use capsular polish as needed. Another important aspect to good data acquisition is ensuring that all dispersive viscoelastic is removed, including the viscoelastic that sometimes forms a

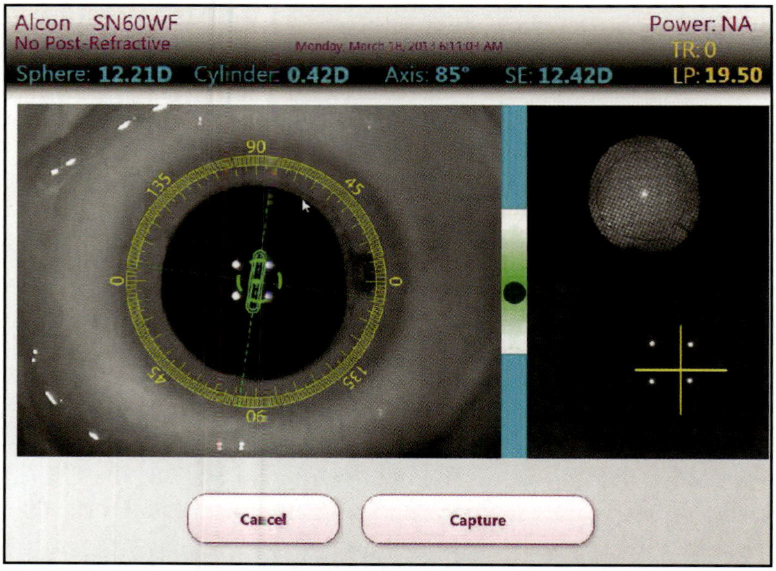

Figure 10-1. Intraoperative aberrometry measures an aphakic wavefront.

shell deep to the corneal endothelium. Once the lens capsule has been cleaned and the dispersive carefully removed, the bag is then filled with a cohesive viscoelastic. By filling the bag and anterior chamber with viscoelastic to the point where it just starts to egress from the main incision, the intraocular pressure is usually left close to 20 mm Hg. An intraoperative tonometer is used to ensure that the pressure is between 15 and 21 mm Hg and can be adjusted accordingly with more or less cohesive viscoelastic.

Once the eye has been prepared to capture the images, it helps to warn the patient that the microscope light is going to turn off, and a small red light will turn on in its place. The patient should maintain fixation on the red target dot during the entire image capture time. The ORA screen has a button labeled "capture" that ideally is not pressed by the assistant until the device is in focus. Usually, the scope is already focused on the anterior chamber, since the surgeon will have just completed the cataract removal. But prior to turning attention to focusing, ensure that the scope is not tilted and that the patient is focused on the alignment target. Make an effort to check that the scope is perpendicular to the patient's visual axis. Topical anesthesia should be used so the patient can control his or her fixation.

Attention can now be turned to the ORA screen. The surgeon's hands are used to gently control the patient's head and also to elevate the eyelid speculum off the globe. On the ORA screen you will find the real-time image of the operative eye and a green alignment circle and target (Figure 10-1).[9] In addition, there are 4 LED reflections that the system must see in order to capture data. The microscope joystick is used in order to grossly position the alignment target within the green circle that is displayed on the wide field of view camera image on the screen. The surgeon can move the patient's head for fine adjustments of the green circle in order to keep the alignment target centered. The alignment target on the screen will turn red to indicate it is not aligned with the central alignment circle, helping to guide the user with the alignment process (Figure 10-2).[9] Once the target is in the alignment circle, it changes from red to green.

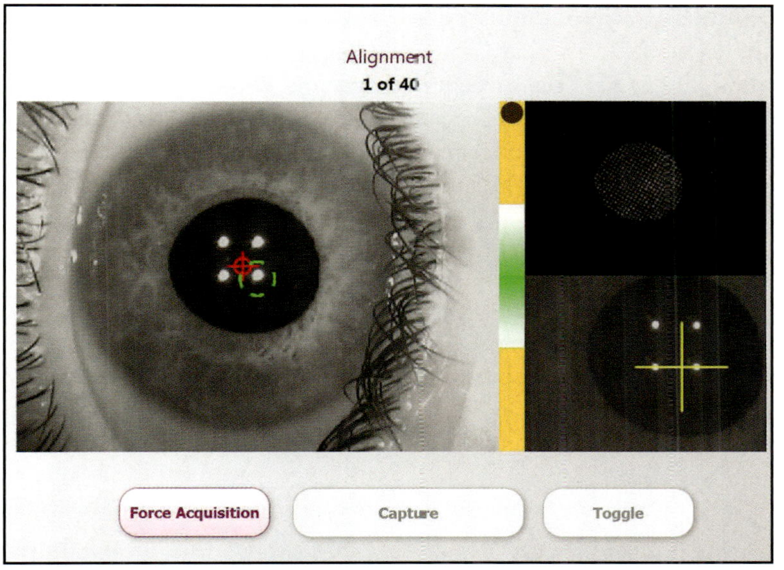

Figure 10-2. After alignment, 40 measurements are taken to give a composite wavefront.

Next, there is a focus ball in the center of the ORA screen that needs to be raised or lowered into the green zone of the focus bar. This is accomplished with the z-axis focus of the microscope foot pedal. Usually, the focus ball is fairly close or even in the center of the green zone just by virtue of the scope having been in focus on the anterior chamber or iris plane during cataract removal. The ORA user's manual does suggest setting the focus to the apex of the cornea, but it seems to work well by simply leaving the focus where it was set at the time of the cataract extraction. If the focus ball is not near the center green zone, it is a good indicator that one of the prior steps has not been optimized, usually the alignment. The focus ball initially can be difficult to fine tune, as small movements from the scope either up or down can often cause major movements of the focus ball. There is a bit of a learning curve to realize that the foot pedal z-axis should only be engaged in small increments when adjusting the focus ball.

Once you have the alignment target centered in the green circle and the focus ball in the green zone of the focus bar, have the assistant give a final rinse to the cornea with balanced salt solution. Remember to elevate the lid speculum so it is not resting on the globe and have the assistant press the capture button. The device takes 40 measurements, which typically takes only several seconds, provided the prior steps have been taken to ensure that alignment and focus are ideal.

ORA: Pearls for Image Capture

- Alignment of the scope should be perpendicular to the iris plane.
- All dispersive viscoelastic should be removed prior to image capture.
- The posterior capsule should be free from posterior subcapsular cataract and as clear as possible.

- ▲ Intraocular pressure confirmed to be close to physiologic with intraoperative tonometer.
- ▲ Thoroughly irrigate the surface so debris and viscoelastic are removed just prior to data capture.
- ▲ Gross alignment can be adjusted with the microscope joystick.
- ▲ Fine tune the alignment by moving the patient's head.

ORA: Data Display

After the ORA device has acquired the data, the screen changes to the display setting. On the display setting, the left portion of the screen shows the preoperative data. Centrally, you will find the measured astigmatism and IOL power with predicted postoperative spherical equivalent. On the right of the screen are the complete refractive findings, which can be used to compare different image capture sets in order to select the surgeon's preferred image group.

ORA: Error Message

Red error messages are occasionally encountered following attempted image capture. The device is programmed to display the red message when there is a large range between the 40 captured images, a dry corneal surface, central air or anterior chamber debris (such as cortex fragments) or posterior vitreous detachment, and in patients with increased higher order aberrations or in any disease that obstructs the path of light to the retina. When this occurs, the user should adjust the variables that can be modified and repeat the image acquisition. Typically, the surgeon will have success by copiously irrigating the cornea and ensuring that the lid speculum is not resting on the globe. At times, the surgical drape has drifted into the field of view of the aberrometer and simply needs to be adjusted out of the field of view of the device.

Obstacles to the device capturing accurate images include the use of iris expansion devices; use in patients with any disease that prevents target fixation (such as macular degeneration); and use in any eye with corneal pathology, such as anterior basement membrane dystrophy, Fuchs dystrophy, keratoconus, or advanced pterygium. As a general principle, any disease with media opacities, such as asteroid hyalosis or advanced vitreous syneresis, that interferes with the wavefront should be a contraindication to using the device for IOL selection. Eyes with a history of radial keratotomy may be inaccurate due to changes in corneal power with changing pressures.

ORA: Reticle Overlay and VerifEye+

The ORA has a reticle display that will overlay the surgical image into the surgeon's ocular. In addition, Alcon has a system called VerifEye+ that gives real-time refractive validation in the microscope ocular. The reticle display amplifies the surgeon's confidence when selecting the axis of cylinder by which to align a toric IOL. The reticle is independent of cyclotorsion caused by the supine position because it is based on the wavefront that is measured during surgery when the cyclorotation would have already taken place. The reticle overlay is based on the intraoperative measurement and therefore already accounts for cyclotorsion as well as anterior and posterior corneal curvatures. The ORA gives the numerical value of the axis on which to place the toric IOL, and this value can then be used to count off the degrees on the reticle display and properly align the toric. Our experience has been that when a patient's corneal steep axis is marked preoperatively, the reticle overlay is very consistent with expected placement. Factors that influence the cylinder axis that have not been accounted for preoperatively (like surgically induced astigmatism and posterior corneal curvature) will be included in the wavefront analysis and thus be accounted for when the toric is aligned by the reticle overlay.

ORA: Pseudophakic Data

ORA can be used in the pseudophakic state to confirm the power of the implanted IOL. This aberrometry measurement is dependent on the IOL position and may not reflect the final postoperative refraction, thus making this measurement more useful in guidance of toric IOLs. When a toric IOL is selected to be implanted, the system automatically will default to the toric screen. The device provides rotation recommendations, allowing the user to achieve the optimal cylinder reduction.

ORA: Challenge with Minimally Invasive Glaucoma Surgery

The intraoperative aberrometer mounts to the inferior-most portion of the operating microscope and reduces the distance between the patient's eye and the scope's objective. The surgeon must be aware of this reduced distance and avoid touching the aberrometer, since it is not sterile; however, a reusable sterile cover is available. In particular, the reduced distance secondary to the added device can be cumbersome when performing intraoperative gonioscopy for minimally invasive glaucoma surgery. There remains enough room to accomplish placement of minimally invasive glaucoma surgery devices safely, but on occasion the proximal end of the delivery instrument or gonio lens can come in contact with the aberrometer. Being attuned to this can reduce the possibility of contaminating the sterile field.

Conclusion

Intraoperative wavefront aberrometry is a valuable tool for the cataract surgeon who seeks to minimize refractive surprises and improve patient safety by reducing the risk of IOL exchanges and laser enhancements. This is especially important for patients who wish some degree of glasses independence following cataract surgery. We are witnessing a growing cohort of active baby boomers who have begun to request refractive cataract surgery and expect the best outcomes.

The intraoperative approach to biometry and refractometry allows measurement of the wavefront after the corneal incisions and measures both the anterior and posterior corneal contributions to the refractive error. Keratometers and topographers assume a standard relationship between the anterior and posterior corneal curvatures, which does not hold true in eyes that are post–refractive surgery. The ORA aberrometer guides not only IOL spherical power selection, but also gives the power and axis of the cylinder. This information aids the surgeon in placement and orientation of toric lenses and also in titrating arcuate incisions. It is important to get the surgical eye as close to physiologic positioning and pressure as possible to ensure data acquisition that mirrors the postoperative state.

Today, the only commercial intraoperative wavefront aberrometer available to surgeons is the ORA, sold by Alcon. Soon the market will have at least one other option for users to consider, and patients will benefit from the improvements that competition will stimulate from both platforms.

Intraoperative aberrometry is one more tool to aid in the refractive cataract surgeon's objective of achieving preoperative refractive targets and getting patients as close as possible to their unaided visual potential.

References

1. Hatch KM, Woodcock EC, Talamo JH. Intraocular lens power selection and positioning with and without intraoperative aberrometry. *J Refract Surg.* 2015;31(4):237-242.
2. Fram NR, Masket S, Wang L. Comparison of intraoperative aberrometry, OCT-Based IOL Formulae, Haigis-L, and Masket Formulae for IOL Power Calculation after Laser Vision Correction. *Ophthalmology.* 2015;122(6):1096-1101.
3. Huelle JO, Katz T, Druchkiv V, et al. First clinical results on the feasibility, quality and reproducibility of aberrometry-based intraoperative refraction during cataract surgery. *Br J Ophthalmol.* 2014;98(11):1484-1491.
4. Lanchulev T, Hoffer KJ, Yoo SH, et al. Intraoperative refractive biometry for predicting intraocular lens power calculation after prior myopic refractive surgery. *Ophthalmology.* 2014;121(1):56-60.
5. Hemmati HD, Gologorsky D, Pineda R II. Intraoperative wavefront aberrometry in cataract surgery. *Semin Ophthalmology.* 2012;27(5-6):100-106.
6. Canto AP, Chhadva P, Cabot F, et al. Comparison of IOL power calculation methods and intraoperative wavefront aberrometer in eyes after refractive surgery. *J Refract Surg.* 2013;29(7):484-489.
7. Koch DD, Ali SF, Weikert MP, Shirayama M, Jenkins R, Wang L. Contribution of posterior corneal astigmatism to total corneal astigmatism. *J Cataract Refract Surg.* 2012;38(12):2080-2087.
8. Krueger RR, Shea W, Zhou Y, Osher R, Slade SG, Chang DF. Intraoperative, real-time aberrometry during refractive cataract surgery with a sequentially shifting wavefront device. *J Refract Surg.* 2013;29(9):630-635.

Chapter 11

Microincisional Cataract Surgery

Mujtaba A. Qazi, MD; Abu-Bakar Zafar, MD; and Jay S. Pepose, MD, PhD

Why the Premium Intraocular Lens Surgeon Should Transition to Microincisional Cataract Surgery

Patient expectations have changed dramatically in recent years. In the past, cataract patients were delighted with the increased contrast sensitivity and reduction of forward light scatter associated with cataract extraction and intraocular lens (IOL) implantation and were satisfied with a change in spectacle correction a month later. Today, many cataract surgery patients anticipate better vision postoperatively than they may have even enjoyed prior to cataract formation, regardless of IOL selection. In effect, irrespective of the choice of a conventional or a premium IOL, many patients expect to experience outcomes consistent with refractive cataract surgery. As a rule, this benchmark is even higher in those patients who have paid the additional expense of premium lifestyle-enhancing, presbyopia-correcting IOLs.

With the convergence of refractive corneal and lens surgeries, satisfying these progressively higher demands requires meticulous and uncomplicated cataract surgery, control and adjustment of corneal astigmatism, and an uneventful postoperative course characterized by rapid visual rehabilitation without potentially devastating complications such as endophthalmitis. In consideration of these stated goals, Table 11-1 lists a number of potential advantages of cataract surgery using an incision of 2 mm or less, which has been termed *microincisional cataract surgery* (MICS).[1] This chapter details the following: the evolution of microincisional surgery; highlights the various steps, instruments, and phaco settings involved; and presents a step-by-step approach to smoothly transitioning to MICS.

Hovanesian JA.
Refractive Cataract Surgery: Best Practices and Advanced Technology, Second Edition (pp 123-140).

Table 11-1
(Potential) Advantages of Microincisional Cataract Surgery

- Watertight wound closure
- Reduced need for suture placement
- Reduced risk of endophthalmitis
- Reduced surgically induced astigmatism
- Reduced iris prolapse
- Improved anterior chamber stability
- Less fluid egress and volume of balanced salt solution utilized (decreased vitreous hydration)
- Increased phaco efficiency requiring lower ultrasound power and shorter time

Background

Modern cataract surgery has transitioned from en bloc extraction techniques, requiring incision sizes greater than 10 mm, to techniques incorporating phacoemulsification (phaco) combined with foldable and injectable IOL insertion through incision sizes less than one-fifth those initially required by Sir Harold Ridley and his contemporaries. With further advancements in phacoemulsification and aspiration equipment, ocular viscoelastic device (OVD), fluidics, and IOL designs, strategies to further reduce incision size have become feasible. An important early step in development was in 1985, when Shearing[2] described a method of bimanual phacoemulsification as a means to further diminish the incision size. By the turn of the 21st century, the concept of MICS, through a sub–2-mm incision, had been introduced,[1] with continued refinement ever since. This transition may become mandatory if we are to eventually progress toward the ultimate goal of accommodating, capsule-filling polymers.

Among the key motivators for these advances has been the elevation of cataract surgery to a full-fledged refractive procedure, along with the advent of foldable IOLs capable of insertion through a sub–2-mm incision. MICS facilitates the goals of the modern refractive lens surgeon, which include minimal and predictable changes in corneal astigmatism, rapid healing and visual recovery, and smaller, stable watertight wound architecture to minimize wound leaks and lower risks of postoperative endophthalmitis. Nowadays, cataract surgery is routinely coupled with limbal relaxing incisions and toric and presbyopic IOL implantation. Reduction of thermal wound injury and corneal edema, control of surgical induction of corneal astigmatism (SIA), and consistency of capsulorrhexis size are key elements of modern-day cataract surgery. Improvement in immediate and long-term postoperative visual acuity and reproducibility of results has gained paramount importance.

A 2008 market survey[3] of 915 surgeons from 5 European countries found that 34% were performing MICS, with the penetrance anticipated to grow to 50%. More of these surgeons utilized coaxial MICS (C-MICS, 27%) than bimanual MICS (B-MICS, 7%), as the development of coaxial MICS systems permitted more natural transition from small incision coaxial surgery to C-MICS with a few simple modifications in surgical techniques. While advances in surgical instrumentation and techniques suggest an easy transition into sub–2-mm incision cataract surgery, there are some basic steps to streamline a successful and complication-free conversion, including understanding of the required fluidics, revision of surgical instruments, adjustment of intraoperative maneuvers, management of corneal astigmatism, and further modification of IOL materials and designs. A stepwise learning process is recommended and outlined in the following section in order to facilitate a smooth transition.

Fluidics of Microincisional Cataract Surgery

Fluid management is a key component of MICS. Higher infusion and vacuum pressure are required for fluid injection and nuclear fragment aspiration through a smaller bore cannula, just as higher suction power is required to sip liquid through a thin vs a thicker straw. Similarly, the amount of volume aspirated at a fixed flow or suction rate through a thin straw is lower than through a large-diameter straw at the same rate. These principles are outlined in Poiseuille's law, which relates the flow through a tube to a function of the radius cubed (r^3) of the tube. A result of this relationship, along with the minimal wound leakage in MICS, is that phacoemulsification is completed using a far lower volume of balanced salt solution (BSS), resulting in less vitreous hydration and corneal edema.

In this regard, MICS phacoemulsification platforms have incorporated gas compressors to increase the infusion pressure and flow. Gas is delivered to the infusion bottle in order to maintain a continuous, high inflow of fluid via higher resistance tubing. This allows for formed and consistent anterior chamber dimensions throughout the procedure. Gas-forced infusion also serves to cool the phaco tip.

Higher vacuum may increase the risk of post-occlusion surge, where flow rates can reach 300 cc/min (6 times normal) when occlusion is broken at high (400 mm Hg) vacuum levels. Therefore, MICS fluidics often involves use of flow restrictors (Figure 11-1) to limit the impact of complete occlusion. Cruise Control, in the Sonic WAVE phacoemulsification platform (STAAR Surgical), places a 2-cm long flow restrictor (see Figure 11-1A) behind a mesh filter that traps the nuclear emulsate. This prevents the narrow 0.3-mm lumen from becoming clogged. Hence, regular aspiration flow occurs below 50 cc/min, but unwanted flow surge above 60 cc/min is limited (see Figure 11-1B), thereby minimizing the inherent risk of capsular capture and tear. Alcon's newest peristaltic system (Centurion) utilizes active fluidics to allow a more consistent physiological intraocular pressure. The system automatically adjusts compression of the fluid bag and pump flow rate to stabilize the anterior chamber.

Some MICS fluidics designs utilize a Venturi pump in place of or in addition to peristaltic pumps. The Venturi pump (Stellaris and Millennium) customizes chamber fluidics using either a flow-based or vacuum-based system. It requires smaller diameter, flow-resistant tubing to generate vacuum as high as 600 mm Hg and steady, low flow (Figure 11-2, top). When vacuum pressure builds during occlusion, resistance to outflow increases such that the anterior chamber remains stable (Figure 11-2, bottom), thereby limiting the possibility of capsular incarceration in the phaco tip. The Stellaris also incorporates a mesh filter.

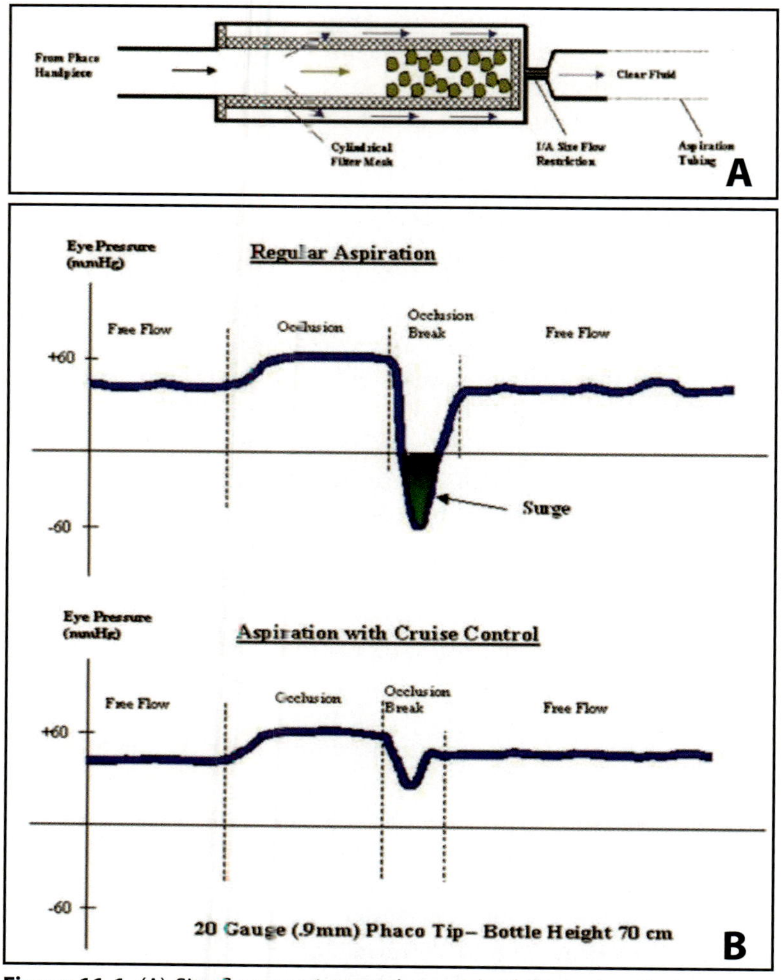

Figure 11-1. (A) Site flow restrictor reduces risk of (B) post-occlusion surge. (Reprinted with permission from STAAR Surgical.)

Thus, higher fluid inflow and vacuum pressures, along with the use of pulsed rather than continuous ultrasound power, promote influx of fragments to the phaco tip, improving followability. Often, the high flow required for MICS fluidics can help break up a fragment engaged at the phaco tip without the use of ultrasound power. The lower power utilization lessens the impact on the corneal endothelium and can result in clearer corneas on the first postoperative day.[4,5]

Incision

Decreasing the incision size has been one of the fundamental advances in modern surgery, including outside the domain of intraocular surgery. Laparoscopic and mini-incisional techniques have been developed for abdominal, cardiothoracic, and gynecological procedures with the aim of limiting tissue trauma and promoting faster

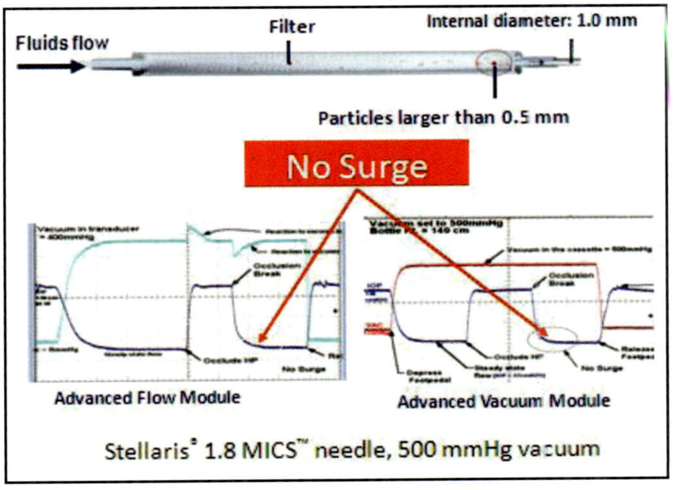

Figure 11-2. Stellaris tubing design and reduction of surge with advanced modules. (Reprinted with permission from Bausch & Lomb.)

healing. For ocular surgeries (see Table 11-1), these principles are extended to make small incisions self-sealing as well. Watertight wound construction is paramount for proper multifocal, Crystalens (Bausch & Lomb), and toric IOL positioning; avoidance of anterior Crystalens IOL vaulting with a resultant myopic shift; and prevention of toric IOL rotation. Watertight incisions may play a significant role in reducing endophthalmitis due to late influx of surface flora.[4] Additionally, smaller incision size prevents egress of viscoelastic (OVD) during capsulorrhexis formation, reducing the risk of errant peripheral migration during this critical step. Smaller incisions limit iris prolapse, especially in cases of intraoperative floppy iris syndrome (IFIS), so that altered pupil contour and suboptimal postsurgical cosmesis can be avoided. Smaller incisions allow for better fluidics control and fragment followability, leading to reduced applied phaco power and improved postoperative visual acuity and corneal optical quality.[5,6]

However, if wound construction is not performed properly, then thermal injury, fluid leakage, induced astigmatism, iris prolapse, and oar-locking of instruments are all possible. In this regard, close attention to incision location, size, shape, and self-sealing ability is required. The authors utilize a posterior clear cornea or "near clear" limbal incision site, so as to avoid conjunctival chemosis and anterior entry of the incision, which can interfere with intraoperative visibility from fluid pooling on the ocular surface or induction of corneal warpage during intraocular maneuvers, respectively. The placement of incisions should generally coincide with comfortable positioning of the hands, avoiding regions with prominent orbital rim structure or proximal to lid speculum wires or blades. The sizing of the incision should match phaco instrument size, to avoid leakage of infusion fluid around the phaco instruments. However, if the incision is too narrow, it will hamper instrument insertion and maneuverability while stretching and distorting the incision. A narrow incision may also impinge the irrigation sleeve in C-MICS, leading to chamber instability and increasing the risk of thermal wound injury. An incision that has been stretched or heated may not seal properly. In order to prevent such complications, surgeons have utilized different incision instruments to assist with reproducible, square wound construction, including trapezoidal steel (Figure 11-3A), sapphire, and diamond

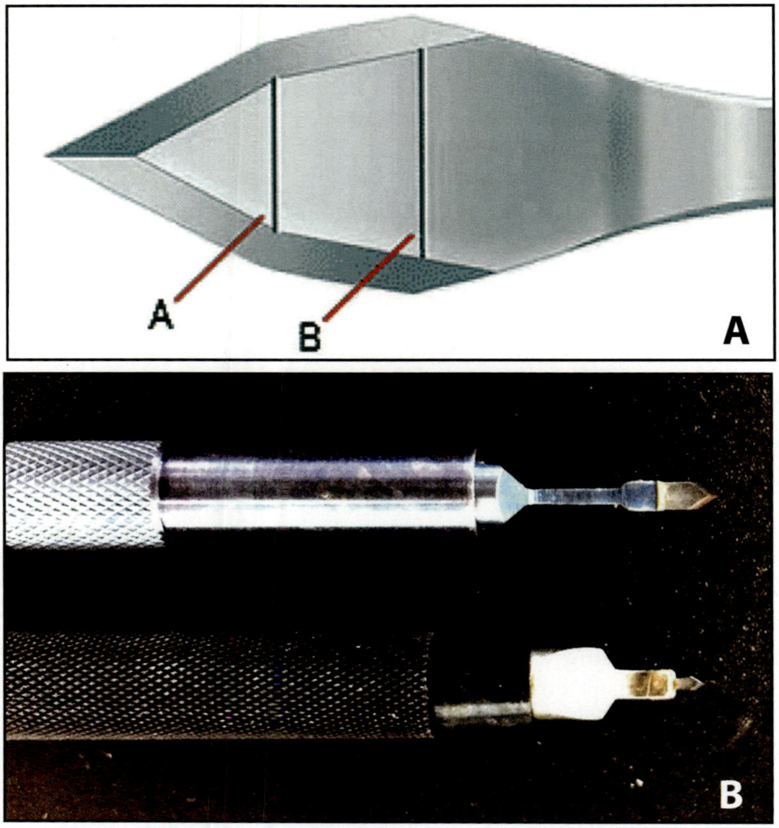

Figure 11-3. (A) Trapezoidal steel, (B) sapphire (top), and diamond (bottom) knives.

knives (Figure 11-3B). The application of femtosecond lasers for use in cataract surgery may further facilitate and standardize MICS incisions.

Typical incision sizes for B-MICS are 1.2 mm for 20-gauge instruments and 1.4 mm for 19-gauge instruments. One incision in B-MICS may need to be enlarged to allow for IOL insertion. C-MICS typically involves a 1.8- to 2.0-mm incision. The incision tunnel can be created by direct entry or in steps. At the end of the procedure, all corneal incisions should be hydrated with BSS and tested to be watertight. Application of fluorescein to the wounds to show that they are Seidel negative is also a sound consideration, particularly for specialty IOLs.

Capsulorrhexis and Hydrodissection

Microincision size requires revision of capsulorrhexis forceps size as well. Several designs have been developed by companies such as Storz, Katena, and MST, using both Utrata-style as well as coapting microincision instruments. Care must be taken during anterior capsulotomy formation to ensure that the micro-forceps do not become oar-locked during lateral or circular movement. This can be avoided by extending the wound slightly as the blade is exiting the incision site, regrasping the rhexis more frequently, and using a rotational wrist motion. Otherwise, there may be contact with the incision borders, translating into corneal distortion and OVD leakage. Such issues may be obviated by use of a femtosecond laser–assisted capsulorrhexis.

As the smaller incision limits OVD leakage, MICS procedures usually have a more controlled chamber. There is, therefore, usually less of a chance of a peripheral tear during MICS capsulorrhexis formation, affording an increased safety margin. However, it is important to wash out some OVD prior to full hydrodissection, as the small incision size and denser OVD may block the egress of fluid, increasing anterior chamber pressure that can then be directed to the posterior capsule, causing capsular blowout.

Ultrasound Power Modulation

Varying the power modulation during phacoemulsification can reduce ultrasound energy exposure to ocular tissues and improve the efficiency of cataract surgery. Pulsing of ultrasound (Table 11-2) and/or adjusting the duty cycle of phaco power on to phaco power off can allow for safer removal of denser nuclei by reducing the overall phaco time, thereby decreasing the risk of endothelial damage and wound burn. Miyoshi and Yoshida[7] demonstrated though ultra-high-speed digital video imaging that micropulse (8 ms on, 4 ms off) allowed for nuclear fragments to remain engaged and rotate at the tip, rather than being pushed away by the ultrasound pulse. The use of torsional phacoemulsification (Infiniti) can additionally diminish the delivered energy and improve followability.[8]

Bimanual Microincisional Cataract Surgery

Bimanual MICS involves 2 microincisions of the same diameter. In addition to the advantages of fluidics with smaller incisions, as outlined previously, this technique allows for greater intraoperative maneuverability, as the irrigation and aspiration hand pieces can be used via either port. This is particularly helpful in subincisional removal of nuclear and cortical material. It also allows for more thorough anterior and posterior capsular polishing, which is important for the stability of hinged-IOLs, such as the Crystalens, and in centration and stability of multifocal and toric IOLs. Bimanual techniques allow the use of irrigating choppers available through many companies such as Katena and MST (Figure 11-4).[9] B-MICS has been espoused for challenging cases,[10] such as for IFIS, miotic pupils, traumatic cataracts, pseudoexfoliation, posterior polar cataracts,[11] vitrectomy,[12] and combined glaucoma cases.

Transitioning to Microincisional Cataract Surgery

The advantages of MICS do not require significant modification of the surgeon's phacoemulsification techniques, whether they range from divide and conquer to horizontal or vertical chopping. In fact, MICS fluidics, greater chamber stability, and pulsed phaco allow for a relatively seamless transition to MICS.

Table 11-2
Coaxial Microincisional Cataract Surgery Settings With Stellaris, 1.8-mm Incision, Gas-Forced Infusion (50 mm Hg), and Venturi Pump

Settings For Dr. Qazi	*Sculpt*	*Segment Removal*	*Epinuclear*	*Irrigation/ Aspiration*
Vacuum (mm Hg)	80	400	400	475
Bottle height	55	95	95	70
Ultrapulse	200 pps, 60 dc	10 pps, 16 dc	10 pps, 16 dc	
Ultrasound power	65	30	30	
Settings For Dr. Pepose	***Sculpt***	***Segment Removal***	***Epinuclear***	***Irrigation/ Aspiration***
Vacuum (mm Hg)	100	400	380	550
Bottle height	65	110	85	50
Ultrapulse	250 pps 50 dc	8 pps, 12 dc	5 pps, 50 dc	
Ultrasound power	65	35	5	

Abbreviations: pps, pulses per second; dc, duty cycle.

During the early transition period to MICS, the authors recommend the following intermediate steps:

1. Use a marked blade for incision construction, in order to control length of tunnel.
2. In order to create a triplanar, self-sealing incision, first create a groove at the posterior clear cornea incision site of approximately half corneal depth using an angled crescent blade. Then insert a steel or diamond keratome to extend the tunnel parallel to the endothelium before diving in to enter the anterior chamber.
3. Use countertraction with a sponge, Colibri forceps, or other instrument at the limbus opposite the incision site to allow for control of incision entry.

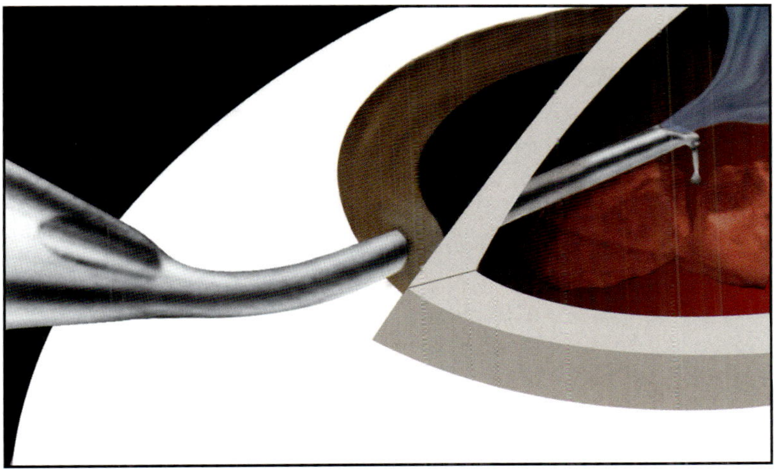

Figure 11-4. Schematic of irrigating chopper.

4. Mark the cornea with a 5.5-mm ring to guide a circular capsulorrhexis tear, as this will assist with rotational wrist movements of the micro-forceps.
5. Initially use a microincision knife to create the main incision, followed by capsulorrhexis and hydrodissection in order to practice these steps with micro-instruments, paying attention to avoid oar locking. Thereafter, the surgeon may expand the main incision to complete small-incision phacoemulsification.
6. Improve bimanual intraoperative maneuvers such as chopping. While this subject is outside the scope of the present chapter, the authors recommend *Phaco Chop: Mastering Techniques, Optimizing Technology, and Avoiding Complications* (David F. Chang, ed., SLACK Incorporated, 1994), which describes a step-by-step approach to learning and refining chopping techniques.
7. Improve bimanual intraoperative maneuvers by using bimanual I/A, initially toward the end of the case for subincisional cortical removal and capsular polish, but later for the entire case. The surgeon should switch the bimanual I/A hand pieces so that both right and left hands improve their dexterity.
8. Modify bottle height and gas-forced infusion during early MICS cases to optimize chamber depth and stability.
9. Routinely use pulsed or hyperpulsed modes during phacoemulsification.
10. Improve bimanual intraoperative maneuvers by polishing the capsule with manual polishers or bimanual I/A tips.
11. Insert IOLs using wound-assist techniques so the wound expansion is limited. This involves abutting the injector cartridge against the corneal incision while creating countertraction using a second instrument in the paracentesis site.
12. If extending the MICS incision for insertion of the IOL, then switch to a larger diameter I/A sleeve to avoid iris prolapse during OVD removal.

Microincisional Cataract Surgery Intraocular Lenses

Wound assist techniques permit insertion of single-piece IOLs, such as the Tecnis (Abbott Medical Optics) and AcrySof (Alcon), via incisions from 2.0 to 2.2 mm. A number of manufacturers have designed IOLs[1,13] to enter MICS incisions without extension of the incision, IOL compression, or wound distortion.

- ▲ AcriFlex MICS 46CSE IOL (Acrimed GmbH)
- ▲ Acri.Tec: CT.Asphina, CT.Spheris, AT.Lisa, AT.Lisa toric, AT.Torbi (Carl Zeiss Meditec)
- ▲ Akreos AO (Bausch & Lomb)
- ▲ CareFlex W20 (Medizintechnik AG)
- ▲ Hoya Y-60H (Hoya Corporation)
- ▲ IOLtech MICS lens (IOLtech and Carl Zeiss Meditec)
- ▲ MicroSlim, Slimflex (PhysIOL)
- ▲ Miniflex (Mediphacos Ltda)
- ▲ Presbysmart Plus (MTO)
- ▲ TetraFlex KH-3500 and ZR-1000 (Lenstec)

Clinical Efficacy With Microincisional Cataract Surgery

Since the advent of MICS, there has been a growing body of literature discussing the clinical efficacy and safety of the procedure. The most recent meta-analyses[14,15] of 14 studies evaluated the outcomes of B-MICS through 1.2- to 1.5-mm incisions vs standard coaxial small-incision cataract surgery (C-SICS) through 2.8- to 3.2-mm incisions. No statistical differences were found in the best-corrected visual acuity (BCVA; $P > 0.05$), SIA at postoperative 1 month ($P = 0.09$), mean endothelial loss ($P = 0.53$), central corneal thickness (CCT) at postoperative 1 month ($P = 0.64$) or 3 months ($P = 0.88$), intraoperative complications ($P = 0.68$), and postoperative complications ($P = 0.30$). B-MICS had the advantage of less SIA at postoperative 3 months ($P = 0.02$) and phaco time ($P = 0.00009$), whereas C-SICS had faster surgery time ($P < 0.00001$) and less early-onset corneal edema ($P = 0.04$).[14,15]

Endothelial Cell Loss, Safety, and Surgical Time

Multiple studies have reviewed the integrity of the endothelium, safety, and surgical time of MICS. Cavallini and colleagues[16] showed that B-MICS (1.4-mm incision) cases used less BSS and had shorter surgical time than C-MICS (2.2-mm incision). With respect to the safety of MICS, Wilczynski and colleagues[17] reported similar postoperative corrected distance visual acuities and interval endothelial cell loss (ECL; mean 9.27% to 9.46%; $P > 0.05$) for C-MICS and B-MICS using the Stellaris platform. A similar study[18] comparing 1.8-mm vs 2.2-mm incision MICS showed comparable uncorrected visual acuity (UCVA), BCVA, astigmatism, and ECL. At day one follow-up, the 1.8-mm incision group had slightly increased incisional corneal thickness but no difference in tunnel morphometric features. Edema resolved in both groups within the same time interval.

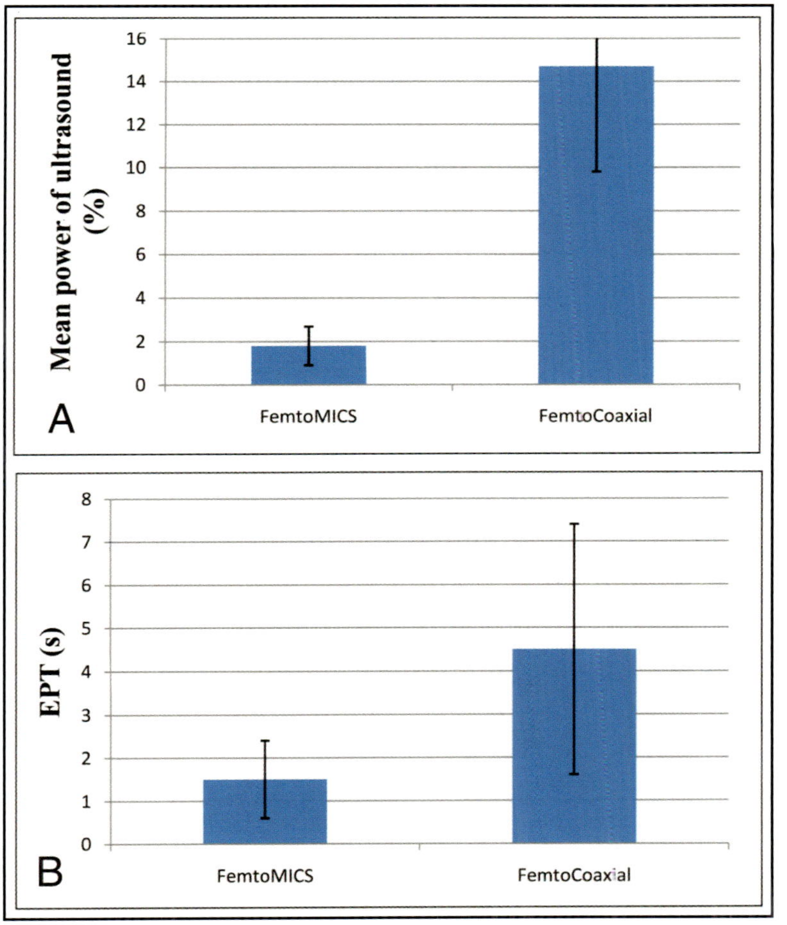

Figure 11-5. (A) Mean ultrasound power and (B) effective phacoemulsification time for microincision cataract surgery. (Reprinted with permission from Alió JL, Soria F, Abdou AA, Peña-García P, Fernández-Buenaga R, Javaloy J. Comparative outcomes of bimanual MICS and 2.2-mm coaxial phacoemulsification assisted by femtosecond technology. *J Refract Surg*. 2014;30(1):34-40.)

Alió et al[4] prospectively compared B-MICS (1.5-mm incision) with traditional coaxial phacoemulsification (2.8-mm incision). B-MICS was associated with a significant reduction in total phaco power (5.28% vs 19.2%), mean effective phaco time (2.19 vs 9.2 s), and vectorial astigmatism (0.43 vs 1.20 diopters [D]). Their group[19] also prospectively compared B-MICS to 2.2-mm coaxial phacoemulsification assisted by femtosecond technology (LenSx, Alcon) for both groups. B-MICS had lower ultrasound power (1.8% vs 14.7%) and phacoemulsification time (1.5 vs 4.5 s). No difference was found in mean postoperative spherical equivalent, corneal thickness, ECL, and macular thickness (Figures 11-5 and 11-6).

A few studies analyzed the impact of different phacoemulsification modes and techniques on safety, paying particular attention to the density of the cataracts. Kim et al[20] evaluated 3 different power modes (burst, pulse, and continuous) for hard cataracts in MICS (1.8 and 2.2 mm) vs C-SICS (2.75 mm). They found no difference in mean

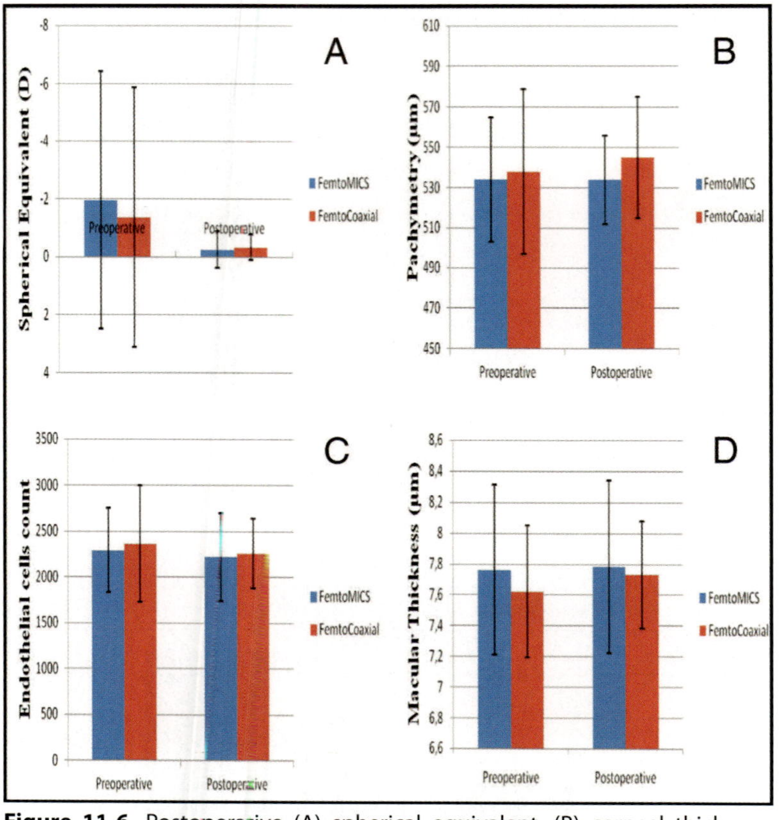

Figure 11-6. Postoperative (A) spherical equivalent, (B) corneal thickness, (C) endothelial cell, and (D) macular thickness values relative to preoperative values in both groups ($P > .05$). (Reprinted with permission from Alió JL, Soria F, Abdou AA, Peña-García P, Fernández-Buenaga R, Javaloy J. Comparative outcomes of bimanual MICS and 2.2-mm coaxial phacoemulsification assisted by femtosecond technology. *J Refract Surg*. 2014;30(1):34-40.)

ultrasound time (UST), cumulative dissipated energy (CDE), BCVA, CCT, or ECL between the 3 incision groups 2 months postoperatively. The 2.75-mm incision group had less incisional corneal edema at 1 week than the other 2 incision sizes. The UST, CDE, incisional corneal thickness, and CCT at 1 week and ECL at 2 months were higher with continuous mode phaco than with the other 2 modes. Another study[21] comparing 1.8-mm C-MICS for hard and soft cataracts found higher ECL in the hard cataracts group (11.37% vs 2.87%) but equal BCVA and SIA at 1 month. Park and colleagues[22] compared phaco-chop, divide-and-conquer, and stop-and-chop phaco techniques in MICS. They showed that the phaco-chop technique showed significantly less UST, CDE, ECL, and BSS use than the other 2 methods for grade 4 cataract densities. There was no significant difference for mild and moderate cataracts among the 3 techniques.

Another concern about MICS is that this technique may require greater surgical experience and skill and, thus, may involve more complications than small-incision cataract surgery (SICS) for the early adapter. Cavallani and colleagues[23] reviewed the visual outcomes and complications of B-MICS performed by surgeons in training. They found comparable visual outcomes and complications rates to those reported in the literature with coaxial cataract surgery.

Early Postoperative Visual Acuity

Several studies have identified early UCVA as a metric to measure the safety and success of cataract surgery, and an indicator of rapid rehabilitation. Saeed et al[24] showed that a greater percentage of patients had UCVA of 20/40 or better at 1 hour after B-MICS compared with conventional phaco (18% vs 2%; $P = 0.02$), although this difference was not significant at later time points. Other studies[25-27] have found similar results, with better UCVA and BCVA on day 1 with MICS compared with SICS, as well as overall lower SIA in the MICS group. Dick[27] reported better UCVA ($P < 0.04$) at day 3, 1 week, and 2 months with MICS in one eye vs SICS in the fellow eye.

Astigmatism and Aberrations

One of the main advantages of MICS is better astigmatism control and aberration neutrality. Elkady and colleagues[28] measured no significant change in corneal astigmatism (-0.80 ± 0.76 D pre, -0.63 ± 0.62 D post; $P = 1.0$) or total corneal root-mean-square (RMS, 2.15 ± 2.51 μm pre, 1.96 ± 2.01 μm post; $P = 1.0$) following MICS. SICS had greater induction of corneal aberrations (oblique astigmatism, secondary oblique astigmatism, and vertical tetrafoil; $P < 0.01$) than 1.2-mm to 1.5-mm B-MICS, as well as greater mean higher-order ($P = 0.023$) and total ($P = 0.007$) aberration RMS.[29] Hayashi et al,[30] using videokeratography, measured higher SIA and showed greater focal corneal flattening corresponding to the incision in a 2.65-mm SICS group vs a 2.0-mm C-MICS group. They also found no difference in regular and irregular astigmatism between 2.0-mm clear cornea and 2.0-mm scleral tunnel cataract surgery, although changes existed when comparing 3.0-mm clear cornea and scleral tunnel incisions, indicating that a 2.0-mm clear cornea incision induced minimal astigmatism (Figures 11-7 and 11-8).[31] Another study found that a 1.8-mm temporal clear cornea incision produced 0.35 D less SIA than a 2.75-mm incision (0.42 D vs 0.77 D).[32]

A few studies[33-35] have also compared astigmatism between C-MICS and B-MICS. No significant difference ($P > 0.05$) was noted in comparing SIA from 1.8-mm C-MICS (0.42 ± 0.29 D) vs 1.7-mm B-MICS (0.50 ± 0.24 D).[33] Von Sonnleithner and colleagues[34] found no significant difference between BCVA, total higher-order aberration, and coma between 1.4-mm B-MICS, 1.8-mm C-MICS, and 2.2-mm SICS. Lastly, Can and colleagues found no significant changes in total and higher-order RMS after both B-MICS and C-MICS.[35]

Posterior Capsule Opacification Formation and Microincisional Cataract Surgery Intraocular Lenses

One of the concerns of microincisional surgery is with regard to the long-term stability of the MICS IOL, particularly in the setting of posterior capsular opacity formation. Numerous studies[36-39] have investigated posterior capsule opacification (PCO) formation rate and grading, via the Automated Quantification of After-Cataract (AQUA) software, with MICS vs SICS IOLs and have found just slightly higher PCO grading

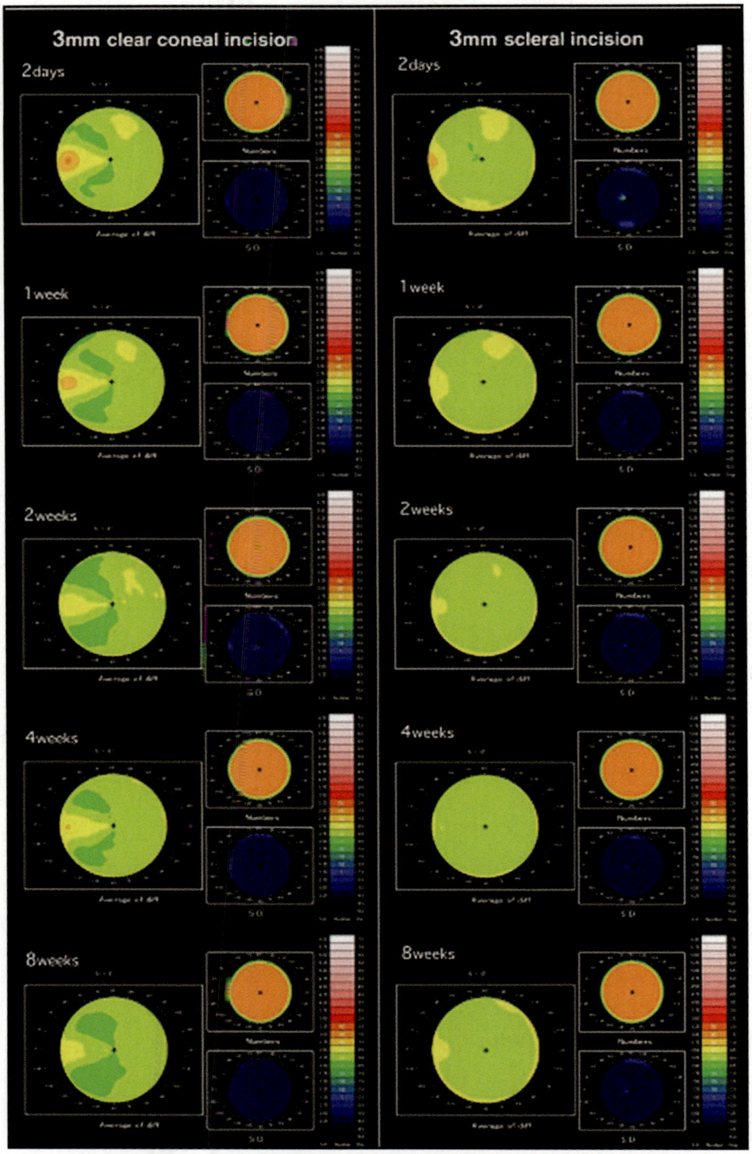

Figure 11-7. Averaged changes in entire corneal shape in (left) the 3-mm clear corneal incision group and (right) the 3.0-mm scleral incision group shown using the average of difference map. At left, in the clear corneal incision group at 2 days after surgery, a wedge-shaped flattening, which corresponds to the incision, and coupled steepening around the flattened area occurred; these changes gradually decreased but persisted for up to 8 weeks. At right, in the scleral incision group, a slight wound-related peripheral flattening was noted at 2 days after surgery, which cleared by 2 weeks. (Reprinted with permission from Hayashi K, Yoshida M, Hayashi H. Corneal shape changes after 2.0-mm or 3.0-mm clear corneal versus scleral tunnel incision cataract surgery. *Ophthalmology*. 2010;117(7):1313-1323.)

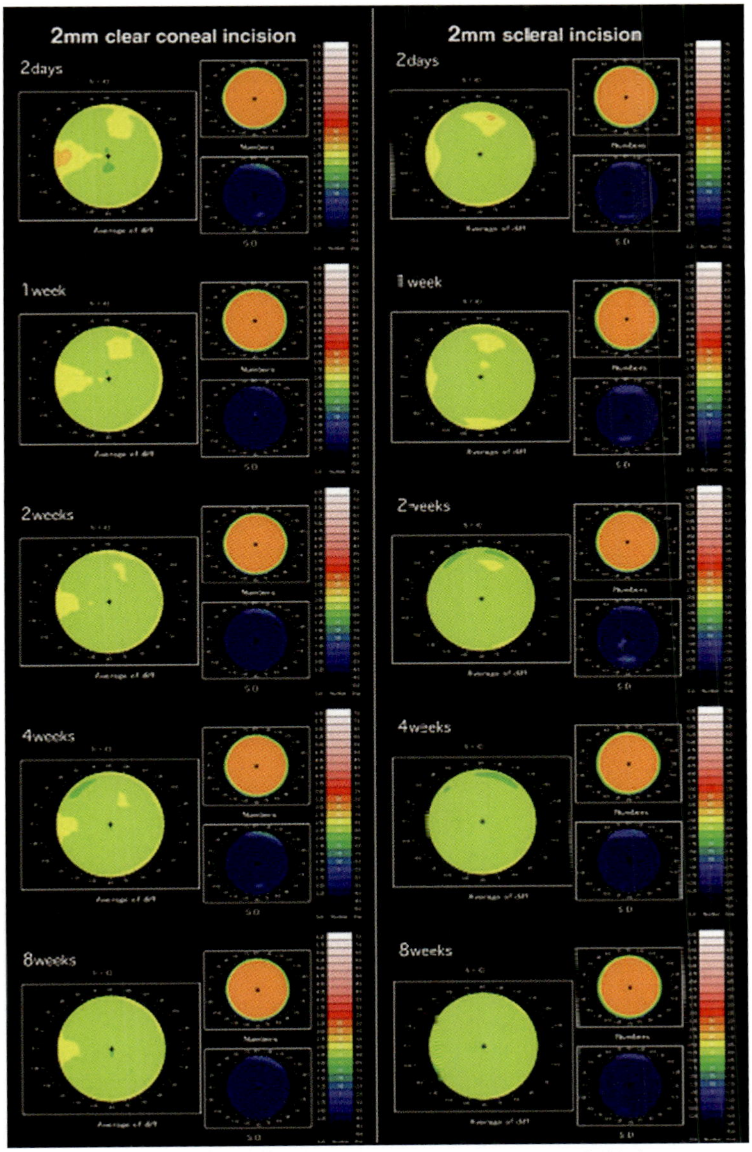

Figure 11-8. Averaged changes in entire corneal shape in (left) the 2.0-mm clear corneal incision group and (right) the 2.0-mm scleral incision groups shown using the average of difference map. At left, in the clear corneal incision group, a wedge-shaped flattening, corresponding to the incision, occurred at 2 days after surgery; this change was markedly reduced at 2 weeks. At right, in the scleral incision group, very slight wound-related peripheral flattening was seen at 2 days after surgery, which disappeared by 2 weeks. (Reprinted with permission from Hayashi K, Yoshida M, Hayashi H. Corneal shape changes after 2.0-mm or 3.0-mm clear corneal versus scleral tunnel incision cataract surgery. *Ophthalmology*. 2010;117(7):1313-1323.)

(1.2 to 2.6 vs 1.9 to 2.1) and neodymium-doped yttrium aluminum garnet (Nd:YAG) capsulotomy rates, but comparable axial stability and amount of decentration, and tilt for up to 3 years postsurgery.

One of the more common MICS lenses used in the United States today is the Akreos MI60 IOL (Bausch & Lomb). Can and colleagues[40] found excellent BCVA, low SIA, contrast sensitivity and glare within normal limits, good centration, and no significant change in total corneal aberrations postoperatively. Approximately 20% of the patients developed PCO, but none required Nd:YAG capsulotomy by the 1-year follow-up period. Selvam and colleagues[41] retrospectively found that approximately 20.1% of patients required a Nd:YAG capsulotomy for PCO in eyes implanted with the MI60 IOL by 3 years follow-up.

Conclusions

MICS is a technique that balances the need for surgical astigmatism neutrality with enhanced safety, greater chamber stability, and improved phacoemulsification efficiency, requiring lower power settings and less overall case time. It offers a potent tool to optimize visual acuity results in all cataract patients, including those choosing lifestyle-enhancing premium IOLs. Future evolution in MICS IOL technology, new surgical tools, and application of femtosecond laser devices may even more rapidly expand the application of MICS to become the standard for cataract surgery.

References

1. Klonowski P, Rejdak R, Alió JL. Microincision cataract surgery: 1.8 mm incision surgery. *Expert Rev Ophthalmol.* 2013;8(4):375-391.
2. Shearing S, Relyea R, Louiza A, Sem A, Routine phacoemulsification through a one-millimeter non-sutured incision. *Cataract.* 1985;2:5-11.
3. Pavlou F. MICS: the European picture. *Ophthalmology Times Europe.* www.oteurope.com/ophthalmologytimeseurope/Cataract+Clinical/MICS-the-European-picture/ArticleStandard/Article/detail/548540. Published September 1, 2008. Accessed January 5, 2017.
4. West ES, Behrens A, McDonnell PJ, Tielsch JM, Schein OD. The incidence of endophthalmitis after cataract surgery among the US Medicare population increased between 1994 and 2001. *Ophthalmology.* 2005;112:1388-1394.
5. Alió JL, Rodriguez-Prats JL, Galal A, Ramzy M. Outcomes of micro incision cataract surgery versus coaxial phacoemulsification. *Ophthalmology.* 2005;112:1997-2003.
6. Alió JL, Agarwal A, Klonowski P. 0.7 mm microincision cataract surgery. In: Alió JL, Fine IH, eds. *Minimizing Incisions and Maximizing Outcomes in Cataract Surgery.* New York, NY: Springer; 2010:13-25.
7. Miyoshi T, Yoshida H. Ultra-high-speed digital video images of vibrations of an ultrasonic tip and phacoemulsification. *J Cataract Refract Surg.* 2008;34:1024.
8. Davison JA. Cumulative tip travel and implied followability of longitudinal and torsional phacoemulsification. *J Cataract Refract Surg.* 2008;34(6):986-990.
9. Alió JL, Klonowski P, Rodriguez Prats JL. MICS instrumentation. In: Alió JL, Fine IH, eds. *Minimizing Incisions and Maximizing Outcomes in Cataract Surgery.* New York, NY: Springer; 2010:25-37.
10. Rose AD. Coaxial and bimanual phacoemulsification: considerations in patient and technique selection. *Tech Ophthalmol.* 2005;3:63-70.
11. Haripriya A, Arvind S, Vadi K, Natchiear G. Bimanual microphaco for posterior polar cataracts. *J Refract Surg.* 2006;32:914-917.

12. Cavallini GM, Pupino A, Masini C, Campo L, Pelloni S. Bimanual microphacoemulsification and Acri.Smart intraocular lens implantation combined with vitreoretinal surgery. *J Cataract Refract Surg.* 2007;33:1253-1258.
13. Klonowski P, Rejdak R, Alió JL. Microincision cataract surgery. *Exper Rev Ophthalmol.* 2013;8(4):375-391.
14. Chen C, Zhu M, Sun Y, Qu X, Xu X. Bimanual microincision versus standard coaxial small-incision cataract surgery: meta-analysis of randomized controlled trials. *Eur J Ophthalmol.* 2015;25(2):119-127.
15. Yu JG, Zhao YE, Shi JL, et al. Biaxial microincision cataract surgery versus conventional coaxial cataract surgery: metaanalysis of randomized controlled trials. *J Cataract Refract Surg.* 2012;38(5):894-901.
16. Cavallini GM, Pupino A, Masini C, Campo L, Pelloni S. Bimanual microphacoemulsification versus coaxial microphacoemulsification: Prospective Study. *J Cataract Refract Surg.* 2007;33:387-391.
17. Wilczynsld M, Supady E, Loba P, Synder A, Palenga-Pydyn D, Omulecki W. Comparison of early corneal endothelial cell loss after coaxial phacoemulsification through 1.8 mm microincision and bimanual phacoemulsification through 1.7 mm microincision. *J Cataract Refract Surg.* 2009;35:1570-1574.
18. Mastropasqua L, Toto L, Vecchiarino L, Di Nicola M, Mastropasqua R. Microcoaxial torsional cataract surgery 1.8 mm versus 2.2 mm: functional and morphological assessment. *Ophthalmic Surg Lasers Imaging.* 2011;42(2):114-124.
19. Alió JL, Soria F, Abdou AA, Peña-García P, Fernández-Buenaga R, Javaloy J. Comparative outcomes of bimanual MICS and 2.2-mm coaxial phacoemulsification assisted by femtosecond technology. *J Refract Surg.* 2014;30(1):34-40.
20. Kim EC, Byun YS, Kim MS. Microincision versus small-incision coaxial cataract surgery using different power modes for hard nuclear cataract. *J Cataract Refract Surg.* 2011;37(10):1799-1805.
21. Wilczynski M, Supady E, Loba P, Synder A, Omulecki W. Results of coaxial phacoemulsification through a 1.8-mm microincision in hard cataracts. *Ophthalmic Surg Lasers Imaging.* 2011;42(2):125-131.
22. Park J, Yum HR, Kim MS, Harrison AR, Kim EC. Comparison of phaco-chop, divide-and-conquer, and stop-and-chop phaco techniques in microincision coaxial cataract surgery. *J Cataract Refract Surg.* 2013;39(10):1463-1469.
23. Cavallini GM, Volante V, Verdina T, et al. Results and complications of surgeons-in-training learning bimanual microincision cataract surgery. *J Cataract Refract Surg.* 2015;41(1):105-115.
24. Saeed A, O'Conner J, Cunnife G, Stack J, Mullhern MG, Betty S. Uncorrected visual acuity in the immediate postoperative period following uncomplicated cataract surgery: bimanual microincision cataract surgery versus standard coaxial phacoemulsification. *Int Ophthalmol.* 2009;29:393-400.
25. Yao K, Wang W, Wu W, Tang XJ, Li ZC, Jin CF. Clinical evaluation on the coaxial 1.8 mm microincision cataract surgery. *Zhonghua Yan Ke Za Zhi.* 2011;47(10):903-907.
26. Orczykowska M, Owidzkaz M, Synder A, Wilczyński M, Omulecki W. Comparative analysis of early distance visual acuity in patients after coaxial phacoemulsification through the micro-incision (1.8 mm) and after standard phacoemulsification through the small incision (2.75 mm). *Klin Oczna.* 2014;116(1):7-10.
27. Dick HB. Controlled clinical trial comparing biaxial microincision with coaxial small incision for cataract surgery. *Eur J Ophthalmol.* 2012;22(5):739-750.
28. Elkady B, Alió JL, Ortiz D, Montalban R. Corneal aberrations after microincisional cataract surgery. *J Cataract Refract Surg.* 2008;34:40-45.
29. Tong N, He JC, Lu F, Wang Q, Qu J, Zhao YE. Changes in corneal wavefront aberrations in microincision and small-incision cataract surgery. *J Cataract Refract Surg.* 2008;34:2085-2090.
30. Hayashi K, Motoaki Y, Hayashi H. Postoperative corneal shape changes: microincision versus small-incision coaxial cataract surgery. *J Cataract Refract Surg.* 2009;35:233-239.
31. Hayashi K, Yoshida M, Hayashi H. Corneal shape changes after 2.0-mm or 3.0-mm clear corneal versus scleral tunnel incision cataract surgery. *Ophthalmology.* 2010;117(7):1313-1323.
32. Wilczynski M, Supady E, Loba P, Synder A, Palenga-Pydyn D, Omulecki W. Evaluation of surgically induced astigmatism after coaxial phacoemulsification through 1.8 mm microincision and standard phacoemulsification through 2.75 mm incision. *Klin Oczna.* 2011;113(10-12):314-320.
33. Wilczynski M, Supady E, Loba P, Synder A, Palenga-Pydyn D, Omulecki W. Comparison of surgically induced astigmatism after coaxial phacoemulsification through 1.8 mm microincision and bimanual phacoemulsification through 1.7 mm microincision. *J Cataract Refract Surg.* 2009;35:1563-1569.
34. von Sonnleithner C, Bergholz R, Gonnermann J, Klamann MK, Torun N, Bertelmann E. Clinical results and higher-order aberrations after 1.4-mm biaxial cataract surgery and implantation of a new aspheric intraocular lens. *Ophthalmic Res.* 2015;53(1):8-14.

35. Can İ, Bayhan HA, Çelik H, Ceran BB. Comparison of corneal aberrations after biaxial microincision and microcoaxial cataract surgeries: a prospective study. *Curr Eye Res.* 2012;37(1):18-24.
36. Hirnschall N, Nishi Y, Crnej A, et al. Capsular bag stability and posterior capsule opacification of a plate-haptic design microincision cataract surgery intraocular lens: 3-year results of a randomised trial. *Br J Ophthalmol.* 2013;97(12):1565-1568.
37. Gangwani V, Hirnschall N, Koshy J, et al. Posterior capsule opacification and capsular bag performance of a microincision intraocular lens. *J Cataract Refract Surg.* 2011;37(11):1988-1992.
38. Schriefl SM, Menapace R, Stifter E, Zaruba D, Leydolt C. Posterior capsule opacification and neodymium:YAG laser capsulotomy rates with 2 microincision intraocular lenses: four-year results. *J Cataract Refract Surg.* 2015;41(5):956-963.
39. Prinz A, Vecsei-Marlovits PV, Sonderhof D, Irsigler P, Findl O, Weingessel B. Comparison of posterior capsule opacification between a 1-piece and a 3-piece microincision intraocular lens. *Br J Ophthalmol.* 2013;97(1):18-22.
40. Can I, Takmaz T, Bayhan HA, Bostancı Ceran B. Aspheric microincision intraocular lens implantation with biaxial microincision cataract surgery: efficacy and reliability. *J Cataract Refract Surg.* 2010;36(11):1905-1911.
41. Selvam S, Khan IJ, Craig EA. Neodymium:YAG laser capsulotomy rate of microincision hydrophilic acrylic intraocular lens. *J Cataract Refract Surg.* 2011;37(11):2080-2081.

Chapter 12

Micro-Invasive Glaucoma Surgery

Savak "Sev" Teymoorian, MD, MBA

Why would a book about refractive cataract surgery have a discussion about glaucoma procedures? The decision on when to remove a cataract and what, if any, concurrent glaucoma surgery to perform plays a significant role in the long-term care of these patients. All cataract surgeons will inevitably take care of patients with glaucoma. It is estimated that 20% to 25% of patients having cataract surgery have some form of glaucoma or ocular hypertension.[1] Of course there are those refractive surgeons who believe that they will not encounter this problem because these patients may not be candidates for premium lenses. However, glaucoma patients still benefit from astigmatic correction, even with a standard monofocal lens, and therefore still fit into a refractive practice.

In fact, the number and percentage of patients with glaucoma will increase in the future for a few reasons. First, the use of advancing technology including optical coherence tomography allows earlier diagnosis of patients and identification of those at risk.[2] Second, the average lifespan of patients continues to increase, and glaucoma is more common with older age.[3-5] What was once a disease requiring management for 10 to 20 years now becomes a challenge lasting 20 to 40 years. The thought process of how to care for these patients has changed from a sprint to a marathon.

In glaucoma patients, it is especially critical to achieve the best refractive outcomes. Glaucoma by definition is an optic neuropathy with associated visual field changes.[6] Glaucoma patients already have or will be having diminished visual fields in the future. It becomes imperative to try to maximize the areas of vision that do remain. Key factors that influence their vision include the use of intraocular pressure (IOP)–lowering eye drops and traditional glaucoma surgery. The use of glaucoma drops help decrease IOP, but at a cost to the corneal surface. It is not uncommon to see patients who have their glaucoma controlled but still have their visual acuity and quality of life decreased

Hovanesian JA.
Refractive Cataract Surgery: Best Practices and Advanced Technology, Second Edition (pp 141-156).

because of the corneal adverse effects of these medications.[7-8] This leads to frustration for providers, because, at best, we are breaking even with the battle against glaucoma, since it can't be reversed, but losing the war on retaining functional vision because of adverse effects of therapy.

The other issue is that gold-standard glaucoma surgery still remains with trabeculectomy and tube shunt surgery.[9-13] These procedures are used only when needed because of the high risk-to-benefit profile.[14] Unfortunately, the perfect storm is created when glaucoma is not controlled earlier in the disease process. Not only do these patients have worsening glaucoma as they get older, but they also are subjected to riskier surgical interventions. The ideal care for glaucoma patients is to avoid these larger surgeries if possible. Any intervention that decreases the need for glaucoma eye drops and either delays the performance or even eliminates traditional glaucoma surgery should be considered. It just so happens this exists, and it comes in the form of cataract surgery.

Cataract surgery is now becoming commonplace, with approximately 3 to 4 million surgeries done every year in the United States. With better procedures and intraocular lens (IOL) technology along with longer lifespans, it becomes an almost inevitable part of a patient's care. Integrating a treatment for glaucoma with a procedure that will naturally be done, like cataract removal, is where micro-invasive glaucoma surgery (MIGS) fits in the paradigm.[15-16]

The key to MIGS is the positive benefit-to-risk ratio. The definition of MIGS is evolving, but the core principles remain the same. This involves any surgical procedure that helps decrease IOP with a risk profile that is less than that seen with trabeculectomy or tube shunt surgery. A secondary requirement is that it is conjunctival-sparing, in order to leave this space undisturbed should there be a need for a more gold-standard surgery.[17] A tertiary requirement is rapid recovery.[18] These guidelines generally lead to ab interno procedures done concurrently with cataract surgery. The hope is to give additional IOP reduction beyond that seen with cataract surgery alone, without much additional risk.[15,16]

The Present and Future of Micro-Invasive Glaucoma Surgery

The landscape of MIGS is rapidly changing. For providers, this means there are products in the pipeline that are under study or development that will become available for implantation in the near future. The technology that is being currently evaluated can be divided into subgroups depending on their anatomical target.

Trabecular Bypass/Schlemm's Canal

These MIGS procedures focus on maximizing the conventional outflow of aqueous through Schlemm canal (SC) by bypassing the trabecular meshwork for 2 reasons. The first is to provide an alternative pathway through the juxtacanalicular section of the meshwork that provides the greatest resistance to flow. The second is to reduce the dependence on the need for aqueous to flow through the disease meshwork.[19] These procedures allow for access of aqueous from the anterior chamber directly to SC.

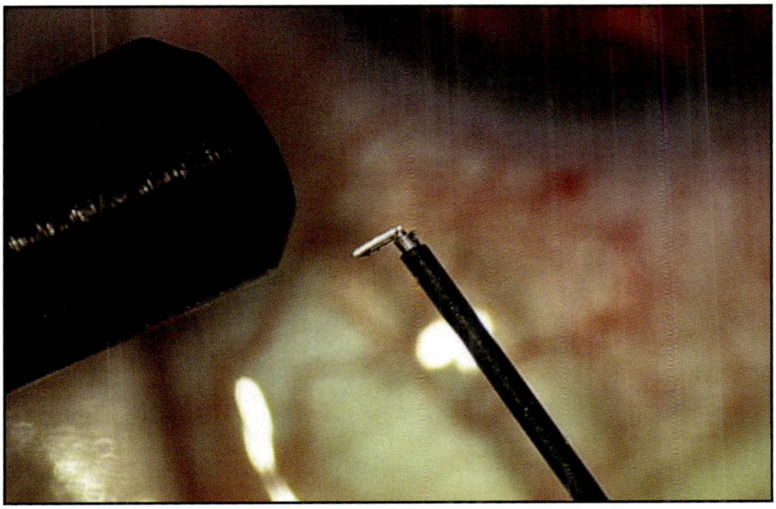

Figure 12-1. External view of iStent Trabecular Micro-Bypass. (Reprinted with permission from Glaukos Corporation.)

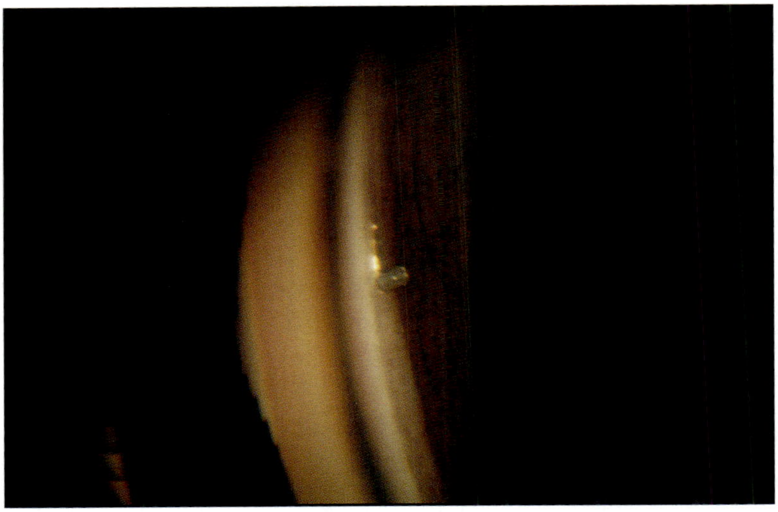

Figure 12-2. Gonioscopic view of iStent in place. (Reprinted with permission from Glaukos Corporation.)

iStent/iStent Inject

The iStent Trabecular Micro-Bypass (Glaukos Corporation) is the first Food and Drug Administration (FDA)–approved stent to be used in conjunction with cataract surgery for those with mild to moderate glaucoma.[20] It is manufactured in both a right and left orientation, allowing the surgeon to point the stent toward the inferonasal quadrant of the surgical eye where the greatest number of collector channels are located[21,22] (Figure 12-1). The tip of the titanium stent is advanced past the trabecular meshwork and into SC, where it is held in place by 3 retention arches (Figure 12-2). Research from the iStent study that compared the use of one iStent in addition to cataract surgery vs cataract

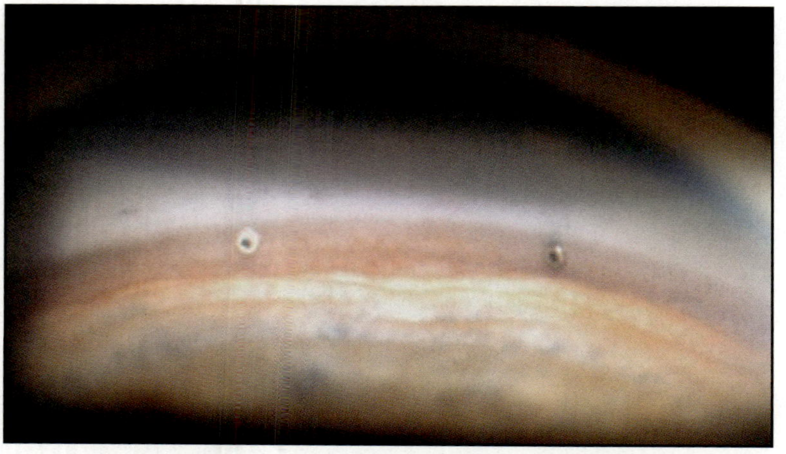

Figure 12-3. Gonioscopic view of 2 stents in place using iStent Inject. (Reprinted with permission from Glaukos Corporation.)

surgery alone met its primary and secondary endpoints. It demonstrated the advantage in IOP reduction using the iStent during cataract surgery.[23]

The iStent Inject, the second generation of this stent, is a 26-gauge injectable system that allows surgeons to place 2 preloaded stents with 1 applicator. The theorized advantages include an easier procedure to position the stent though an injection action and also place multiple stents in rapid progression[24] (Figure 12-3). It is currently under investigational trials.

Hydrus

The Hydrus Microstent (Ivantis Inc) is intended to be used as a scaffold placed into SC to enhance aqueous outflow through that pathway.[25] The injector system helps direct the 8-mm, crescent-shaped, flexible stent into place[26] (Figure 12-4). It is intended for those with mild to moderate glaucoma and is still under investigational trials.

Trabectome

The Trabectome (NeoMedix) is an externally powered unit that uses electrosurgical pulses to bypass through the trabecular meshwork and open the inner wall of SC. Once the instrument is guided into SC, a foot-operated switch is used to turn the pulse, which results in the removal of the tissue at the instrument tip[27] (Figure 12-5). This creates a direct path for aqueous to flow from the anterior chamber to the collector channels by SC. The Trabectome is FDA approved at this time and available for use in patients.[28]

Ab Interno Trabeculotomy

Recent innovations in trabeculotomy procedures allowing for it to be performed through an ab interno approach places this surgical intervention under the MIGS category. The first is gonioscopic-assisted transluminal trabeculotomy. After performing goniotomy to create an opening from the anterior chamber to SC, a suture is guided 360 degrees around the canal. The ends of the threaded object are then pulled from the eye, creating the circumferential opening of the canal.[29]

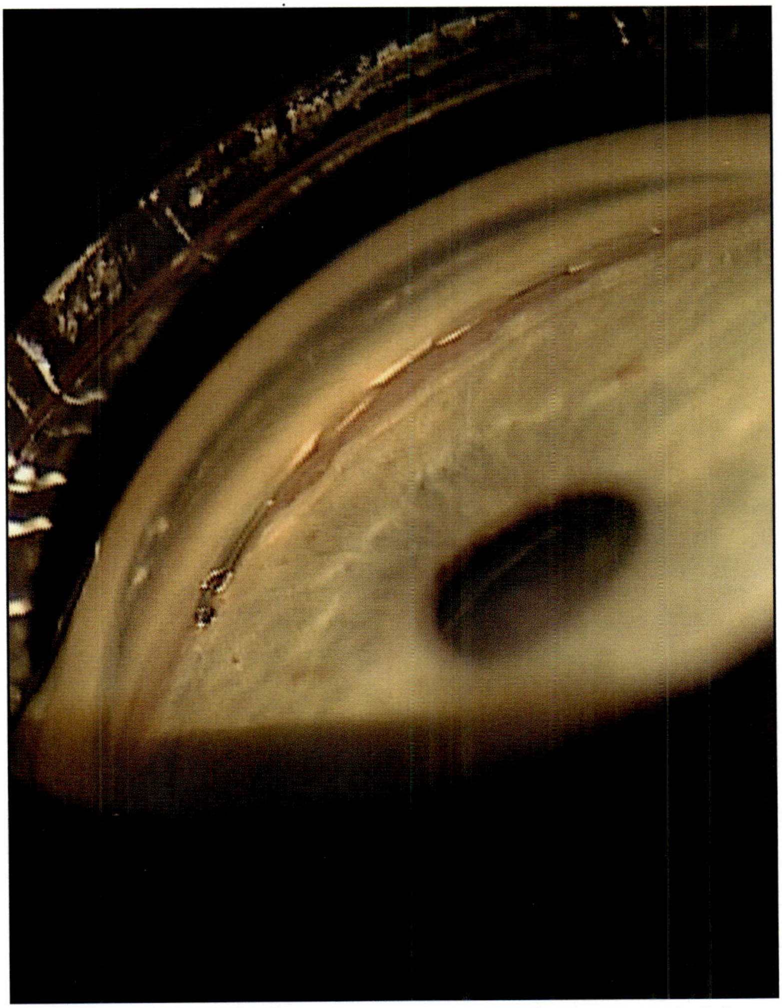

Figure 12-4. The Hydrus Microstent dilates and scaffolds SC in 3 clock-hours of the eye's natural outflow channel. (Reprinted with permission from Ivantis Inc and Jason Jones, MD.)

The second approach is the use of the Trab360 (Sight Sciences) instrument. It is a hand-held instrument that uses a sharp tip to enter SC. Then, a medical-grade polymer is advanced through the space by rotating the wheel on the instrument (Figures 12-6 and 12-7). Removal of the instrument from the eye then pulls open the area of the canal that the polymer had passed. The polymer can then be recoiled back into the instrument, and then the remaining area of SC can be opened if desired by the surgeon.[30]

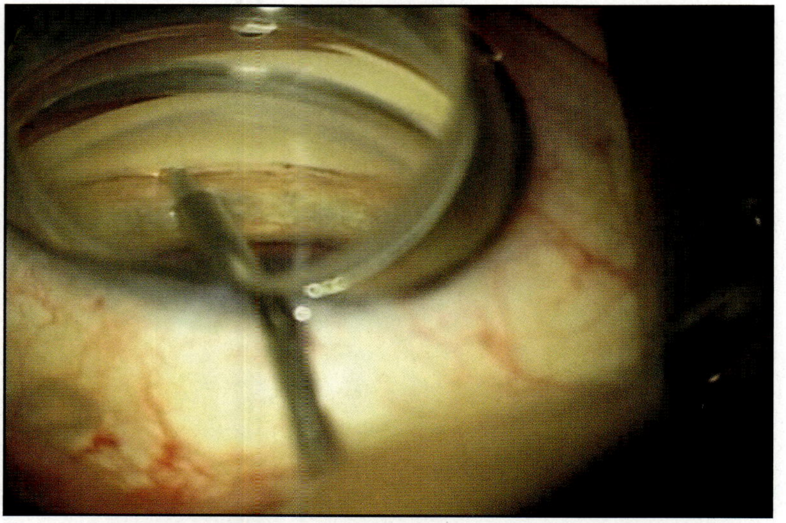

Figure 12-5. View through goniolens of Trabectome handpiece in SC removing trabecular meshwork. (Reprinted with permission from NeoMedix Corporation.)

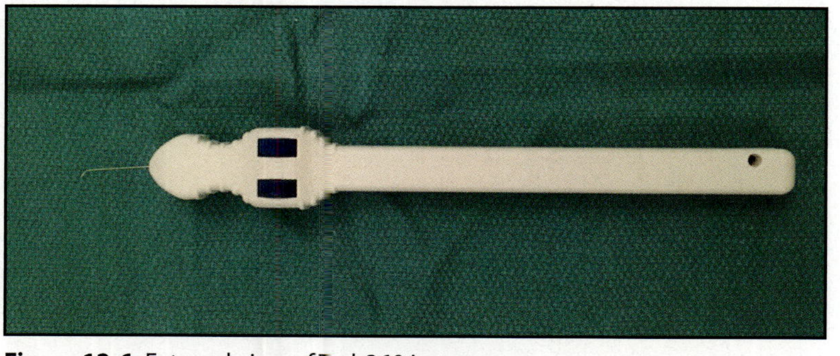

Figure 12-6. External view of Trab360 instrument.

Suprachoroidal/Supraciliary Space

These procedures also aim to divert aqueous away from the meshwork and SC but do so by allowing flow from the anterior chamber to the suprachoroidal/supraciliary space, for similar reasons. They take advantage of the negative pressure that is naturally created in the eye to permit aqueous outflow.

CyPass

The CyPass Micro-Stent (Alcon) is a 6-mm, polyimide device with fenestrations that is placed into the supraciliary space using an applicator that deploys it into position[31,32] (Figures 12-8 and 12-9). It is the second FDA-approved stent and is commercially available.

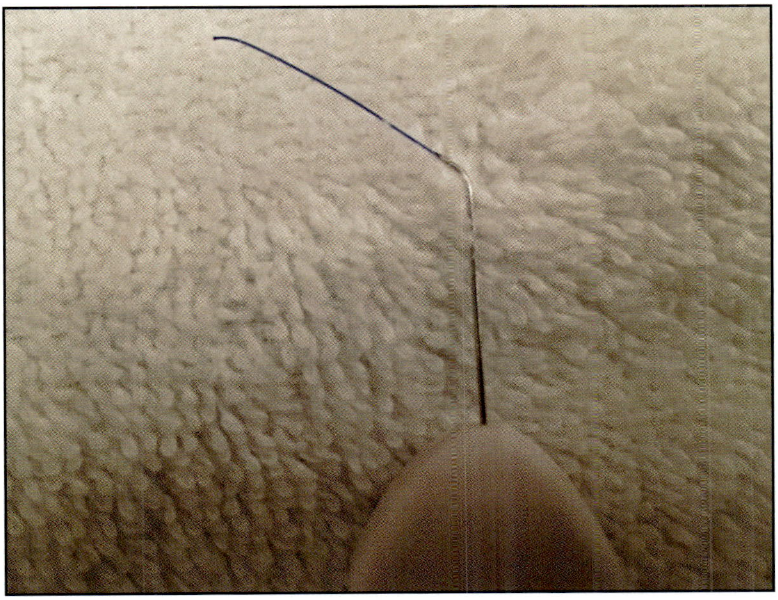

Figure 12-7. External view of medical grade polymer extending out from Trab360 instrument.

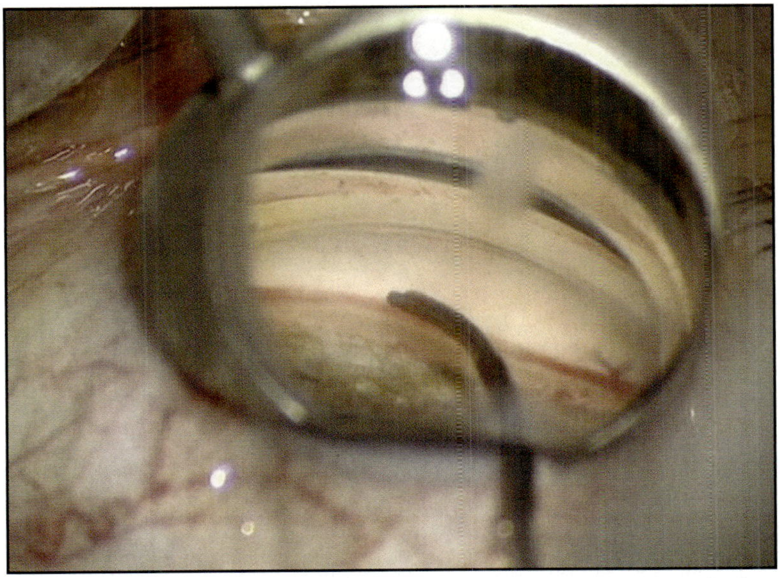

Figure 12-8. Gonioscopic view of CyPass inserter in the eye prior to deployment of Micro-Stent. (Reprinted with permission from Alcon.)

iStent Supra

The iStent Supra (Glaukos), the third generation of this device, centers on placing a 4-mm device with an injector through an ab interno approach into the suprachoroidal space[33] (Figure 12-10). It is under investigational trials.

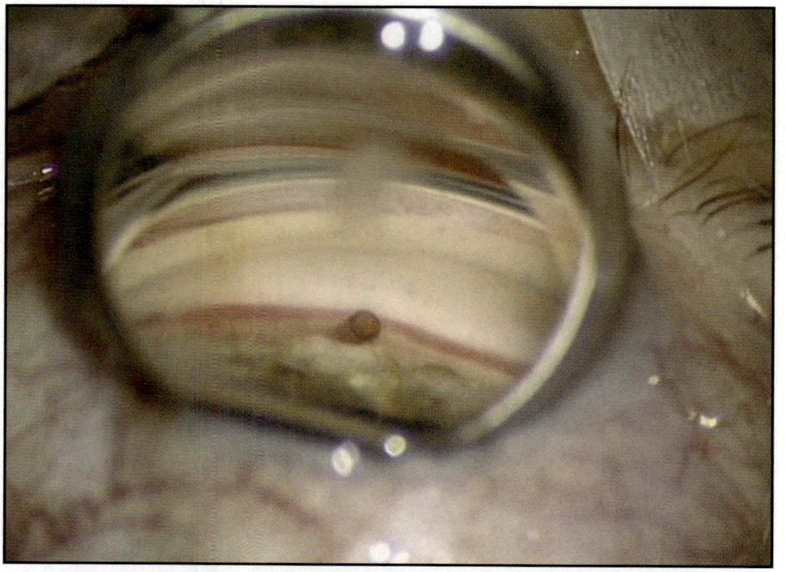

Figure 12-9. Gonioscopic view of CyPass Micro-Stent in place. (Reprinted with permission from Alcon.)

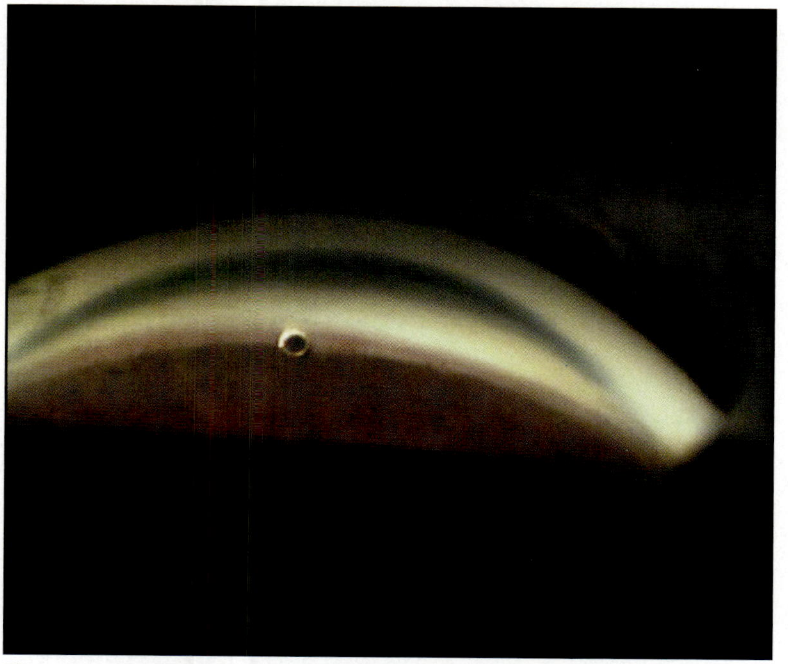

Figure 12-10. Gonioscopic view of iStent Supra in place. (Reprinted with permission from Glaukos Corporation.)

Subconjunctival Space

These surgical interventions attempt to create a new pathway for aqueous drainage, similar to those seen with trabeculectomy and tube shunt surgeries. They divert flow

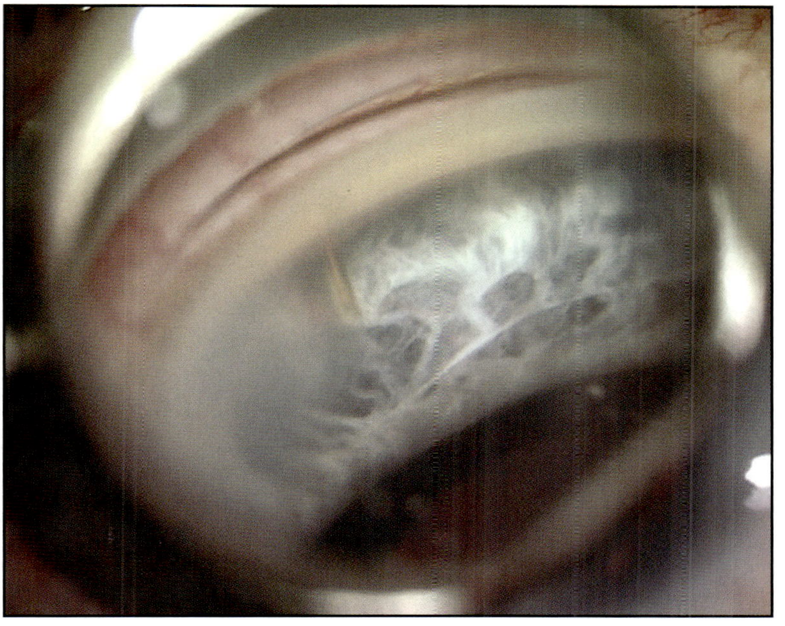

Figure 12-11. Gonioscopic view of Xen implant in place. (Reprinted with permission from Allergan.)

from the anterior chamber to the subconjunctival space. This approach decreases the need for aqueous to transcend through the trabecular meshwork and also any section of diseased tissue in SC.

Xen

The Xen implant (Allergan) is a 6-mm gelatin tube that is placed into the subconjunctival space with an ab interno approach (Figure 12-11). It is inserted through an inferotemporal incision and implanted in the superonasal quadrant 3 mm posterior to the limbus. It does involve the creation of bleb, and as such benefits from the use of mitomycin C. There are 3 versions of various lumen size, but the Xen 45 is at the forefront.[34] It is FDA approved.

InnFocus

The InnFocus MicroShunt (InnFocus) is a flexible, 9.5-mm tube that is placed from the subconjunctival space to the anterior chamber through a needle track using an ab externo approach.[35] This device does involve the need to cut a small piece of conjunctival tissue and benefits from the use of mitomycin C.[36] Unlike a trabeculectomy, it doesn't require the need to dissect sclera or perform an iridectomy. It is under investigational study.

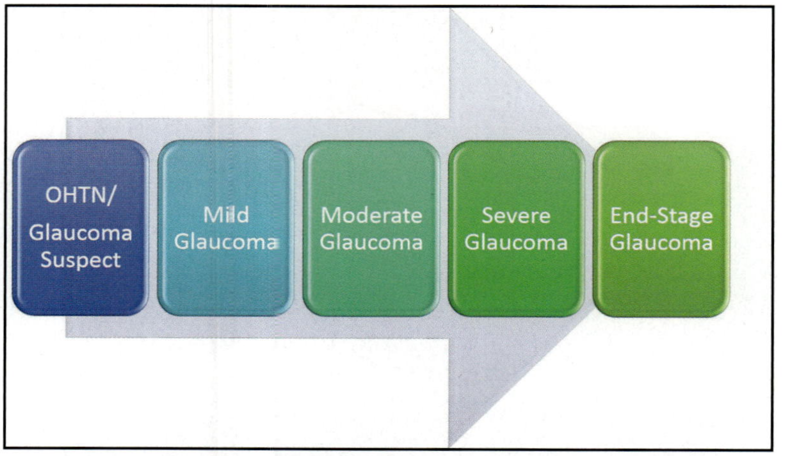

Figure 12-12. The spectrum and progression of glaucoma disease.

The Physician Decision to Add Micro-Invasive Glaucoma Surgery to Cataract Surgery

The decision-making process when considering the use of MIGS during cataract surgery involves 2 questions. The first is whether the patient will benefit from IOP reduction. Certainly any patient that is currently under glaucoma eye drop therapy should be considered for a MIGS procedure. This includes those who have already had prior glaucoma surgery. One long-term goal for these patients is to decrease or hopefully eliminate the reliance on eye drops, which may eliminate their adverse effects. The fewer the number of drops, the better likelihood of achieving this target. The other goal is to prolong or possibly prevent the need for eventual trabeculectomy or tube shunt surgery.

There are also other patients to consider besides those on drops. This includes patients who are currently under therapy with laser trabeculoplasty only. The thought process in this select set of patients is that future repeat laser applications may be needed. The use of MIGS along with cataract surgery may decrease the IOP enough that an additional laser procedure may not be needed if the previous laser procedure's effectiveness wears off. The other patient who may benefit from MIGS is the high-risk ocular hypertension patient. Consider a patient with higher IOP, thinner pachymetry of his or her cornea, and positive family history of glaucoma with larger cup-to-disc ratios. Although by definition not currently classified as a glaucoma patient, this patient is clearly at risk in the future. The use of MIGS may prevent the need for glaucoma drops, or at least delay the eventual use of drops or other glaucoma surgery.

The second question is whether the patient is a good candidate for this procedure. This decision making revolves around analyzing risk vs benefit and also identifying contraindications to MIGS. Treating glaucoma patients involves understanding that glaucoma is a spectrum of disease. This includes those with ocular hypertension or glaucoma suspects on one end through those with end-stage glaucomatous damage (Figure 12-12). The physician needs to weigh the benefits of MIGS with its possible risks. As the relative risks of MIGS remain low compared with traditional glaucoma surgery, there is a trend to using this technology in patients earlier in disease staging. This is opposite to those

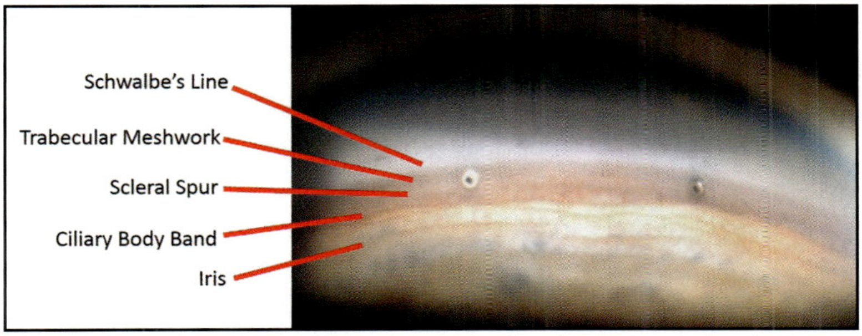

Figure 12-13. Gonioscopic view of angle landmarks. (Reprinted with permission from Glaukos Corporation.)

with more advanced or aggressive disease, who would benefit from traditional glaucoma surgery.

Contraindications to the MIGS procedure also need to be identified and evaluated. Patients whose angle anatomy drifts away from the standard and more predictable forms of primary open angle, pseudoexfoliation, or pigment dispersion glaucoma should be considered with caution. The reason MIGS procedures are advantageous is their low adverse-effect profile. When a patient presents with anatomy that differs from those that are more standard, then the predictability and subsequent risk profile changes. These conditions include chronic angle closure with peripheral anterior synechia, traumatic glaucoma with recession, and neovascular glaucoma.[37,38] Careful consideration needs to be undertaken in these patients about the use of MIGS.

These contraindications to surgery highlight the need for careful preoperative examination, including gonioscopic examination. Physicians considering the use of MIGS, just like with any other surgery, need to understand the anatomical landmarks (Figure 12-13). It is important to have the skill set to properly identify them, including the trabecular meshwork. However, at first surgeons may not be comfortable in that space if they are far removed from their training experience with angle surgery. In such instances, it is best for physicians to be reacquainted with the anatomical landmarks. This can include reviewing normal anatomy through gonioscopic examination in clinic and practicing looking at the angle during surgery with normal patients. The most critical step in any angle surgery is a good understanding and view of the targeted tissue.

Discussing Micro-Invasive Glaucoma Surgery With Patients

As with any other disease physicians take care of, it is important for patients to understand their disease process in order to have the ability to understand and consent for treatment. The discussion about the use of MIGS during cataract surgery is no different. One approach is to describe the care of glaucoma patients as like starting a long journey from Point A to Point B. Point A is now, and Point B is the end of life, with the goal of functional vision (Figure 12-14). The fastest road would be the straight line between these points. Unfortunately, there are usually obstacles in the way that require deviation from this path. The angle and degree of deviation early in the journey has a significant impact on the length and ultimate outcome. For patients with an earlier glaucoma diagnosis,

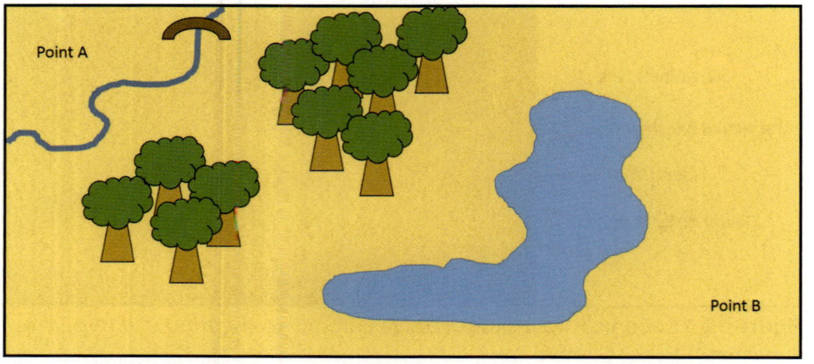

Figure 12-14. The journey in the care of a glaucoma patient from Point A (start) to Point B (end).

treatment and compliance lead to better outcomes. More importantly, this helps to possibly avoid major obstacles that can interfere with successful care. These obstacles might include the adverse effects of drop therapy and risks of traditional surgery. This is why the timing of cataract surgery and the possible use of MIGS becomes critical.

Cataract surgery is becoming the first-line glaucoma surgery for several reasons. The first being that for most patients, the IOP decreases after cataract surgery. The expected amount of reduction increases with higher preoperative IOP. The addition of MIGS can help further decrease the postoperative IOP. This allows patients to stay more on the path to Point B, as opposed to taking a serpentine route closer to obstacles as IOP deviates toward dangerous levels.

Some patients still do progress in their disease process after cataract surgery, and more traditional glaucoma surgery is needed. However, the removal of a cataractous lens helps prime the eye for more predictable and hopefully successful traditional glaucoma surgery. Performing a trabeculectomy or tube shunt surgery is technically easier in a pseudophakic than a phakic patient. In pseudophakics, the anterior chamber is deeper.[39] This allows a wide area of safe placement of tube shunts and also EX-Press Glaucoma Filtration devices (Alcon) used in trabeculectomy. The concern for causing intraoperative trauma to the native lens is eliminated. It also prevents having to deal with a quickly progressing, visually significant cataract that occurs once intraocular surgery is done. A source of frustration for phakic patients with traditional surgery can be the accelerated development of a cataract despite achieving even the best of IOP control.[40] This then forces the patients and surgeons to earlier cataract surgery, and with that comes additional obstacles in the journey. The rate of failure in prior traditional glaucoma surgery can be as high as 75% in just 2 years.[41] This occurs partly due to the creation of inflammation in the eye when cataract surgery is done. The best approach to avoid glaucoma surgery is to avoid inflammation. Therefore, for many reasons, it is advisable for a patient to be pseudophakic earlier in the journey, as it helps stay away from trouble areas.

For these reasons, intervening at the right time with the correct treatment can help our patients get to their goal of reaching Point B (Figure 12-15). The use of MIGS when performing cataract surgery can decrease or eliminate the use of eye drops. It can also prolong or possibly avoid the need for more risky glaucoma surgery. Once the patient understands the possible obstacles facing him or her in the future, then he or she can

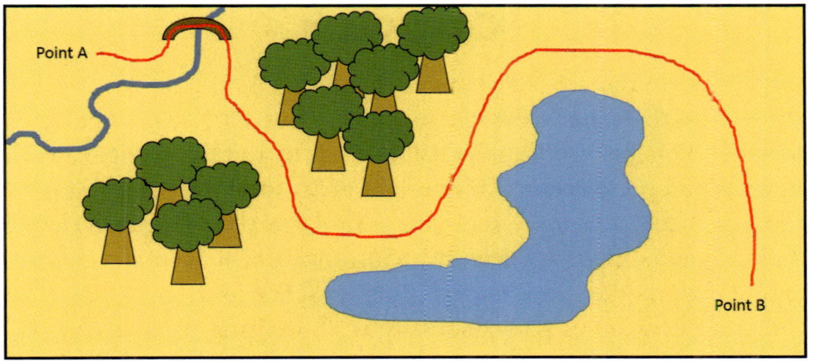

Figure 12-15. The successful route in the care of a glaucoma patient.

make the decision and give consent to surgery. The physician in this example has covered the risks, benefits, alternative, and indications to the use of MIGS with cataract surgery.

The Influence of Cost and Coverage for Micro-Invasive Glaucoma Surgery

As with any other surgical procedure, the cost of the intervention to the patient and society is important. For a majority of these stents, they are still under investigation. Their cost will need to be determined and evaluated.

In the United States, the FDA has approved the use of single iStent at the time of cataract surgery. Coverage for this application is approved by Medicare along with most major providers. International studies, however, have shown additional benefits to implantation of more than one iStent.[42] Any off-label use of multiple stents would need to be discussed with patients both in terms of medical care but also cost. One approach would be have the patient sign an advanced beneficiary note if implantation of more than one stent is considered in his or her care.

There is also coverage for the use of Trabectome. It is covered in both phakic and pseudophakic patients. This procedure can be done as a stand-alone or combined with cataract extraction. Reimbursement helps cover the cost of this procedure over time. There is a cost to each individual pack used in every case, and also an initial capital expense to buying the Trabectome unit, much like a phacoemulsification unit.

In terms of costs to society, earlier diagnosis and intervention in glaucoma paves the way for better clinical outcomes. This can lead to major cost savings in the long term. Better results lead to more functional vision. The possession, or lack, of functional vision can have a major influence on a person's productivity in society. It also decreases the costs that would have come with any additional medical and surgical procedures that were avoided.[43]

Conclusion

It is a privilege to take care of glaucoma patients. As physicians, we are allowed to not only take part in their journey with this disease but also have a significant influence on their outcome. This places the responsibility on us to take complicated issues about treatment options and present them in the right order to achieve the best possible results. As cataract surgery becomes a more standard part of everyone's medical care, the strategic use of it in glaucoma patients is critical. It can improve their quality of life by helping avoid major obstacles that attempt to derail our patients' journey.

The present and future of glaucoma care is an exciting time, as the MIGS era has arrived. We will have not only more but also a wider range of surgical procedures in our armamentarium to fight this disease. As research continues and studies are completed, ophthalmologists will need to alter their treatment options to suit the unique needs of each patient. The ability to combine a low-risk MIGS procedure with one that will almost inevitably occur, like cataract surgery, is a prime example. The best clinical results routinely come with planning and executing at the right time. It is important for ophthalmologists to take advantage of these opportunities to help our patients achieve the best quality of life with the least risk.

References

1. Centers for Medicare and Medicaid Services. *2002-2007 Medicare Standard Analytical File.* Baltimore, MD: Centers for Medicare and Medicaid Services, US Department of Health and Human Services; 2007.
2. Bussel II, Wollstein G, Schuman JS. OCT for glaucoma diagnosis, screening and detection of glaucoma progression. *Br J Ophthalmol.* 2014;98(Suppl 2):ii15-19.
3. Arias E. *United States Life Tables, 2010.* National Vital Statistics Reports. Washington, DC: US Department of Health and Human Services; 2014.
4. Quigley HA. Number of people with glaucoma worldwide. *Br J Ophthalmol.* 1996;80:389-393.
5. West S. Epidemiology of cataract: accomplishments over 25 years and future directions. *Ophthalmic Epidemiol.* 2007;14:173-178.
6. Allingham RR, Damji KF, Freedman SF, Moroi SE, Rhee DJ, Shields MB. *Shields Textbook of Glaucoma.* 6th ed. Baltimore, MD: Lippincott Williams & Wilkins; 2010.
7. Baudouin C, Pisella PF, Fillacier K, et al. Ocular surface inflammatory changes induced by topical antiglaucoma drugs: Human and animal studies. *Ophthalmology.* 1999;106:556-563.
8. Noecker RJ, Herrygers LA, Amwarudin R. Corneal and conjunctival changes caused by commonly used glaucoma medications. *Cornea.* 2004;23:490-496.
9. Lander J, Martin K, Sarkies N, Bourne R, Watson P. A twenty-year follow-up study of trabeculectomy: risk factors and outcomes. *Ophthalmology.* 2012;119(4):694-702.
10. Gedde SJ, Schiffman JC, Feuer WJ, et al. Treatment outcomes in the tube versus trabeculectomy (TVT) study after five years of follow-up. *Am J Ophthalmol.* 2012;153(5):789-803.
11. AGIS Investigators. The Advanced Glaucoma Intervention Study (AGIS): 9. Comparison of glaucoma outcomes in Black and White patients within treatment groups. *Am J Ophthalmol.* 2001;132(3):311-320.
12. Christakis PF, Kalenak JW, Zurakowski D, et al. The Ahmed versus Baerveldt study: one-year treatment outcomes. *Ophthalmology.* 2011;118(11):2180-2189.
13. Budenz DL, Barton K, Feuer WJ, et al. Treatment outcomes in the Ahmed Baerveldt Comparison Study after 1 year of follow-up. *Ophthalmology.* 2011;118(3):443-452.
14. Gedde SJ, Herndon LW, Brandt JD, et al. Postoperative complications in the tube versus trabeculectomy (TVT) study during five years of follow-up. *Am J Opthalmol.* 2012;153(5):804-814.
15. Choi D, Suramethakul P, Lindstrom RL, Singh K. Glaucoma surgery with and without cataract surgery: revolution or evolution? *J Cataract Refract Surg.* 2012;38:1121-1122.

16. Chang RT, Shingleton BJ, Singh K. Timely cataract surgery for improved glaucoma management. *J Cataract Refract Sug.* 2012;38:1709-1710.
17. Jea SY, Mosaed S, Vold SD, Rhee DJ. Effect of a failed trabectome on subsequent trabeculectomy. *J Glaucoma.* 2012;21(2):71-75.
18. Saheb H, Ahmed II. Micro-invasive glaucoma surgery: current perspectives and future directions. *Curr Opin Ophthalmol.* 2012;23(2):96-104.
19. iStent Product Information. Glaukos Corporation. www.glaukos.com/iStent. Accessed July 15, 2015.
20. Glaukos iStent trabecular micro-bypass stent FDA approval information. US Food and Drug Administration. www.fda.gov/MedicalDevices/ProductsandMedicalProcedures/DeviceApprovalsandClearances/Recently-ApprovedDevices/ucm312053.htm. Updated January 17, 2014. Accessed July 17, 2015.
21. Zhou J, Smedley GT. A trabecular bypass flow hypothesis. *J Glaucoma.* 2005;14(1):74-83.
22. Zhou J, Smedley GT. Trabecular bypass: effect of Schlemm canal and collector channel dilation. *J Glaucoma.* 2006:15(5):446-455.
23. Samuelson TW, Katz LJ, Wells JM, Duh YJ, Giamporcaro JE; US iStent Study Group. Randomized evaluation of the trabecular micro-bypass stent with phacoemulsification in patients with glaucoma and cataract. *Ophthalmology.* 2011;118(3):459-467.
24. Bahler CK, Hann CR, Fjield T, Haffner D, Heitzmann H, Fautsch MP. Second-generation trabecular meshwork bypass stent (iStent inject) increases outflow facility in cultured human anterior segments. *Am J Ophthalmol.* 2012;153(6):1206-1213.
25. Samuelson T, Tetz M, Pfeiffer N, Ramirez M, Scharioth G, Vass C. One year results of an intra-canalicular microstent for IOP reduction in open angle glaucoma. Paper presented at: AAO Annual Meeting; November 2012; Chicago, IL.
26. Gulati V, Fan S, Hays CL, et al. A novel 8 mm Schlemm's canal scaffold reduces outflow resistance in a human anterior segment perfusion model. *Invest Ophthalmol Vis Sci.* 2013;54(3):1698-1704.
27. Nguyen QH. Trabectome: a novel approach to angle surgery in the treatment of glaucoma. *Int Ophthalmol Clin.* 2008;48(4):65-72.
28. Minckler DS, Baerveldt G, Alfaro MR, Francis BA. Clinical results with the Trabectome for treatment of open-angle glaucoma. *Ophthalmology.* 2005;112(6):962-978.
29. Grover DS, Godfrey DG, Smith O, et al. Gonioscopy-assisted transluminal trabeculotomy, ab interno trabeculotomy: technique report and preliminary results. *Ophthalmology.* 2014;121(4):855-861.
30. Trab360 Product Information. SightSciences. http://sightsciences.com. Published 2016. Accessed January 5, 2017.
31. Ianchulev T, Ahmed IK, Hoeh HR, et al. Minimally invasive ab interno suprachoroidal device (CyPass) for IOP control in open-angle glaucoma. Poster presented at: AAO Annual Meeting; October 2010; Chicago, IL.
32. Craven ER, Khatan A, Hoeh H, et al. Minimally invasive, ab interno suprachoroidal micro-stent for IOP reduction in combination with phaco cataract surgery. Poster presented at AAO Annual Meeting; October 2011; Orlando, FL.
33. Glaukos Corporation. Multicenter investigation of the Glaukos Suprachoroidal stent model G3 in conjunction with cataract surgery [clinical trial NCT01461278]. http://clinicaltrials.gov/ct2/show/NCT01461278. Updated March 23, 2016. Accessed January 5, 2017.
34. Varma R. Ab interno stent procedures. In: MY Kahook *MIGS: Advances in Glaucoma Surgery.* Thorofare, NJ: SLACK Incorporated; 2014:57-62.
35. Acosta AC, Espana EM, Yamamoto H, et al. A newly designed glaucoma drainage implant made of poly(styrene-b-isobutylene-b-styrene): biocompatibility and function in normal rabbit eyes. *Arch Ophthalmol.* 2006;124(12):1742-1749.
36. Batile J, Frante F, Alburquerque R, et al. One year follow-up of a novel minimally invasive glaucoma drainage implant. Abstract presented at: AAO Annual Meeting; November 2012; Chicago, IL.
37. Spiegel D, Garcia-Feijoo J, Garcia-Sanchez J, Lamielle H. Coexistent primary open-angle glaucoma and cataract: preliminary analysis of treatment by cataract surgery and the iStent trabecular micro-bypass stent. *Adv Ther.* 2008:25(5):453-464.
38. iStent Trabecular Micro-Bypass Stent [package insert]. Laguna Hills, CA: Glaukos Corporation; 2010.
39. Su PF, Lo AY, Hu CY, et al. Anterior chamber depth measurement in phakic and pseudophakic patients. *Optom Vis Sci.* 2008;85(12)1193-1200.
40. AGIS Investigators. The Advanced Glaucoma Intervention Study: 8. Risk of cataract formation after trabeculectomy. *Arch Ophthalmol.* 2001;119(12):1771-1779.
41. Husain R, Liang S, Foster P, et al. Cataract surgery after trabeculectomy. The effect on trabeculectomy function. *Arch Ophthalmol.* 2012;130(2):165-170.

42. Belovay GW, Naqi A, Chan BJ, Rateb M, Ahmed II. Using multiple trabecular micro-bypass stents in cataract patients to treat open-angle glaucoma. *J Cataract Refract Surg.* 2012;38(11):1911-1917.
43. US Centers for Disease Control and Prevention. Vision Health Initiative. www.cdc.gov/visionhealth/basic_information/vision_loss.htm. Updated September 29, 2015. Accessed January 5, 2017.

Chapter 13

The Toric Intraocular Lens
Successful Strategies

Adi Abulafia, MD and Warren E. Hill, MD

Experienced surgeons generally agree that the toric intraocular lens (IOL) is an excellent beginning for those looking to add premium lenses to their practice. A large cataract surgery keratometry database shows that greater than 60% of patients have 0.75 diopters (D) of corneal astigmatism or more (Figure 13-1). Stepping up to lens-based surgery as a refractive procedure, with potentially more than half of patients as instantly eligible candidates, is a wonderful introduction.

Corneal astigmatism can be corrected by 4 different methods (Table 13-1). A widely used approach involves limbal relaxing incisions (LRI). LRIs have the advantage of being inexpensive and relatively easy to do. However, LRIs are considered more for the reduction of astigmatism to some acceptable amount rather than precise correction. LRIs also have a limited effective range, with most surgeons reserving them for 1.50 D of corneal astigmatism or less.

Popularized by Dick Mackool, an innovative variation on the theme of incisional surgery is the use of paired, full-thickness penetrating incisions. By this method, 2 standard phacoemulsification incisions are made 180 degrees apart on the steep axis. The amount of correction is mostly a function of the incision width and location. When guided by a preoperative axial topographic power map, full-thickness penetrating incisions are also effective when the areas of steepening on either side of the corneal vertex are not in a perfectly straight line. Like LRIs, these are also easy to carry out, but they require each surgeon to develop an individual nomogram.

Bioptics is another approach for the correction of corneal astigmatism. By this method, a LASIK flap is cut prior to cataract surgery, which is combined with a myopic target refraction. After the postoperative refraction has stabilized, LASIK is undertaken to correct the residual refractive astigmatism and any remaining spherical equivalent.

Hovanesian JA.
Refractive Cataract Surgery: Best Practices and Advanced Technology, Second Edition (pp 157-166)

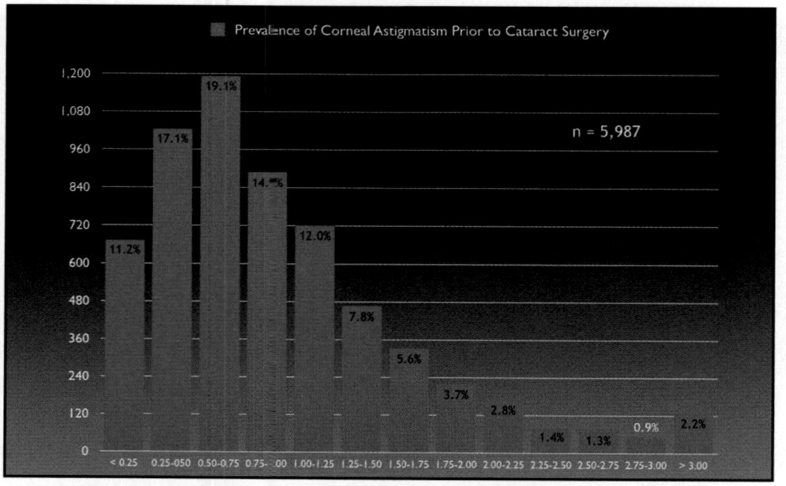

Figure 13-1. Distribution of anterior corneal astigmatism for a patient population undergoing routine cataract surgery.

Table 13-1
Comparison of the Various Methods for the Correction of Corneal Astigmatism

Procedure	*Advantage*	*Disadvantage*	*Patient Cost*	*Physician Reimbursement*
LRIs	Simple, familiar	Lacks precision	+2	+2
Paired incisions	Simple	Individual nomogram development required	+2	+2
LASIK	Precise	Requires second procedure	+3 to +4	+2 to +3
Toric IOL	Precise	Currently lacks higher correction	+2	+2

This has the advantage of offering a relatively precise correction but has the disadvantage of requiring 2 separate procedures, along with 2 opportunities for complications and 2 separate charges to the patient. In general, bioptics is not widely used.

For many surgeons, the correction of corneal astigmatism using a toric IOL has the advantage of requiring a single procedure, and with careful planning, it can be very accurate. If the physician normally charges for LRIs, the physician charge for a toric IOL may be comparable. Because toric IOLs generally come in 0.75 D power steps, implanting a toric IOL can be accomplished with almost the same level of precision as the spherical power of the intraocular lens. In the United States, toric IOLs are available to correct up to 4.00 D of corneal astigmatism. However, in many other countries, it is possible to correct a much wider range of corneal astigmatism using innovative solutions such as toric IOLs that are custom manufactured to the individual needs of a specific patient.

The Measurement of Corneal Astigmatism

If you ask 5 surgeons the best way to measure corneal astigmatism preoperatively, you may get 6 different answers. Of course, the best method is the one that delivers the least amount of residual postoperative astigmatism. In general, this requires that we know 2 components: the power difference between principal meridians (which are generally orthogonal, unless the astigmatism is irregular) and the orientation of the steep meridian.

A common misconception that often leads surgeons in the wrong direction is the assumption that the measurement of corneal astigmatism should be the same with multiple instruments. It is helpful to keep in mind that different devices often measure different areas of the astigmatic cornea and may also employ different algorithms. Expecting manual Ks, Placido-based simulated Ks, slit-scanning Ks, Scheimpflug Ks, and the various forms of autokeratometry to all give the same answer is unrealistic. Measurements by 3 or more different instruments will typically produce 3 or more different values. What works best is to first develop a plan.

Aside from the incision location and the surgically induced astigmatism, toric calculators are mostly looking for 2 items. First is the correct identification of the steep meridian, and second is the power difference between principal meridians. This information may actually be different from what we get with a set of Ks. Recall that the toric calculator does not care as much about the absolute powers as it does about the difference between them. Added accuracy comes when we try to think like the toric calculator.

Step 1

Using a topographic or tomographic axial power map, we first look to see how the power is distributed across the anterior cornea within the central 3 to 4 mm. Regular astigmatism is represented by a pair of symmetrical astigmatic power lobes straddling the corneal vertex (often referred to as a *bow tie*), with both lobes being aligned along the same meridian (Figure 13-2). If a line is drawn through the center of each lobe and the corneal vertex, where this line intersects the axis scale in the periphery is, by definition, the steep meridian. If the power distribution on the other side of the corneal vertex is not the same, the astigmatism is asymmetric, and if a single meridian cannot be drawn through both lobes, it is irregular. Early in the process, this simple method forces us to carefully look at the cornea when making a decision about the appropriateness of a toric IOL. If the steep meridian cannot be identified, each lobe is aligned with a different meridian, or things are quite asymmetric, the patient may not be a toric IOL candidate.

A topographic axial power map is considered a primary instrument for determining the steep meridian. A primary instrument is one that is well suited to a given task and always provides the correct information when presented in a specific way.

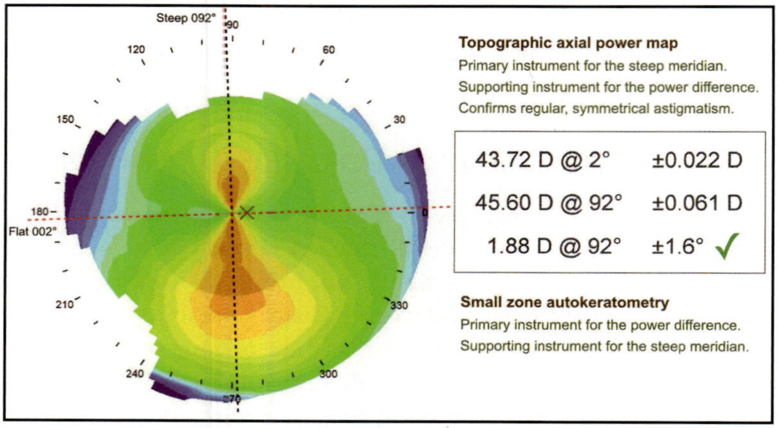

Figure 13-2. Axial curvature topographic map demonstrating mostly regular astigmatism within the central 3.5 mm of the corneal vertex. A manually determined steep meridian validates the steep and flat meridians by autokeratometry, which provides the power difference between meridians.

Step 2

Following the identification of the steep meridian, next we need to determine the power difference between the principal meridians (ie, steep and flat). Here, we use this manually determined steep meridian from the topographic axial power map to validate the power difference. This is often best done using small zone autokeratometry for eyes that have not had prior refractive surgery (see Figure 13-2). Be cautious about using any form of simulated Ks for this exercise, especially for low magnitudes of astigmatism. We look to see that the steep meridian on Ks is the same as what we know to be correct after looking at the topographic axial power map. This is a key concept.

If we are certain about the steep meridian, but the autokeratometer is telling us something different, then the Ks by keratometry are most likely being measured in an incorrect location. This is not uncommon when the power distribution is irregular. When this kind of disconnection occurs, everything stops until the discrepancy can be resolved. One approach is to settle this discrepancy by manual keratometry by setting a manual keratometer to the previously determined steep meridian, taking a measurement, then rotating the *same drum* 90 degrees and taking a measurement. In this way, we are measuring the power difference; the actual numbers are not as important.

Single-Angle and Double-Angle Plots for Astigmatism Data Presentation

Data regarding corneal astigmatism, residual astigmatism prediction errors, etc, can be graphically represented on single and double-angle plots. The traditional single-angle plot is laid out like we see it in the phoropter, in that way the against-the-rule (ATR) eyes are laid separately (Figure 13-3A). The double-angle plot takes the with-the-rule (WTR) eyes and moves them to the left, and it takes the 150 to 180 degrees group of ATR eyes

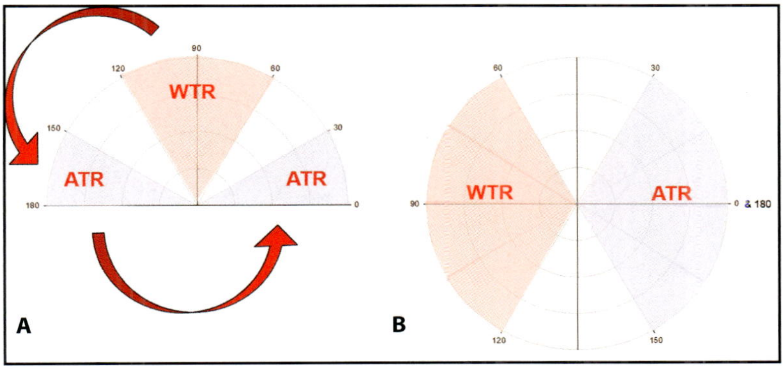

Figure 13-3. (A) Single-angle vs (B) double-angle plots for astigmatism data presentation.

and moves it to the right. All the WTR eyes are grouped to the left, and all the ATR eyes are grouped to the right (Figure 13-3B).

The Posterior Cornea

The anterior and posterior corneal surfaces each contribute to the total corneal astigmatism. Standard keratometry, and corneal topographers that use a Placido image, are based on anterior corneal measurements and have traditionally been used to measure corneal astigmatism for determining the correct axis and cylinder power needed for a toric IOL, based on the assumption that the posterior cornea induces minimal refractive astigmatism and can therefore be ignored.[1-3] Using a standardized corneal refractive index, most commonly 1.3375, these devices assume a fixed posterior-anterior corneal curvature ratio to calculate total corneal power and astigmatism.

The relationship between the anterior and posterior cornea first described in 1890 by Javal (*Javal's rule*) and was later simplified in 1988 by Grosvenor et al and confirmed by several authors for diverse populations as well as for pseudophakic eyes.[4-12] The role of the posterior cornea in assessing the net corneal astigmatism in toric IOL calculations was highlighted in 2012 by Koch, who questioned the validity of the way in which we were measuring the amount of corneal astigmatism for toric IOL calculations.[13]

Koch et al analyzed 715 corneas of 435 consecutive patients and found that about half (50.9%) of the corneas had anterior WTR astigmatism; however, 86.6% of the corneas were steep vertically along the posterior surface.[14] Since the posterior cornea acts as a negative lens, the effect of the posterior cornea will cause anterior corneal measurements to underestimate the total corneal astigmatism on the horizontal meridian. Thus, using only anterior corneal measurements for toric IOL calculations tends to lead to ATR prediction errors of the postoperative residual astigmatism, which could end up with overcorrection of eyes with WTR astigmatism and undercorrection of eyes with ATR astigmatism[9-11] (Figure 13-4).

Several studies have recently reported that methods of calculation that account for posterior corneal astigmatism might be more appropriate for toric IOL calculations. Those methods apply nomograms, coefficients of adjustment, direct measurements of

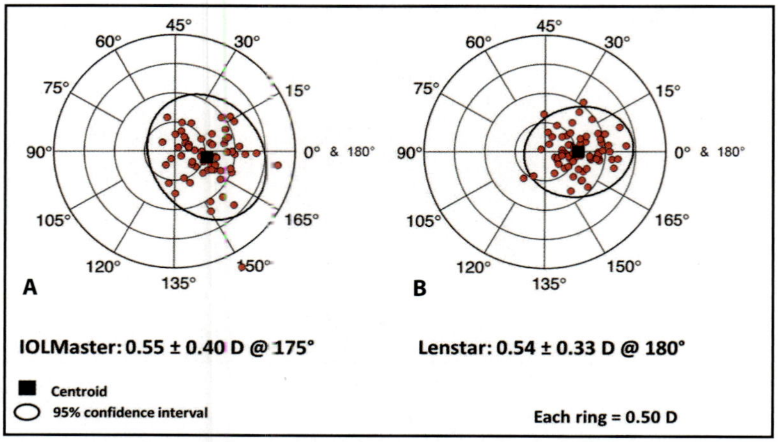

Figure 13-4. Double-angle plots of errors in predicted residual astigmatism using an effective lens position–based calculator with (A) a partial coherence interferometry device and (B) an optical low-coherence reflectometry device. (Reprinted with permission from Abulafia A, Barret GD, Kleinmann G, et al. Prediction of refractive outcomes with toric intraocular lens implantation. *J Cataract Refract Surg*. 2015;41(5):936-944.)

the posterior cornea, ray tracing approach using combined keratometry and tomography data, intraoperative aberrometry, and mathematical models.[15-23]

Surgically Induced Astigmatism

Surgically induced astigmatism typically refers to the amount of the change in the corneal astigmatism induced by the corneal incisions during cataract surgery. A free online tool at www.SIA-calculator.com is available to determine this value as a mean (average), median (lessens the influence of outliers), and centroid value for each surgeon. In years past, most surgeons used a mean absolute value for surgically induced astigmatism. Beginning with the introduction of the Barrett toric calculator in 2014, the improved accuracy of using a centroid value became known. Many surgeons are now using a centroid value for surgically induced astigmatism with the new Alcon and AMO toric calculators.

The Barrett Toric Calculator

The Barrett toric calculator employs the Universal II formula to calculate both the spherical equivalent dioptric power of a toric IOL for a desired refraction and the required amount of cylinder power correction at the corneal plane based on an estimated effective lens position.[21,22,24] Using only anterior corneal measurements, this calculator predicts the posterior corneal astigmatism using theoretical and regression models. Therefore, this calculator should be used only with data based on anterior corneal measurement.

The Barrett toric calculator has been shown to have a lower median absolute and centroid error in the prediction of residual astigmatism than other toric calculators as well

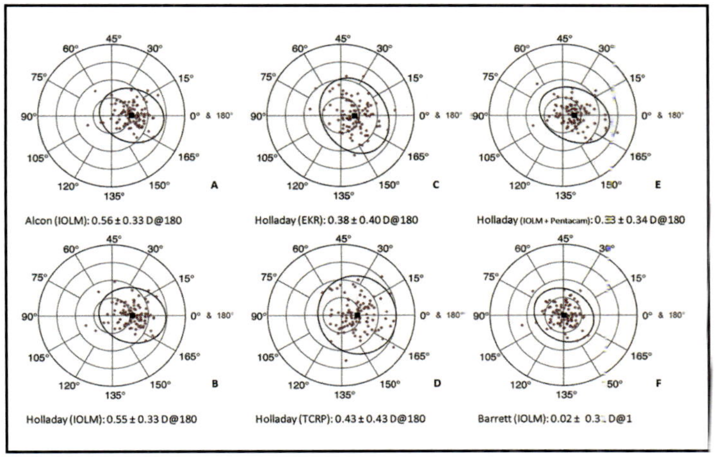

Figure 13-5. Double-angle plots of errors in predicted residual astigmatism. (A) The Alcon toric calculator using IOLMaster measurements, (B) the Holladay toric calculator using IOLMaster measurements, (C) the Holladay toric calculator using the Pentacam equivalent keratometer reading (4.5 mm) Ks, (D) the Holladay toric calculator using the Pentacam total corneal refractive power Ks, (E) the Holladay toric calculator using a vector summation of the IOLMaster measurements combined with the posterior corneal measurements by the Pentacam, and (F) the Barrett toric calculator using IOLMaster measurement. (Reprinted with permission from Abulafia A, Hill WE, Franchina M, Barrett GD. Comparison of methods to predict residual astigmatism after intraocular lens implantation. *J Refract Surg.* 2015;31(10):699-707.)

as compared with direct measurement of the posterior corneal curvature (Figure 13-5); it is available online on the American Society of Cataract and Refractive Surgery and Asia Pacific Association of Cataract and Refractive Surgeons websites.[21-23]

Corneal Marking

Marking the eye for toric IOL alignment is another potential source of error for inexperienced surgeons. Accurate alignment is required for minimizing postoperative residual astigmatism, since a one-degree error in the meridian of alignment of the toric IOL will reduce the astigmatic correction by approximately 3%.

One potential pitfall in correctly marking the cornea is cyclotorsion, which frequently occurs in both the supine position and with near fixation. This can be avoided by preoperatively marking the eye with the patient in an upright position, fixating with the contralateral eye at a straight ahead, distant target.

There are several manual eye marking techniques. The most commonly described is a 2-step procedure: 1) preoperatively marking the eye at the horizontal meridian (3- and 9-o'clock positions), which can be done using a handheld marking pen, a bubble marker, a pendular marker, a marker on the end of a tonometer, or a coaxial thin slit beam of the slit-lamp. Drying the limbal area to be marked, as well as the inferior fornix, before applying the ink marks will help to minimize ink smear; 2) intraoperatively aligning these marks with a secondary device with angular graduations, such as the Mendez gauge, and then marking the limbus or the cornea at the desired angle of alignment using a surgical marking pen or a needle.

Although meticulous manual marking is considered by most to be accurate, it is still very much user dependent, time consuming, and prone to ink washout and smear.[25] Accuracy can be enhanced by also referencing a preoperative anterior segment that displays anatomic landmarks, such as limbal vessels together with imaging software to identify the desired meridian.[26]

More sophisticated imaging modalities for toric IOL alignment are now available, including Callisto Eye with Z Align (Carl Zeiss Meditec), TrueGuide software (TrueVision 3D Surgical, Inc.), and VERION Digital Marker (Alcon). These modalities use a high-contrast digital reference image to determine the appropriate meridian and provide intraoperative registration and eye-tracking, based on various landmarks such as iris features, limbal and scleral vessels, and scleral pigmentation to enable digital intraoperative surgical guidance and alignment of toric IOLs, without the need for preoperative or intraoperative ocular marking. Finally, intraoperative aberrometry systems are available that provide an integral solution for toric IOLs' power calculation and alignment.[20]

Placement of the Toric Intraocular Lens

With the capsular bag and anterior chamber inflated with viscoelastic, the toric IOL is implanted in much the same way as its single-piece counterpart. However, the toric IOL must ultimately be aligned with the previously placed corneal alignment marks.

First, the lens is stabilized approximately 10 to 15 degrees counterclockwise from its final position with a second instrument, and all viscoelastic is then removed from both behind the IOL and from the anterior chamber. Gently, the IOL is rotated clockwise until the reference marks on each side of the optic are oriented in a line with the previously placed alignment marks on the cornea. Sometimes it may be necessary to inject a little balanced salt solution under the capsulorrhexis edge to gently separate the posterior aspect of the optic from the posterior capsule, so that the lens rotates without interacting with the lens capsule, which could lead to a capsular tear.

Once the toric IOL has been properly aligned against the corneal alignment marks, using the irrigation/aspiration tip, gentle pressure is used to "seat" the IOL against the posterior capsule. This allows for an interaction between the posterior capsule and the acrylic material of the posterior surface of the IOL, which prevents subsequent rotation.

Residual Refractive Astigmatism

If there is significant residual postoperative astigmatism, one of the more common causes is that the toric IOL has not been optimally aligned, either by a miscalculation or intraoperative error. A free online tool is available to make this determination at www.astigmatismfix.com, which will calculate both the optimal meridian of alignment and the resultant change in the refractive astigmatism. Insights are also provided into the amount of toric correction. If there is remaining residual astigmatism, but the refractive axis has been flipped, there is too much toricity. If the remaining residual astigmatism is near the intended meridian of alignment, there is too little toricity. Most find this online tool to be an indispensible part of the postoperative assessment of all toric IOL cases.

Conclusion

The toric lens is a perfect introduction to premium IOLs. Selecting candidates is relatively straightforward, and uncorrected distance vision for most patients allows for spectacle independence. All that is needed in addition to surgery for standard IOLs is a topographer and well-reasoned plan for each of the component parts of measurement, calculation, marking, and placement.

References

1. Lee H, Chung JL, Kim EK, Sgrignoli B, Kim TI. Univariate and bivariate polar value analysis of corneal astigmatism measurements obtained with 6 instruments. *J Cataract Refract Surg.* 2012;38:1608-1615.
2. Hill W, Osher R, Cooke D, et al. Simulation of toric intraocular lens results: manual keratometry versus dual-zone automated keratometry from an integrated biometer. *J Cataract Refract Surg.* 2011;37:2181-2187.
3. Potvin R, Gundersen KG, Masket S, et al. Prospective multicenter study of toric IOL outcomes when dual zone automated keratometry is used for astigmatism planning. *J Refract Surg.* 2013;29:804-809.
4. Javal E. *Mémoires d'ophtalmométrie annotés et préédés d'une introduction.* Paris, France: G. Masson; 1890.
5. Grosvenor T, Quintero S, Perrigin DM. Predicting refractive astigmatism: a suggested simplification of Javal's rule. *Am J Optom Physiol Opt.* 1988;65:292-297.
6. Remon L, Benlloch J, Furlan WD. Corneal and refractive astigmatism in adults: a power vectors analysis. *Optom Vis Sci.* 2009;86:1182-1186.
7. Tong L, Carkeet A, Saw SM, Tan DT. Corneal and refractive error astigmatism in Singaporean schoolchildren: a vector-based Javal's rule. *Optom Vis Sci* 2001;78:881-887.
8. Alpins NA. New method of targeting vectors to treat astigmatism. *J Cataract Refract Surg.* 1997;23:65-75.
9. Auger P. Confirmation of the simplified Javal's Rule. *Am J Optom Physiol Opt.* 1988;65:915.
10. Lam AK, Chan CC, Lee MH, Wong KM. The aging effect on corneal curvature and the validity of Javal's rule in Hong Kong Chinese. *Curr Eye Res.* 1999;18:83-90.
11. Teus MA, Arruabarrena C, Hernández-Verdejo JL Sales-Sanz A, Sales-Sanz M. Correlation between keratometric and refractive astigmatism in pseudophakic eyes. *J Cataract Refract Surg.* 2010;36:1671-1675.
12. Bae JG, Kim SJ, Choi YI. Pseudophakic residual astigmatism. *Korean J Ophthalmol.* 2004;18:116-120.
13. Koch DD. Corneal optics for IOL selection: cracking the code. Paper presented at: American Society of Cataract and Refractive Surgery Annual Meeting; April 23, 2012; Chicago, IL.
14. Koch DD, Ali SF, Weikert MP, Shirayama M, Jenkins R, Wang L. Contribution of posterior corneal astigmatism to total corneal astigmatism. *J Cataract Refract Surg.* 2012;38:2080-2087.
15. Koch DD, Jenkins RB, Weikert MP, Yeu E, Wang L. Correcting astigmatism with toric intraocular lenses: effect of posterior corneal astigmatism. *J Cataract Refract Surg.* 2013;39:1803-1809.
16. Goggin M, Zamora-Alejo K, Esterman A, van Zyl L. Adjustment of anterior corneal astigmatism values to incorporate the likely effect of posterior corneal curvature for toric intraocular lens calculation. *J Refract Surg.* 2015;31:98-102.
17. Preussner PR, Hoffmann P, Wahl J. Impact of posterior corneal surface on toric intraocular lens (IOL) calculation. *Curr Eye Res.* 2015;40(8):809-814.
18. Savini G, Naeser K. An analysis of the factors influencing the residual refractive astigmatism after cataract surgery with toric intraocular lenses. *Invest Ophthalmol Vis Sci.* 2015;56:827-835.
19. Hoffmann PC, Wahl J, Hutz WW, Preussner PR. A ray tracing approach to calculate toric intraocular lenses. *J Refract Surg.* 2013;29:402-408.

20. Hatch KM, Woodcock EC, Talamo JH. Intraocular lens power selection and positioning with and without intraoperative aberrometry. *J Refract Surg.* 2015;31:237-242.
21. Abulafia A, Barrett GD, Kleinmann G, et al. Prediction of refractive outcomes with toric intraocular lens implantation. *J Cataract Refract Surg.* 2015;41:936-944.
22. Abulafia A, Hill WE, Franchina M, Barrett GD. Comparison of methods to predict residual astigmatism after intraocular lens implantation. *J Refract Surg.* 2015;31(10):699-707.
23. Abulafia A, Koch DD, Wang L, et al. A novel regression formula for toric IOL calculations. Paper presented at: European Society of Cataract and Refractive Surgeons Congress; September 5-9, 2015; Barcelona, Spain.
24. Barrett GD. An improved universal theoretical formula for intraocular lens power prediction. *J Cataract Refract Surg.* 1993;19:713-720.
25. Popp N, Hirnschall N, Maedel S, Findl O. Evaluation of 4 corneal astigmatic marking methods. *J Cataract Refract Surg.* 2012;38:2094-2099.
26. Cha D, Kang SY, Kim S-H, Song J-S, Kim H-M. New axis-marking method for a toric intraocular lens: mapping method. *J Refract Surg.* 2011;27:375-379.

Chapter 14

Limbal Relaxing Incisions

R. Bruce Wallace III, MD and
John A. Hovanesian, MD, FACS

Restoring multifocal vision with a predictable and safe procedure is now a reality. The steps to success include all of the topics discussed in this text, with astigmatism correction being an essential ingredient. All manufacturers of presbyopic intraocular lenses (IOL) have either developed or are in the process of designing toric models to correct corneal cylinder. As we have learned from our results with monofocal toric IOLs, toric presbyopic IOLs show great promise. Until the option is widely available, surgeons will continue to depend on corneal reshaping to reduce astigmatism with spherical IOLs. Even when toric versions of presbyopic IOLs become available in the United States, corneal procedures may still be used because of cost and inventory issues. This chapter will focus on the use of peripheral corneal relaxing incisions, commonly referred to as *limbal relaxing incisions* (LRI), which have been shown to safely and predictably provide permanent astigmatic correction.[1]

Origin of Limbal Relaxing Incisions

LRIs are probably the friendliest and most cost-effective refractive procedures we can offer our patients. There's no expensive laser, no central corneal or intraocular trauma, and perforations are rare in healthy corneas. So why is it that many cataract surgeons are not yet using LRIs? Some of us are not convinced that they are reliable, especially if instruments were purchased and results were disappointing. For many, just the awkwardness of incisional corneal surgery along with an uncomfortable change in routine for surgeon and staff have placed LRIs in a negative light. Yet judging by the swell in attendance at teaching events like LRI wet labs at the last few American Academy of

Hovanesian JA.
Refractive Cataract Surgery: Best Practices and Advanced Technology, Second Edition (pp 167-176).

Ophthalmology and American Society of Cataract and Refractive Surgery meetings, LRI popularity continues to grow.

We owe a great deal of thanks to early pioneers who promoted the benefits of combining astigmatic keratotomy with cataract surgery many years ago. A partial list would include Drs. Gills, Hollis, Osher, Maloney, Shepherd, Koch, Thornton, Gayton, Davison, and Lindstrom. Dr. Robert Osher has advocated peripheral relaxing keratotomy at the time of cataract surgery since 1983, learning the principles of the technique from Dr. George Tate.[2]

I have had the pleasure to teach LRI techniques for over 20 years. During these training sessions, I have learned the steps necessary to convince cataract surgeons that LRIs can be an important part of refractive cataract surgery. Before a cataract surgeon transitions to the routine use of LRIs, he or she must understand the benefits, be confident in the system of treatment, and be confident with his or her technique.

Astigmatism in Three Dimensions

In order to reduce unwanted astigmatism, the surgeon must lead the way in his or her practice to develop a systematic approach to surgical correction. Reducing astigmatism begins with effective preoperative assessment. Most cataract surgeons depend on trained technicians to perform preoperative astigmatism measurements, which include refraction, keratometry and videokeratography, or corneal topography. Unfortunately, most technicians do not think about astigmatism in 3 dimensions because these measurements only generate numbers or 2-dimensional color maps. For technicians and surgeons to be effective in astigmatism control, it is helpful to understand and visualize astigmatism, especially corneal astigmatism, in 3 dimensions. Such terms as the *flat axis*, the *steep axis*, and *coupling* become easier to grasp when thinking of corneal shapes rather than numbers or colors.

To determine whether your office staff perceives astigmatism in 3 dimensions, try this experiment. Ask your best-trained technicians to imagine that the oblong curvatures of an American football represent the astigmatic corneal surfaces of a patient's eye with the curvature in one axis steep, the other flat. Imagine that the football is lying flat on the ground horizontally. Would that resemble with-the-rule or against-the-rule astigmatism? If they answer with-the-rule, they are correct and are probably thinking about astigmatism in 3 dimensions. With this fundamental understanding of what the term *regular astigmatism* means, all members of the surgical team will find astigmatism correction easier to understand.

Surgical Planning

The goal for astigmatism control should be the creation of a resultant cylinder of 0.5 diopter (D) or less at any axis. Most patients enjoy good unaided visual acuity with this degree of astigmatism.[3] Some studies suggest a benefit to leaving some amount of residual against-the-rule cylinder so that uncorrected near vision after cataract surgery is improved.[4] However, surgical practices using multifocal IOLs and/or monovision will not find this to be an advantage, because of the compromise of the loss of distance visual acuity with amounts over 0.5 D of cylinder.[5]

One of the more challenging tasks that the surgeon faces is deciding which astigmatic preoperative measurements should be used when planning a surgical correction. Do we depend on the cylinder diopters and axis from the refraction, the keratometry, or do we always need to perform corneal topography? One study showed the frequency of poor correlation of all 3 methods of measurement, especially with less than 2.0 D of astigmatism.[6] Fortunately, unlike correction of spherical refractive errors, astigmatism correction is more forgiving, especially when treating moderate to low levels.

One way to plan surgical correction of astigmatism is to initially assess the refraction and the keratometry simultaneously. If good correlation exists as to the amount of cylinder and axis, the surgical planning for astigmatism correction during cataract surgery is fairly straightforward. If, however, there is poor correlation (even though keratometry should be more reliable), surgical correction can be less predictable, even with corneal topography. This is where the art of astigmatism correction applies. The surgeon needs to also judge the relative reliability of the astigmatic information. If, after careful consideration, there is doubt as to a reasonable surgical plan, the astigmatism correction should be postponed until after cataract surgery and adequate time for incision healing.

The recent improvements in computerized corneal topography provide more dependable preoperative astigmatic parameters and also signal important warnings, such as irregular astigmatism and forme fruste keratoconus. More reliable keratometry readings from biometers such as IOLMaster Series 700 (Carl Zeiss Meditec) and Lenstar LS 900 (Haag-Streit) continue to replace traditional manual keratometry.

Posterior Astigmatism

As Douglas Koch first pointed out, 87% of eyes have posterior corneal astigmatism that is not measured by keratometers, optical biometry devices like the IOLMaster or Lenstar, or Placido-based topographers. This posterior astigmatism has an optical effect similar to adding 0.5 D of against-the-rule astigmatism (ie, a cornea that is steeper at 180 degrees than it appears on the above measurements). This posterior corneal astigmatism does not drift with age, so for surgical planning, we can add this astigmatism to that measured by the traditional techniques mentioned previously.[7]

Another effect we may want to consider when planning surgery is the predictable drift of astigmatism with age described by Hayashi.[3] Among the aged cataract surgery population, most patients will over 10 years have an axis shift of their astigmatism toward the horizontal axis amounting to about 0.4 D.

So how do we incorporate these 2 effects into surgical astigmatism planning? Most experts advocate the following approach:

- ▲ When correcting *with-the-rule astigmatism* (corneas steep near 90 degrees), correct 0.5 to 0.7 D *less* than measured on the corneal surface.
- ▲ When correcting *against-the-rule astigmatism* (corneas steep near 180 degrees), correct 0.5 D *more* than measured on the corneal surface.
- ▲ When correcting *oblique* astigmatism, make no changes.

A perhaps oversimplified way of looking at these corrections is to simply ignore the surgically induced astigmatism (SIA) of a temporal (180 degrees) clear corneal astigmatism, assuming the surgeon's average SIA is about 0.5 D.

Many current online astigmatism planning tools do not automatically make these adjustments for posterior corneal astigmatism, so surgeons must manually account for them in planning. However, intraoperative wavefront aberrometry measurements do not require adjustment, because these devices measure the optics of the entire eye, including the posterior cornea.

Here are 2 examples of compensating for posterior corneal astigmatism in an LRI procedure.

Example 1: A patient's IOLMaster reading shows keratometry values of 44.00 at 90 degrees and 43.20 at 180 degrees or about 0.8 D steep at 90 degrees. The surgeon plans a temporal clear corneal incision that will typically induce 0.5 D of flattening at 180 degrees. In this case, the phaco incision's SIA of 0.5 D will negate all but 0.1 D of the patient's presumed posterior corneal astigmatism of 0.6 D steep at 180 degrees.

Keratometric astigmatism: 0.8 D at 90 degrees

+ Posterior cornea: -0.6 D at 90 degrees (same as 0.6 steep at 180 degrees)

+ Surgically induced correction: +0.5 D at 90 degrees (same as 0.5 D flattening at 180 degrees)

= Astigmatism to correct: -0.7 D at 90 degrees

In this case, the resultant astigmatism might be corrected by 2 paired 30-degree corneal arcs, centered at 90 degrees.

Example 2: A patient's IOLMaster reading shows keratometry values of 43.00 at 180 degrees and 42.00 at 90 degrees or about 1.0 D steep at 180 degrees. The surgeon plans a temporal clear corneal incision that will typically induce 0.5 D of flattening at 180 degrees. In this case again, the phaco incision's SIA of 0.5 D will negate all but 0.1 D of the patient's presumed posterior corneal astigmatism of 0.6 D steep at 180 degrees.

Keratometric astigmatism: 1.0 D at 180 degrees

+ Posterior cornea: +0.6 D at 180 degrees

+ Surgically induced correction: -0.5 D at 180 degrees

= Astigmatism to correct: -1.1 D at 90 degrees

In this case, the resultant astigmatism might be corrected by 2 paired 35-degree corneal arcs, centered at 180 degrees.

Limbal Relaxing Incision Treatment Systems

A systematic approach to LRI use improves results. A number of LRI nomograms have been developed by Gills, Lindstrom, Nichamin, and myself. I first used Dr. Nichamin's excellent nomogram and then modified it to slant more toward one incision for lower levels of cylinder (Figures 14-1 and 14-2). Since we make our LRI incisions so far in the corneal periphery, paired incisions were not found to be as important for postoperative corneal regularity as traditional astigmatic keratotomy made at the 7-mm optical zone. An advantage of Nichamin nomograms and their modification is that treatment is planned in degrees of arc rather than cord length. With corneal diameters

The "NAPA" Nomogram

Nichamin Age & Pachymetry-Adjusted Intralimbal Arcuate Astigmatic Nomogram

Louis D. "Skip" Nichamin, M.D. ~ Laurel Eye Clinic, Brookville, PA

WITH-THE-RULE

(Steep Axis 45°-145°)

PREOP CYLINDER	Paired Incisions in Degrees of Arc			
(Diopters)	20-30 yrs old	31-40 yrs old	41-50 yrs old	51-60 yrs old
0.75	40	35	35	30
1.00	45	40	40	35
1.25	55	50	45	40
1.50	60	55	50	45
1.75	65	60	55	50
2.00	70	65	60	55
2.25	75	70	65	60
2.50	80	75	70	65
2.75	85	80	75	70
3.00	90	90	85	80

AGAINST-THE-RULE

(Steep Axis 0-40°/140-180°)

PREOP CYLINDER	Paired Incisions in Degrees of Arc			
(Diopters)	20-30 yrs old	31-40 yrs old	41-50 yrs old	51-60 yrs old
0.75	45	40	40	35
1.00	50	45	45	40
1.25	55	55	50	45
1.50	60	60	55	50
1.75	65	65	60	55
2.00	70	70	65	60
2.25	75	75	70	65
2.50	80	80	75	70
2.75	85	85	80	75
3.00	90	90	85	80

When placing intralimbal relaxing incisions following or concomitant with radial relaxing incisions, total arc length is decreased by 50%

Figure 14-1. The NAPA nomogram.

varying and the fact that we make arcs, not straight line incisions, degree measurements are universally more accurate.

More recently, planning LRIs with computer programs has become popular, similar to the toric IOL calculator offered by Alcon. The AMO LRI calculator (LRIcalculator.com) designed by Eric Donnenfeld and the PalmScan AP2000 (Micro Medical Devices) modified by Rafi Israel are now available.

For lower levels of astigmatism (less than 2.0 D), selecting the axis of cylinder can be challenging. I look at all axis measurements but usually select ones from computerized corneal topography. Sometimes, especially with smaller cylinder corrections, there is poor correlation of axis with refraction, K readings, and topography. Many times when I encounter this situation with first eyes for cataract surgery, I will postpone the LRI and

LIMBAL RELAXING INCISIONS – R. Bruce Wallace, III, MD

INSTRUMENTS:
- Diamond knife: Trifacet 600m preset depth, single foot plate
- Marker: Mendez axis ring
- Forceps: 0.12 calibre

PROCEDURE:
- Place axis ring around limbus
- Mark axis with forceps
- Mark limits of intended incision(s) with forceps
- Remove axis ring
- Dry marks with cellulose sponge
- Fixate globe with forceps
- Perform incision(s) direct toward fixation

NOMOGRAM

Assuming all cataract incisions are performed temporally and are relatively astigmatically neutral:

FOR WITH-THE-RULE AND OBLIQUE ASTIGMATISM:

Astigmatism (in diop)	40 – 50yo	50 – 60yo	60 – 70yo	70 – 80yo	80+yo
1.00 – 1.50	60°(1)	50°(1)	50°(1)	40°(1)	30°(1)
1.50 – 2.00	70°(1)	70°(1)	70°(1)	60°(1)	60°(1)
2.00 – 2.50	60°(2)	60°(2)	60°(2)	70°(1)	70°(1)
2.50 – 3.00	70°(2)	70°(2)	70°(2)	60°(2)	60°(2)
3.00 – 4.00	80°(2)	80°(2)	80°(2)	70°(2)	70°(2)

FOR AGAINST-THE-RULE ASTIGMATISM:

Astigmatism (in diop)	40- 50yo	50 – 60yo	60 – 70yo	70 – 80yo	80+yo
1.00 – 1.50	60°(1)	50°(1)	40°(1)	40°(1)	30°(1)
1.50 – 2.00	70°(1)	60°(1)	60°(1)	60°(1)	40°(1)
2.00 – 2.50	60°(2)	80°(1)	80°(1)	70°(1)	60°(1)
2.50 – 3.00	70°(2)	70°(2)	70°(2)	60°(2)	60°(2)
3.00 – 4.00	80°(2)	80°(2)	80°(2)	70°(2)	70°(2)

(1) – denotes one(1) incision
(2) – denotes two(2) incisions

When using nomogram, if age/astigmatism at dividing point:
- choose shortest incision length
- choose one incision over two

Figure 14-2. Dr. Wallace's nomogram.

measure the postoperative cylinder.[9] If there is visually disturbing postoperative astigmatism, I will perform LRI centered on the axis of the postoperative refraction the same day the patient returns for cataract surgery in the fellow eye.

Some surgeons concerned about cyclotropia will mark the 6 and 3 or 9 o'clock limbal axis at the slit lamp, prior to surgery. For lower levels of astigmatism, this may just offer little benefit. Yet for higher levels (over 2.0 D) marking the limbus may be worthwhile. An instrument to mark the horizontal axis while the patient is sitting up in the preoperative area, the Bakewell Marker (Mastel Precision), may be more convenient than marking at the slit lamp.

Questions arise concerning IOL power modifications with LRIs. With low to moderate levels of cylinder (0.50 to 2.75), corneal coupling equalizes the central corneal power so there is less chance the IOL power selection will be inaccurate. Longer LRI incisions for higher cylinder (> 3.0 D) may create a radial keratotomy effect and produce unwanted postoperative hyperopia. Increasing the IOL power 0.5 to 1.0 D may be necessary in these cases.

Instrumentation

Simplification of instruments and techniques improves efficiency and comfort with the procedure. There are many excellent LRI instrument sets available from Mastel, Rhein, Katena, ASICO, and others. I designed the Wallace LRI Kit with Duckworth and Kent and Storz. This kit includes the following:

- ▲ Pre-set single foot plate trifacet diamond knife (600 microns)
- ▲ Mendez axis marker
- ▲ 0.12 caliber forceps

The trifacet diamond is less likely to chip. The Mendez marker has actual numbers on the dial to help guide the surgeon to the proper axis mark. (This orientation guide is valuable because the biggest fear besides a perforation is placing the incision on the wrong axis.) All of these instruments are made of titanium to increase longevity.

Patient Counseling

Similar to preoperative discussion of the new refractive IOLs, informing patients about the option of surgical treatment for astigmatism has become a common event in many cataract practices. We start by describing the optical disadvantages of astigmatism and the relative effectiveness and low risk surrounding LRIs. In the United States, when charging most Medicare patients an additional out-of-pocket fee for LRIs, an advance beneficiary notice should be filed.

Technique

A surgeon's LRI technique will vary, depending on the instruments used for the procedure. For the routine I use, the instruments are as follows:

- ▲ Do before phaco after wetting the cornea
- ▲ Mark the axis (Mendez ring and 0.12 forceps)
- ▲ Mark the incision borders (Mendez ring and 0.12 forceps)
- ▲ Fixate the globe (0.12 forceps)
- ▲ Advance the knife toward fixation (usually toward the surgeon)

Try to insert the knife into the peripheral corneal dome (approximately 1.5 mm from the actual limbus) as perpendicular as possible (Figures 14-3 and 14-4). Maintain this blade orientation, and with moderate pressure complete the LRI by "connecting the dots" on the cornea and twirling the knife handle to make an arcuate incision using the limbus as a template. (Available on YouTube is a video to provide stepwise direction for at-home wet lab training for LRIs on porcine eyes. LRIs are some of the best-suited procedures for surgical training in a wet lab environment.)

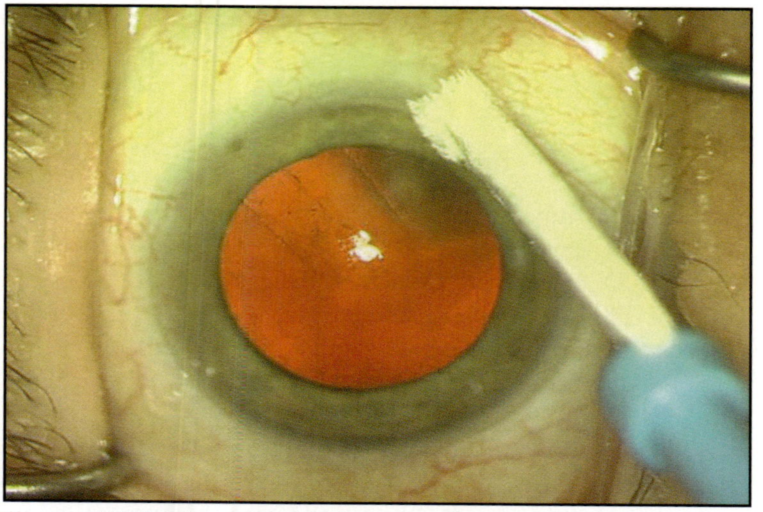

Figure 14-3. The three peripheral corneal reference marks are dried with a surgical sponge.

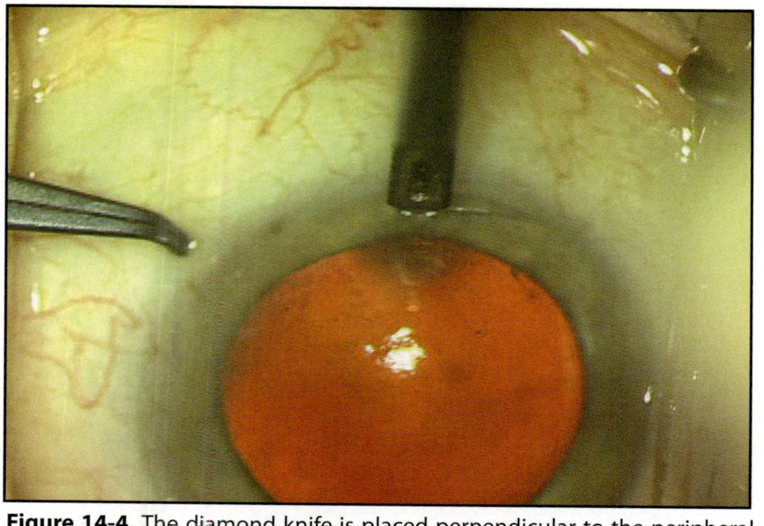

Figure 14-4. The diamond knife is placed perpendicular to the peripheral cornea and the LRI is performed by advancing the knife toward the fixation forceps, "connecting the dots" of the corneal marks.

Postoperative Care

For many years, we added a nonsteroidal anti-inflammatory drug to our postoperative cataract surgery regimen to offer corneal analgesia. We now use a nonsteroidal anti-inflammatory drug routinely for all cataract surgery patients, pre- and postoperation, mainly to help reduce inflammation and the incidence of cystoid macular edema. A topical fourth-generation fluoroquinolone and steroid (Pred Forte [prednisolone acetate]) are also part of routine medication for cataract surgery. We do not patch the eye after LRI but do apply Betadine 5% on the cornea preoperation and immediately postoperation.

Measuring Results

A number of methods are available to measure our results with LRIs. Computer software, such as the Holladay II Surgical Outcomes Assessment Program, include postoperative astigmatic analysis. Surgically induced refractive change and vector analysis are often used to demonstrate astigmatic change. A simpler way to follow results is just to measure the amount of postoperative cylinder at any axis. If a patient has 0.75 D or less of postoperative astigmatism, he or she is likely to be happy with the result.

Femtosecond Laser–Assisted Cataract Surgery

Femtosecond laser–assisted cataract surgery continues to grow as an option for upgrading modern cataract surgery, especially when paired with multifocal and accommodating IOL. An important ingredient in the value femtosecond laser–assisted cataract surgery provides is the peripheral corneal incisions the femtosecond laser can create to reduce corneal astigmatism. The same rules governing LRIs created with a diamond blade also apply to those created with a femtosecond laser: the longer, deeper, and closer to the corneal apex the incisions are, the greater they will modify astigmatism. However, there is another dimension unique to femtosecond LRIs; incisions can be created but not manually opened. Femtosecond laser astigmatic incisions also may be purely intrastromal, with no component of the photodisruption as superficial as the Bowman membrane. Either of these 2 approaches will achieve less astigmatic correction for a given incision length and depth than a traditional LRI opening to the ocular surface. Advocates of these techniques suggest that if the ocular surface is undisturbed, they cause less surface irritation and perhaps less dry eye than traditional LRIs. Most find that the unopened or intrastromal incisions will create about two-thirds of the correction that the same-sized traditional incision would create. For example, if paired 30-degree arcs are expected to correct 1.0 D of cylinder on the steep axis, if left unopened, these same incisions would correct about 0.67 D.

Some surgeons create femtosecond LRIs and initially leave them unopened, with the intention of re-checking residual astigmatism with intraoperative aberrometry at the conclusion of surgery or with manifest refraction in the postoperative clinic setting. In either case, if residual steepness is found at approximately the axis of the unopened laser LRI, the incision can then be fully opened with a blunt instrument, either in surgery or at the slit lamp. This enhancement procedure will generally deliver the full astigmatic correction that the incisions are capable of, or in the previous example, about 1.0 D.[10]

The Future of Limbal Relaxing Incisions

Like phacoemulsification, LRI instruments and techniques will continue to evolve. As we follow LRI results with imaging, such as more sophisticated corneal topography and wavefront aberrometry, modifications such as adjustments in blade depth and optic zone diameter will help us improve. One study published in the *Journal of Cataract and Refractive Surgery* demonstrated the long-term stability of LRIs.[11] Competition with toric IOLs and combinations of bioptics with corneal laser and light-adjustable IOLs may reduce LRI popularity. Regardless, any improvement in methods to reduce unwanted astigmatism will continue to be an important part of successful refractive cataract surgery.

References

1. Carvalho MJ, Suzuki SH, Freitas LL, Branco BC, Schor P, Lima AL. Limbal relaxing incisions to correct corneal astigmatism during phacoemulsification. *J Refract Surg.* 2007;23(5):499-504.
2. Osher RH. Consultations in refractive surgery. *J Refract Surg.* 1987;3(6):240.
3. Hovanesian JA. Preoperative and surgical factors that correlate with the highest patientreported satisfaction with multifocal IOLs. Paper presented at: American Society of Cataract and Refractive Surgery Annual Symposium, April 17-21, 2015; San Diego, CA.
4. Verzella F, Calossi A. Multifocal effect of against-the-rule myopic astigmatism in pseudophakic eyes. *J Refract Corneal Surg.* 1993;9:58-61.
5. Sawusch M, Guyton D. Optimal astigmatism to enhance depth of focus after cataract surgery. *Ophthalmology.* 1991;98:1025-1029.
6. Wallace RB. On-axis cataract incisions: where is the axis? *1995 ASCRS Symposium of Cataract, IOL and Refractive Surgery Best Papers of Sessions.* 1995;Nov:67-72.
7. Koch D, Ali S, Weikert M, Shirayama M, Jenkins R, Wang L. Contribution of posterior corneal astigmatism to total corneal astigmatism. *J Cataract Refract Surg.* 2012;38(12):2080-2087.
8. Hayashi K, Hirata A, Manabe S, Hayashi H. Long-term change in corneal astigmatism after sutureless cataract surgery. *Am J Ophthalmol.* 2011;151(5):858-865.
9. Wallace RB. Reducing astigmatism. In: Wallace RB, ed. *Refractive Cataract Surgery and Multifocal IOLs.* Thorofare, NJ: SLACK Incorporated; 2001:167-172.
10. Hovanesian JA, unpublished data.
11. Lim R, Borasio E, Ilari L. Long-term stability of keratometric astigmatism after limbal relaxing incisions. *J Cataract Refract Surg.* 2014;40:1676-1681.

Chapter 15

Integrating Monovision Into Presbyopic Intraocular Lens Surgery

J. E. "Jay" McDonald II, MD and Garth Rotramel, BA, SPHR

The purpose of this chapter is to provide you, the practitioner, with a hands-on method for successfully making pseudophakic aspheric advanced monovision a working piece of your presbyopic cataract repertoire.

Background and History of Monovision

Today, the average person is using a personal digital assistant (PDA) 30 to 60 hours a week. The point of focus is no longer a book. Reading glasses and bifocals are a poor and debilitating choice. Future patients will no longer tolerate these archaic appliances. The need for the monovision platform for near and far has never been greater. Every lens replacement surgeon needs the ability to give his or her patient a spectacle-free ability to function in today's world.

Thirty years of clinical, optical, and surgical practice have taught me that the prescription people comfortably function with is not always identical to what comes out of the phoropter. My eyes were opened to the fact that the patient's best fit is much more powerful and important than a person's 2 individual prescriptions. In fact, in treating presbyopia, visual function can be expanded greatly by learning and appreciating the power of bilateral integrative visual function.

Prior to the development of the intraocular lens (IOL), we used contact lenses to reduce size disparity to within 7% of the phakic eye, and the uniocular aphakic patient was visually "made whole."

Monovision soft contact lens fitting provided the plano presbyope the appreciation of not having to raise the chin in order to type, read, order from a menu, or work on a

Hovanesian JA.
Refractive Cataract Surgery: Best Practices and Advanced Technology, Second Edition (pp 177-188). © 2017 SLACK Incorporated.

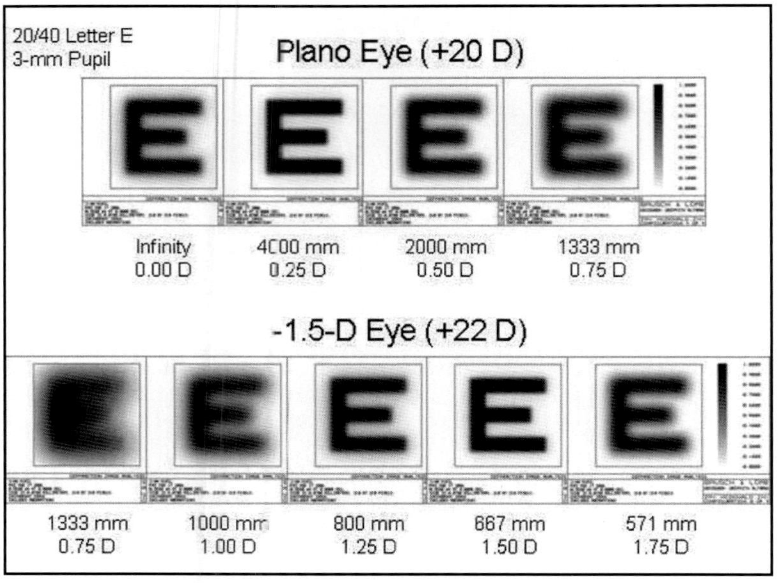

Figure 15-1. Range of visual acuity with monovision. (Reprinted, with permission from Chang DF. *Mastering Refractive IOLs: The Art and Science*. Thorofare, NJ: SLACK Incorporated; 2008.)

factory line. Pilots, finish carpenters, and office workers no longer had to rely on bifocals or trifocals to visually function.

Incisional refractive surgery allowed us to give an even greater enhanced near/far vision complement for the presbyope—yes, a new more complete freedom from any optical appliance. Fifteen years ago, as we began laser vision correction, I never blinked an eye in encouraging my presbyopic patients to do *monovision*, a term I continue to feel grossly under-describes the huge advantages it offers our patients when extricating themselves from their dysfunctional natural lenses by embarking on their remaining life's journey with the IOL.

In 1998, Greenbaum reported using intraocular monovision in his postoperative cataract patients by targeting -2 50 myopia in their nondominant eye and targeting plano in their dominant eye.[1] He was successful in producing happy postoperative cataract patients who could read without spectacle correction.

Currently, in our practice, by using aspheric IOLs, we precisely target a separation of only -1.25. This is almost universally successful, as the difference in intraocular images is minimal. Stereopsis is preserved in the 40- to 60-second range. More importantly, by using monofocality rather than splitting the image with multifocality, we maximally preserve, for the patient's lifetime, the highest quality of optical and visual potential. In Figure 15-1, we can see the progression of the uniocular image from near to far.

The fact is, the patient over age 60 years rarely has a pupil greater than 3.2 mm.[2] This small pupil creates the continual depth of focus that, as demonstrated in Figure 15-1, produces a bilateral clarity of vision from 24 inches to infinity. This small amount of refractive separation is well accepted by every patient but the most strongly eye dominant person.[3] Currently being validated is a quantitative ocular dominance testing device that will help us broaden our scope of identifying, on a spectrum, a person's relative tolerance to what we shall call *blended vision*.[4]

Monovision provides a highly successful mechanism to deliver spectacle independence for our presbyopic patients. Doing so requires considerable additional evaluation, as well as staff and doctor skill refinements. Additional testing, new staff counseling, and the surgeon's ability to eliminate astigmatism—both intra- and postoperatively—is demanded. Thus, entering the presbyopic surgical arena, whether using accommodative, multifocal, or advanced aspheric monovision, must be undertaken seriously. However, the reward of spectacle independence for the patient and doctor more than warrants this extra energy by the doctor and staff and expenditure by the patient.

The Centers for Medicare and Medicaid Services Ruling No. 05-01 provides a mechanism so that a patient can be responsible for payment of that portion of the physician's charge for a presbyopia-correcting IOL exceeding the physician's charge for a conventional IOL following cataract surgery. In 2005, after several meetings and discussions with Kevin Corcoran, a longtime respected reimbursement consultant, our practice arrived at a proper charge and fee evaluation for the process leading to spectacle independence through pseudophakic monovision. Unlike the multifocal and accommodative lenses, there is not a significant charge for the lens products involved, thus making the charge more affordable for our patients while allowing for great satisfaction. Corcoran and associates are happy to provide the forms and information surrounding this at their website (www.corcoranccg.com).

In our community, we have not only been able to afford the increased time and resources required to implement these services in our clinic, but we have been able to save our patients thousands of dollars in out-of-pocket costs related to premium lens products. The out-of-pocket expense of a costly multifocal lens is avoided. At the same time, the surgeon's additional staff time, skill set, and increased postoperative time is covered by a justifiable out-of-pocket amount commensurate with a multifocal IOL use.

Why Monofocality Versus Multifocality?

The answer to this question requires a long and detailed process that involves my personal journey of several years working through the current knowledge of the neurocognitive processes involved in binocular vision. I owe this awareness to many colleagues directly or indirectly involved in the visual sciences as well as clinicians, most notably Randolph Blake, PhD; Martin Mainster, MD, PhD; Patricia Turner, MD; Griffith Altmann, MS, MBA, Director of Global Product Strategy for Intraocular Lens Products at Bausch & Lomb; Richard Lindstrom, MD; and Jack Holladay, MD. I believe very strongly that as a given patient ages, he or she incurs normal deterioration of his or her visual processes and often visual pathology; the contrast sensitivity deficit created by the use of multifocality may, in fact, become material in his or her visual function (Figure 15-2).

For further discussion and a more detailed description of aspheric monovision and its optical and neurocognitive superiority to current multifocal techniques of presbyopic IOL correction, I refer you to Chapters 77 and 78 written on this subject in *Mastering Refractive IOLs: The Art and the Science* by Dr. David F. Chang.[5,6]

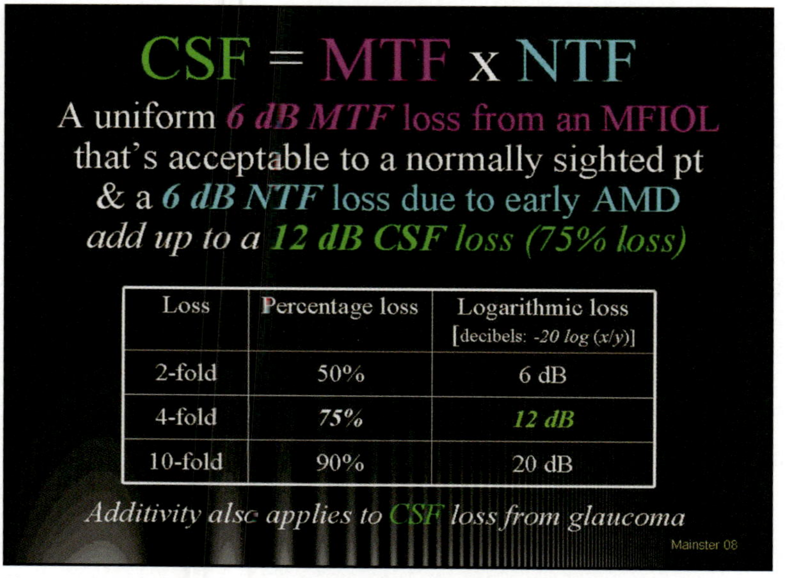

Figure 15-2. Using a multifocal IOL decreases the reserved visual sensitivity of the neurotransfer function. A person with a normal reserve may not notice this diminution. The additional loss of early maculopathy, however, may deplete the neurotransfer function to a level that is very noticeable clinically. These losses are logarithmic, not linear. AMD = age-related macular degeneration, CSF = contrast sensitivity function, MFIOL = multifocal intraocular lens, MTF = modulation transfer function, NTF = neurotransfer function, pt = patient. (Reprinted with permission from Martin A. Mainster, PhD, MD, FRCOphth.)

From a very practical standpoint, monovision, from day 1, provides the surgeon and patient the best alternative. By utilizing a pair of spectacles, monovision always affords the patient and the surgeon the best "fall-back position." The patient's optical neuroprocessing bases are never compromised. The patient has instant access to a full binocular complement of vision by simply utilizing a pair of spectacles. Similarly, night vision can be instantly restored to its fullest visual potential by supplementation with a pair of spectacles. Thus, when the surgeon uses aspheric monofocal presbyopic IOL correction, he or she never backs him- or herself or his or her patient into a potentially visually compromised situation.[7]

Integrating Monovision Option Into the Presbyopic Premium Channel

Delivering spectacle independence using monovision requires the same precise patient education, staff attention and awareness, and accurate biometrics and surgical skill sets as any other form of presbyopic surgery. It requires a complete complement of staff and physician skills.

Table 15-1
Additional Tests Required

▲ Stereopsis	▲ Ocular dominance
▲ Blur suppression	▲ Corneal topography
▲ Phorias	▲ Pupil size

Part I: Educating Patients

Most patients today are not aware that cataract surgery presents their best opportunity to finally rid themselves of spectacle dependence. In our practice, many patients think of LASIK, not lens or cataract surgery, as the surgery pathway to becoming glasses-independent. When the patient calls for a cataract evaluation appointment, we introduce the fact that many times spectacle independence can be an outcome, and we tell them we are going to include some information in his or her packet. This information is general and mentions in a very undetailed manner the options available, one of which is *continuous vision*, our wording for monovision.

When the patient arrives for his or her appointment and our staff technician does his or her intake history and general medical examination, the question is asked again: "Are you interested in hearing about spectacle independence?" Multifocal, accommodative, and continuous vision are described. The advantages and disadvantages of each are presented in a fairly simple manner. If the patient has a strong preconception that he or she wants one or the other, this issue is addressed. We tend to let the patient describe his or her predetermined prejudice. We present the fact that all of the choices can work, but they are in their infancies and are marginal compared with 20-year-old vision. In addition, if astigmatism is found to be present, we explain that modification or elimination is necessary if one wants to achieve spectacle independence. At this time, the patient usually asks about cost. If so, the cost of each option is presented. Since monovision does not require the purchase of a much more expensive IOL, we explain that this savings can be passed on to the patient.

How Is the Charge for Astigmatism Addressed?

Astigmatism correction is a necessary component for the success of any premium choice, and generally the patient will need to have 0.5 diopter (D) or less to be successful.[8] Because correcting astigmatism is a surgical procedure not covered by insurance or Medicare, and because it may require an enhancement about 20% of the time, there is a significant cost to this enhancement process. This cost is in addition to the cost of continuous vision or blended vision. Most patients with astigmatism are aware of their condition and, in fact, we find they easily accept this component and its cost. Remember, these patients have had their spectacle prescription altered by their optometrists due to their astigmatism throughout their lifetime of eyeglass purchases.

How Is the Charge for Monovision Addressed?

If one selects advanced aspheric monovision, or, as we refer to it, *blended vision* or *continuous vision*, the patient incurs a global charge. These tests are listed in Table 15-1.

The documentation of this is available at Corcoran's Web site (www.corcoranccg.com). The additional testing is coded as a *super refraction,* as well as an assessment of additional cognitive skills that enhance or detract from the success of monovision. Topography reveals whether there is any corneal impediment to blended vision success, as each eye after cataract surgery must individually deliver a noncompromised image in order for the cortical component of blended vision to work. The one thing I do not do is a contact lens trial. I have found even the process of putting in the contact lens discourages the patient, as well as the fact that at least a 3-week period of successful contact lens all-time wear is required in order for the patient to neuroadapt.

We have found adapting to IOL monovision is easier than monovision with contact lens. We have never done contact lens trials of monovision to predict IOL monovision success, just as we never used spectacle monovision trials to predict the success of contact lens monovision.

What Are the Compromises of Monovision?

Binocular IOL monovision is great but not perfect. There is some loss of best acuity in low contrast. With the use of PDAs as well as computer screens for near, the higher screen vs paper contrast provides acceptable near component with a lower-power near. There is some small loss of measurable stereopsis, but this is inconsequential when viewing a PDA or computer screen. We find those with strong preoperative stereopsis maintain a strong tendency for high-level stereopsis postoperatively and adapt easily. If a patient expresses some anxiety about adaptation, at each point of the examination, he or she is reassured that almost anyone can adapt. The results can always be reversed by, at worst, wearing a pair of glasses. I also hold in reserve, and use occasionally, the removal of the near eye correction with, almost always, a mini-radial keratotomy (usually 2 incisions, sometimes 4), as described in Chapter 16 of this book. Surgeons not comfortable with incisional surgery for myopia can always use laser vision correction as their fallback position, or simply a pair of reading glasses. The reassurance that aspheric monovision can be removed with a simple refractive procedure, when said with assurance, is the most important comfort factor for the person undergoing spectacle-independence surgery. The willingness to do so releases almost all of the patient's anxiety. This refractive touch-up is much easier for me and less anxiety producing for the patient than having to go back and remove a multifocal lens in order to reverse a multifocal lens choice. The actual occurrence of this in our practice is less than 0.01%.

The Surgeon's Role

By the time the patient reaches the doctor, most of the questions have been answered by the highly trained tech. The patient has made his or her choice, and I usually end up spending less than 5 minutes of my time answering questions. I explain that our eyes are like television cameras and that, in actuality, "we see with our brain."

If the patient expresses doubt about his or her being able to adapt to blended vision, I show him or her how with one eye occluded we see our nose, but with both eyes open we do not. I may also add that if we truly saw with our eyes, our world would jiggle up and down with every step we took. I reassure them that 95% of people will adapt, and if they do not, they can always wear a pair of glasses or have their monovision surgically reversed. We are talking about, at most, a -1.25 surgical procedure.

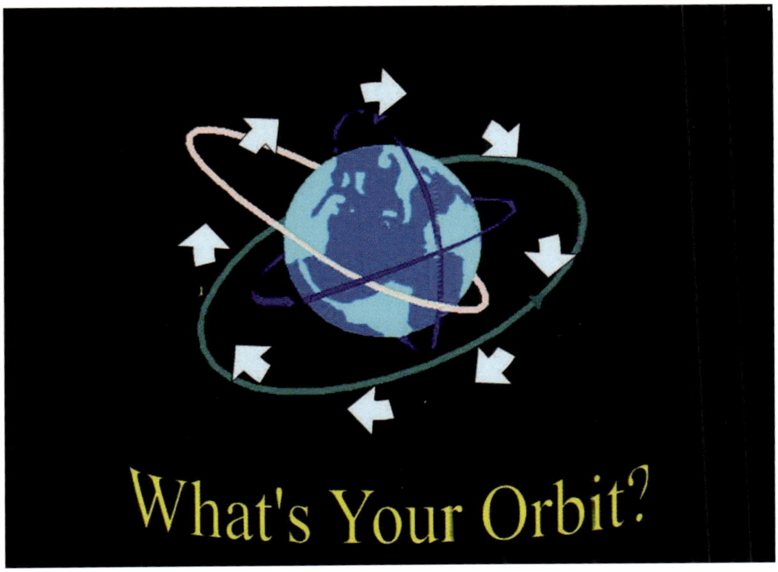

Figure 15-3. What's your orbit?

The fact that everyone over age 45 years in our office does monovision with contacts or IOLs helps give the patient the confidence that he or she has made an excellent choice. At this point, I will stress that if he or she has chosen monovision instead of a more expensive choice (in our practice, an accommodative lens), he or she has not made a less desirable decision nor has he or she shortchanged him- or herself through this choice. I often interject that this is what I did with my mother, my wife, my sister, my brother-in-law, and my aunts, and that they all are happy with their outcomes. I also use this point to again remind the patient that it is not the vision of a 25-year-old, and he or she may still require or feel more comfortable driving at night or doing intense close work with glasses. My goal is 80/80; 80% of the time, 80% of my patients do not wear glasses.

The importance of the doctor's confidence in his or her product, and that he or she can deliver, cannot be overemphasized. In fact, each person in the office must be confident about the fact that blended vision is a successful avenue that delivers happy patients. Figure 15-3 depicts our orbit of presbyopic cataract lens correction. Notice how many phases of what we call *patient touch* are involved. Each staff touch has the ability to coach this person's motivation and confidence to succeed, usually by his or her own personal experience.

Part II: The Implementation

The Refractive Orbit

Until this point, you have heard in a didactic manner how I, as a surgeon, see this process. However, as you turn your attention to integrating monovision into your practice, start by looking at your *sphere of patient contact* as an orbit. So, "What's your orbit?"

The concept is recognizing that your practice currently has a usual and customary way of interacting with patients. We call this our orbit; the goal here is to, as a team, document, with as much detail as possible, every touchpoint you have with a patient as he or she walks through the preoperative process. You will want to be detailed, because once you have recorded your current processes accurately, you will be able to show how the new processes being integrated are simply adjustments to the things you already do vs major change initiatives. Given the human tendency to resist change, you will likely find this approach helpful as you introduce the process to your staff.

The next step in light of each touchpoint you have identified is to consider possible opportunities to begin a conversation regarding options for spectacle independence after cataract surgery. The objective is to raise patient awareness of the existence of such opportunity. In the beginning phase of integration, you will want to focus on touchpoints such as including information about spectacle independence in the paperwork that is mailed to cataract patients. You may want to have your front desk confirm that the patient received the information about options for spectacle independence as he or she arrives for his or her preoperative appointment. Eventually, you will find the conversation about spectacle independence through cataract surgery permeating the fabric of your practice. Early on, when cataracts are first diagnosed, perhaps long before surgery is indicated, the patient is made aware of advances in technology that make spectacle independence a positive part of the process of leaving the world of a deteriorating natural lens. To some degree, this conversation will actually begin to define your practice, potentially differentiating you from others who practice ophthalmology in your community.

I have outlined some specific points in our orbit related to moving the conversation about spectacle independence forward. While every person along the way plays a role, the ophthalmic technician is pivotal to the overall process.

Upon arrival, the patient goes through a preoperative interview, which is focused on simply gathering medical history and information about current medications (this is a normal part of the preoperative process). The interviewer notes, "I see you have indicated interest in options for spectacle independence (or not)." The interviewer simply gets the thoughts of the patient as related to spectacle independence. The interviewer provides only a basic description of options, noting the fact that (depending on certain variables), "The cost per eye could be as little as what one pair of glasses would cost for the rest of your life" or "For some people, if you have significant astigmatism, the cost would be more, but that is something the technician will test for and discuss with you today." Many people are aware or have been told by the optometrist they have astigmatism. The big point is that we are beginning a conversation with the patient a little bit at a time as the process unfolds.

In our practice, we have a registered nurse from our own ambulatory surgery center do this interview, combining history and physical and anesthesia questions during this process. We have found that the connection between the registered nurse at preoperation all the way through surgery day is helpful and comforting—very personalized care—and the doctors like the upfront awareness of red flags related to the patient's health (eg, need for surgery clearance from the primary care physician). This step could be less medically focused if a practice simply wants to build the conversation prior to starting the preoperative process.

At the end of the preoperative interview, we show the Eyemaginations loop, educating the patient about cataract surgeries, monovision, accommodating lenses, and multifocal lenses (about 5 minutes). At the end of the video, the patient is introduced to the technician, who proceeds with preliminary tests (eg, standard diagnostic testing related to preoperative cataract).

Following the preliminary testing (refraction auto/K's/IOLMaster [Carl Zeiss Meditec]), the technician simply affirms or confirms the patient's indicated interest in knowing about options and costs for reduced dependence on glasses and introduces the fact that he or she will be talking more about these options as he or she works through the preoperative visit (just another opportunity to affirm patient's interest) and then proceed to examination lane. The technician injects affirming statements, such as, "You may have noticed I don't wear spectacles, as I have continuous vision and love it."

At examination lane, the technician starts gathering preoperative information. During the phoropter work, if the presence of astigmatism is noted, there should be a discussion of what astigmatism is and how it affects vision, a demonstration with a phoropter, and an example of vision with and without astigmatism correction, noting that in order to achieve spectacle independence we must get rid of the astigmatism, which is possible through surgical correction at the time of cataract surgery. So in these cases, there is a decision for the patient to make, and the cost for astigmatism correction is discussed. If there is no significant astigmatism, the technician can take the opportunity to share the good news (ie, the patient has no astigmatism, there is no need to correct it, this keeps the cost down).

Either way, the technician tells the patient we will focus on gathering results of a number of other (standard) tests, and when we have all of this together, we will discuss options in more detail. This is because certain options tend to be better, depending on what we learn with these tests. After the basic preoperative testing is completed, the technician discusses options with the patient; this discussion will be tailored to each patient based on preoperative findings to that point (eg, astigmatism greater than 2.00 D indicates a discussion about toric lens with monovision—other options would not apply). No astigmatism or little astigmatism would open the door for monovision or enhanced monovision (we use the phrase continuous vision), and the applicable respective costs would be discussed. Following this discussion, the technician states, "You may already be leaning toward a certain option, but at this point, if you would like to pursue any option for reduced dependence on glasses, we will need to do some testing that is specific to these options. This is not covered by your insurance. The cost is high for these tests. You do not have to choose a specific option at this point, but you will need to have these tests performed regardless of which option you choose, and each option includes this cost."

Once nonstandard testing is completed, the patient is made ready for the doctor to enter examination lane (eg, dilated). The doctor typically *blesses* or suggests that the posterior chamber IOL may not be the best option; but generally, the surgeon is not spending inordinate amounts of time educating patients about available options. This has been handled by the technician, as he or she has walked the patient along the way.

The doctor discusses the findings, gives a blessing or recommendation, and then makes the surgical plan.

Then it is time to schedule the surgery, at which time the patient's decision is reviewed and documented, and the patient signs the proper forms (eg, Notice of Exclusion from Medicare Benefits) related to options and acknowledging out-of-pocket expenses for the noncovered services. The surgery scheduler states, "These fees can be paid today or on the day of your surgery," which will elicit questions regarding financing options from patients who are not prepared to pay on the day of surgery.

Guiding Principles: Developing the Scripting/Message Process

In the larger scheme of this process, we find that our clinic staff, regardless of their function, is called on to approach each interaction with patients as an actor or guide. It is advisable to literally script the message. The point of this exercise is for your staff members to work at saying just the right thing at just the right time in just the right way to allow your patients to understand that you "get it" (ie, you are engaged with them enough to understand what they really want). The following 4 guiding principles will be helpful in the scripting process.

Function as a Guide in the Transformative Process Related to Spectacle Independence After Cataract Surgery

In the role as guide, we want to raise the aspiration of our patients to a higher place, not focus on the product. In the context of their vision, many patients need our help to envision what reduced dependence on glasses means. Many truly cannot imagine the freedom of waking up without needing to put on glasses just to get out of bed. So we talk about spectacle independence in terms that help the patient to visualize the possibilities. Every person who touches the patient along the way, from the optometrist who diagnoses a cataract for the first time to the scheduler making the preoperative appointment to the technician working up the cataract patient, should carefully consider what words he or she will use to have this conversation.

Focus Distinctly on the Benefit Available Through Monovision Versus Lens Design

As previously mentioned, in guiding the patient, every staff member should be deliberate in choosing words that communicate the benefit available through spectacle independence after cataract surgery. The goal would be to focus statements in a context that the patient can imagine (with our help.) Certainly most people plan to wake up each morning and get out of bed and do various activities around the house, so our statements should be geared to such a context and tuned precisely by listening to interactions with patients (eg, do they use a computer? Are they in an assisted living facility in which they fear losing their glasses?). The fact that today, and in the future, our world revolves around our PDA is especially powerful in helping the patient visualize their potential freedom from spectacles. The blue-collar worker who can use machinery, drills, and screwdrivers without spectacles is benefitted as much as the office worker.

Walking the patient through his or her day and pointing out the frequency with which he or she uses near to intermediate distance vision opens almost every patient's eyes to the benefit of monovision. While some will say, "I don't mind wearing glasses," many will think about the possibility and find it appealing, especially for as little as the cost of a pair of glasses, for the rest of their lives.

Open the Conversation About Spectacle Independence as Early and as Often as Possible

We should look for every possible opportunity to open the conversation about spectacle independence. At the first diagnosis of cataract, in the preoperative packet we mail to the patient, when scheduling the preoperative appointment, in virtually every context where we mention cataract surgery, we should be informing patients about the existence of these options. As we make this a regular part of the conversation, we will find, over time, the patient will be more educated about these options and will actually initiate the discussion. We know word of mouth is the most effective marketing tool we have, so as we "produce" more patients with spectacle independence, we will begin to be defined by that reality from the public's perception. We will begin to see people coming to the practice because other doctors only do "regular" cataract surgery.

Prepare to Guide the Patient Beyond Surgery Day

It is important that we learn to anticipate patient responses and to then prepare to help the patient through the process of visual recovery. We know, for example, the near vision eye is likely to be the first eye for surgery; therefore, we know the patient will not have clear distance vision (it is the near/intermediate range). The point here is to celebrate and encourage the patient because we know "getting the reading vision is the hardest part." At every step along the way, if we can prepare the patient for what we anticipate (because he or she does not have the experience we have), he or she will be more comfortable (because we remove the potential for unknown as much as possible). I know with refractive surgery (eg, LASIK) there is that moment with the microkeratome when things go dark for the patient. I have heard many patients afterward comment on how they were glad to have been told multiple times to expect that, because it was not so frightening as it would have been. The biggest fear factor is related to things that are unknown. So, in cataract surgery, when we come to the point of describing the procedure or explaining the preoperative process or the individual nature of the healing process, we anticipate and guide the patient along the way.

Our goal is to always have happy patients. Setting and managing expectations is the key to happy patients. We must consider part of preoperative care as coaching. In every aspect of our practice, each staff member's actions are described as that of a coach. The adaptation to a new pair of glasses many times involves coaching. The transformation to spectacle independence involves coaching, and when a patient reaches a difficult hurdle, this is when coaching is needed the most. The less-than-happy patient can be brought along to acceptance. Listening to the patient's issue and acknowledging his or her disappointment, many times, is all it takes. We almost always err on the side of myopia. We always have done so because the corneal approach to making someone less myopic is always easier and better. Frequently, it is a matter of reducing the amount of myopia rather than totally eliminating it. Occasionally, in doing the near eye first, we fall short, and the patient ends up plano. We will do the second eye for near, essentially "flipping" the near and far eye. In a study performed in our clinic, we found that success with monovision was independent of whether the dominate eye ended up to be the near or far eye.

Conclusion

Monovision is a natural process, and if for some reason intervention is required, whether spectacle or surgical, the fallback position always leaves the patient with the highest possible optical contrast result. Future visual additive technologies are a possibility. As our patients age and their vision gradually decreases, monofocality always preserves their highest contrast potential. Remember, advanced aspheric monofocal blended vision does the following:

- ▲ Preserves a lifetime of quality of vision.
- ▲ Capitalizes on our age-related decreasing pupillary aperture, yielding an increasing depth of focus.
- ▲ Affords the easiest and safest fallback position for the patient (pair of spectacles) and for the surgeon (incisional or laser vision correction).

References

1. Greenbaum S. Monovision pseudophakia. *J Cataract Refract Surg.* 2002;28(8):1439-1443.
2. Nakamura K, Bissen-Miyajima H, Oki S, Onuma K. Pupil sizes in different Japanese age groups and the implications for intraocular lens choice. *J Cataract Refract Surg.* 2009;35(1):134-138.
3. Handa T, Mukuno K, Uozato H, et al. Ocular dominance and patient satisfaction after monovision induced by intraocular lens implantation. *J Cataract Refract Surg.* 2004;30(4):769-774.
4. Yang E, Blake R, McDonald JE II. A new interocular suppression technique for measuring sensory eye dominance. *Invest Ophthalmol Vis Sci.* 2010;51(1):588-593.
5. McDonald JE II, Deitz DJ. Monovision with aspheric IOLs. In: Chang DF, ed. *Mastering Refractive IOLs: The Art and Science.* Thorofare, NJ: SLACK Incorporated; 2008:291-294.
6. McDonald JE II, Deitz DJ. Neuroadaptation to monovision. In: Chang DF, ed. *Mastering Refractive IOLs: The Art and Science.* Thorofare, NJ: SLACK Incorporated; 2008:295-301.
7. McDonald JE II. Why I am not implanting multifocals. *Cataract & Refractive Surgery Today.* 2010;Feb:69-71.
8. Rubin M. Perspectives in refraction. *Surv Ophthalmol.* 1996;40(6):491-499.

Chapter 16

Multifocal Implants

Farrell (Toby) Tyson, MD, FACS

First Patients to Choose

When getting started with multifocal intraocular lenses (IOL), it is just as important to choose the right patient as it is which type of multifocal. Many surgeons start out their multifocal careers in disappointment by choosing a medical outlier for their first patient. Your multifocal patients should be some of your happiest patients, because you are "cherry picking" them from the start.

Initial evaluation should start with your basic biometry before you enter the examination room. This helps you lead the discussion with patients in an efficient manner. First, evaluate the amount of astigmatism. The keratometric astigmatism magnitude should be under 1 diopter (D) to start with. This low level of astigmatism is generally well tolerated by patients with multifocals and may not require enhancements. Next, evaluate the type of astigmatism. If the astigmatism is asymmetric, then exclude this patient, as even future enhancements will be difficult. Small amounts of symmetric astigmatism can easily be dealt with by wound placement, small limbal relaxing incisions (LRI), or femtosecond laser astigmatic incisions.

Multifocal IOLs do well in a large range of axial lengths. When starting out, I would recommend staying in the more normal ranges. This is due to the inherent loss of IOL power accuracy at the extremes, which leads to a higher likelihood of IOL surprise, which is poorly tolerated in multifocal IOLs. Low hyperopes are some of the best initial patients for multifocals, because you are taking a patient with poor uncorrected distance and near vision and giving them both. The bar is low with these patients. High hyperopes would seem like equally easy patients to satisfy, but effective lens position is harder to predict in these smaller eyes, which can lead to a refractive surprise. This can

Hovanesian JA.
Refractive Cataract Surgery: Best Practices and Advanced Technology, Second Edition (pp 189-198). © 2017 SLACK Incorporated.

be equally true of high myopes. Caution must be used in selecting low myopes for multifocals. Their uncorrected preoperative near vision is usually pretty good and at a set focal length. Operating on a low myope may give him or her the best of both worlds but may also change his or her near working distance and magnification. Careful preoperative counseling is necessary for success.

Basic eye pathology needs to be assessed next. The majority of your multifocal patients are going to be in your cataract age group. This same group of patients usually has some dry eye issues. The extent of their dry eyes needs to be evaluated and treated first, before multifocal implantation. Most patients' conditions are easily controlled with artificial tears, gel, or punctual plugs. If further treatment is necessary, cyclosporine ophthalmic drops can be very beneficial. If the dry eye symptomatology does not abate with treatment, then monofocal implantation should be considered. Ocular surface disease causes a loss of contrast and an increase in glare, which is incompatible with multifocal IOLs.

Endothelial health should be evaluated. Moderate to severe guttata should be avoided, as it leads to loss of contrast sensitivity. The presence of pseudoexfoliation or zonular instability should be ascertained. In early cases, these patients should be excluded, but with greater experience they may be successfully treated with the use of 3-piece multifocals and/or capsular tension rings. The concern being short- and long-term lens stability and centration.

Posterior pole evaluation should be relatively benign. Make sure to look for small epiretinal membranes. They have a tendency to cause trouble in your multifocal patients. A preoperative macular optical coherence tomography evaluation may save you hours of headaches by evaluating retinal structure. In addition, a flicker pattern electroretinogram can elucidate potential problems by evaluating retinal function. Active diabetic retinopathy or macular drusen/degeneration are additional red flags. To achieve initial success with multifocal IOLs, one needs to limit the number of possible complications.

Setting Up Expectations

Setting the expectations for patients may be the most difficult part of multifocal IOL implantation for the beginning surgeon. This is because most surgeons have not been trained to interact personally with patients or in the past have deferred this task to surgery counselors or technicians. Multifocal patients have high demands from the beginning. They expect more because they are paying more. These expectations include the fact that they want real interaction with their surgeon. This is your chance to set the stage and manage expectations. If you don't, the patient is always going to be disappointed, because they walk in expecting perfect vision at all distances.

We have all heard the phrase, "under promise and over deliver." That is easier said than done. I like to start by letting the patient know that there is nothing perfect in life, especially cataract surgery, but the technology has come a long way and we can now help provide a fuller range of vision. I let them know not to expect 18-year-old eyes. On the other hand, I like to have them hold a reading card at the appropriate working distance and show them what they can reasonably expect of their postoperative near vision and where.

Different multifocals perform differently at different near focal lengths and under different conditions. This allows you to tailor the lens to the patient's lifestyle. A good general opening question is "What do you like to do?" This helps you realize whether the individual is detail-oriented, a reader, or a more intermediate-task individual. One of the more defining traits is computer use. This task can steer your choice considerably. The ReSTOR (Alcon) aspheric 4.0 lens has a near focal length of 33 cm, the Tecnis ZMAOO and ZMBOO (Abbott Medical Optics) multifocal lenses have a near focal length of 37 cm, and the ReSTOR aspheric 3.0 lens has a focal length of 44 cm. The newer ReSTOR aspheric 2.5 lens has focal length of 50 cm. The low add Tecnis multifocals ZKBOO (2.75) and ZLBOO (3.25) have respective focal lengths of 50 cm and 44 cm. All of these aspheric multifocals provide excellent distance vision.

Dysphotopsias are probably the most important part of the preoperative discussion. If they aren't addressed before the surgery, they will surely be after the surgery. Luckily, this current generation of multifocals has made great strides in reducing the perceived glare and halos at night by reducing the spherical aberrations in the ocular system. In addition, the migration toward lower add powers that require fewer rings has further reduced the perceived glare and halos of this category of IOLs. Many patients are now aware of premium lenses from their friends, with varying degrees of success and failure. It is appropriate to address the fact that older style multifocals did have significant glare issues.

Cerebral adaptation is difficult to convey to patients in scientific terms. I find it best to explain it to them through analogy. I tell them cataract surgery is like getting a new ring. "At first, you know it is there, and you look at it and play with it. Over time, though, you almost forget it is on, but if you look for it you can still see it. The same is true with your vision. Immediately after cataract surgery, everything is going to be brighter and more vibrant. At night, you might notice some rings and halos around lights. Over the next 3 months, that usually diminishes and goes away, but if you look for them, you can still find them."

Cerebral summation has been shown to improve both distance and near vision by at least 1.5 lines of acuity. Therefore, I inform my patients not to expect much of their vision after the first eye, that it takes both eyes for the brain to truly utilize multifocal IOLs. This statement lowers their expectations between surgeries and allows for the second surgery to be performed in hesitant patients. Cerebral summation is very effective in masking the deficiencies of a single eye.

Preoperative Measurements

Multifocal IOL implantation requires not only accurate preoperative measurements but reproducible ones. Good outcomes are achieved when variability is minimized, and this can be done through optimization of your IOL power calculation formulas. Corneal topography should be performed on all multifocal candidates to rule out asymmetric astigmatism that could be masked on a manual or an optical biometry A-scan keratometer.

Axial length measurements are critical to success. This measurement should be obtained with either an immersion ultrasound unit, IOLMaster (Carl Zeiss Meditec),

Lenstar (Haag-Streit), or other optical biometer. These methods are noncontact, accurate, and reproducible. Contact ultrasonography should not be used, as it allows for too much variability in axial length measurements.

Keratometry can come from a manual keratometer, corneal topographer, IOLMaster, Lenstar, or other method. One method should be chosen in a practice to maintain consistency so that IOL power calculation optimization can be performed accurately. Most practices have chosen to use an automated method to reduce the variability between different technicians.

Pupil size should be measured in both light and dark conditions. In the past, small pupils would rule out the use of ReZoom (Abbott Medical Optics) IOLs, as the reading benefit was lost. Now, patients with large photopic pupils may benefit from the Tecnis multifocal's full diffractive optic in providing reading vision at large pupil sizes. The ReSTOR aspheric 4.0/3.0/2.5 become distance dominant at larger pupil sizes. Some patients present with very small and poorly dilating pupils. These patients lose the aspheric correction of the current multifocals due to the small pupil size and may have limited multifocality. These individuals would do better with a monofocal and probably will still have good depth of field due to the pinhole effect.

Corneal aberrometry can be obtained with some of the newer diagnostic equipment, such as the OPD III (Nidek), iTrace (Tracey), and Galilei (Ziemer). By obtaining the corneal spherical aberration, one can better match the appropriate multifocal IOL to minimize the total postoperative spherical aberration. Studies have shown that contrast sensitivity increases and glare decreases as spherical aberration is minimized. The average corneal spherical aberration in the cataract patient population is +0.27 microns.[1,2] This can vary significantly from patient to patient and eye to eye, especially if refractive surgery has been previously been performed. The ReSTOR aspheric 4.0/3.0 lenses correct for 0.1 microns of spherical aberration, whereas the ReSTOR 2.5 lens corrects for 0.2 microns of spherical aberration. The Tecnis multifocal family corrects for 0.27 microns of spherical aberration. This difference in value allows the surgeon to custom match the IOL to the patient's cornea for reduced glare and halos and better contrast sensitivity.

Angle kappa, the measurement between the pupillary center and the optical axis, has become more important in the assessment of potential multifocal IOL patients. As angle kappa increases, there has been a correlation with unhappy multifocal patients.[3] Patients with large angle kappas, greater than 0.4 mm or 2.8 degrees when using a penlight,[4] should avoid multifocal implantation.

Contraindications

Multifocal IOLs place a greater demand on the optical system of the eye. Therefore, there are some pathologies that are incompatible with the current multifocal IOLs. Most surgeons will not implant multifocal IOLs when any maculopathies are present. While early macular degeneration may show good postoperative visual potential, the disease course is known to be progressive. This contrast-reducing disease combined with a contrast-reducing lens platform is not the best combination. An aspheric monofocal IOL would be a better choice.

Diabetes, if well controlled without retinopathy, would not be a contraindication. If retinopathy is present and control is questionable, then multifocals should be avoided. Once again, we have to be considering how the retina is going to be not just 1 month postoperatively but 10 years postoperatively.

Glaucoma is another relative contraindication. If the patient has significant glaucomatous damage, then the macula has already lost some of it contrast sensitivity. In these glaucoma patients, a multifocal IOL would be contraindicated. Since the advent of better screening and treatment of glaucoma, many patients present with well-controlled intraocular pressures and no glaucomatous damage. These well-controlled glaucoma patients, with appropriate counseling, should have the option of multifocal IOLs.

Any corneal pathology that might reduce contrast sensitivity or induce glare should be avoided. Corneal scarring and gross dystrophies are relatively easy to diagnose. It is the more subtle changes that can be a problem postoperatively if left undiagnosed. Careful attention should be made for anterior basement membrane disease and mild corneal guttata; both can worsen postoperatively and severely degrade the performance of multifocal IOLs. Any evidence of keratoconus or pellucid marginal degeneration on corneal topography is a contraindication for multifocal IOLs.

When first starting with multifocal IOLs, all previous corneal refractive surgery patients should not be implanted with multifocal IOLs. Over time and experience, certain patients may benefit from multifocal IOLs only after thorough counseling. All radial keratometry patients are contraindicated from multifocal IOLs due to their refractive instability. Prior hyperopic LASIK or photorefractive keratectomy (PRK) patients should not receive any of the current multifocal IOLs, as it would exacerbate the spherical aberration and cause increased glare and halos. In addition, it would be mixing a multifocal cornea with a multifocal lens, which do not work well together. Previous myopic LASIK or PRK patients have increased corneal spherical aberration. In these patients, refractive surprise is more common due to the change in corneal curvature affecting the effective lens position in our current formulas. If a multifocal IOL is to be used in post myopic LASIK or PRK patients, the Tecnis multifocal IOL family would be the better choice, as it corrects the greatest amount of spherical aberration of the current generation of multifocal IOLs.

Intraocular Lens Selection and Targeting

The good news is that we have options. The bad news is that no one lens can do it all yet. The first step is to match the technology to the patient's lifestyle. The current multifocal IOLs all have very good distance vision, so the key is to ask which is more important to the patient: near or intermediate vision. The ReSTOR aspheric 4.0 and Tecnis ZMA/BOO both have exceptional near vision, whereas the ReSTOR 3.0/2.5 and Tecnis ZK/LBOO have better intermediate vision than near.

If the patient is a heavy computer user, then the ReSTOR 2.5 or Tecnis ZKBOO have a higher probability of providing spectacle-free usage of the computer. The Tecnis ZMA/BOO patients do very well on the computer without glasses, but it cannot be guaranteed. The ReSTOR aspheric 4.0 patients will not be able to use the computer without moving the monitor toward them substantially. The ReSTOR 3.0 and Tecnis ZLBOO

Table 16-1
Multifocal/Accommodating Optimized IOLMaster Constants

Manufacturer	Crys-talens AO	ReSTOR 3.0/4.0/3.0	Re-STOR 2.5	Tecnis ZMA00	Tecnis ZLB00 ZKB00 ZMB00
A Const	119.0	118.9	119.1	119.1	118.8
SRK II A Const	118.4	119.13	119.8	120.0	119.87
SRK/T A Const	118.5	119.01	119.5	119.5	119.53
Haigis a0	1.156	-0.385625	1.66	-1.75013	-1.0130.998
a1	0.4	0.1973	0.4	0.2424	0.1994
a2	0.1	0.204217	0.1	0.2661	0.242239
Hoffer Q pACD	5.38	5.6461	5.82	5.8028	5.8978
Holladay SF	1.54	1.84 83	2.07	2.061.49	2.1200

are a good compromise between computer and reading vision. This is easily explained when looking at the different IOLs' working distances.

Since the extended range of add powers has become available to the multifocal category, several surgeons have advocated using different add powers in different eyes. This is not true mixing and matching, as we used to see by mixing dissimilar technologies, but now we are using identical distance optics with slightly differing near adds. There have been different strategies to implement this. The most common is to place the lower add multifocal in the dominant eye. If the patient is happy with his or her near vision, place the similar add power in the fellow eye. On the other hand, if he or she feel his or her near vision is too weak in the first eye, then the second eye should receive a larger add power.

Pilots, truck drivers, and patients in any other occupation who cannot tolerate nighttime glare or halos should not receive any multifocal. If nighttime near vision is important, then the Tecnis multifocal family would be the best choice. This can be seen in flight attendants, who need to be able to read labels in dim light. The ReSTOR aspheric family becomes distance dominant in dim light, which prevents good reading under such circumstances but reduces glare and halos.

When starting with multifocals, I suggest starting with an automated biometry system such as the IOLMaster. It is able to obtain your keratometry, axial length, anterior chamber depth, and white-to-white readings for you, and then integrate some of them into a variety of IOL calculation formulas. Initially use the built-in Holladay I or Holladay II formula, as they are ideal for average-length eyes. As you expand your patient base into the extremes, you may consider the Hoffer Q for smaller eyes and the SRK/T for larger eyes. In Table 16-1, you will see some optimized IOL constants for the different formulas and the different lenses. After implanting 25 of your own patients, you can further optimize these values based on your results.

When targeting monofocal IOLs, we usually aim for a little minus in case we are off a little hyperopically. With multifocals it is a little different. The ReSTOR aspheric 4.0 and the Tecnis ZMA/BOO are best targeted for plano. If forced to choose between a little minus or a little plus, target a little minus. Leaving the patient a little minus allows for easier enhancement with LRIs or LASIK/PRK. The ReSTOR aspheric 3.0/2.5 has the same A-constant as the ReSTOR aspheric 4.0, but it is best to aim for a little minus. This is because you do not want the near focal point greater than arm's length. The Tecnis ZK/ZLBOO does best when aiming for a little minus to plano. Some discussion has been given to mini monovision with multifocals. When starting out, I would recommend matching the 2 eyes to get the best cerebral summation.

Intraoperative Pearls

Incision location can be used to reduce against-the-rule astigmatism when operating from the temporal aspect. This will usually result in a reduction of about 0.25 D. Beyond that, corneal relaxing incisions need to be planned accordingly or deferred until a month postoperatively when the eye has stabilized.

Capsulorrhexis size should be approximately 5.5 mm to allow for a slight overlapping of the optic. This helps with better centration. If using a femtosecond laser, the capsulorrhexis is better to be pupil-centered than bag-centered. This allows for easier centration of the optic to align pupil-centered, which has been thought to be superior to an optical axis–centered multifocal IOL. This is because you obtain more constructive interference in a pupil-centered orientation than an optical axis–centration if they are different. An overlapping capsulorrhexis helps diminish temporal dysphotopsias common with square-edge acrylic IOLs (Figure 16-1). This also allows for easier explantation in the future, if necessary. Be careful not to make the capsulorrhexis too small, because capsular phimosis may occur, resulting in decentration of the optic.

Good cortical cleanup will help prevent posterior capsular opacification, which can quickly reduce the quality of vision in multifocal IOLs. Multifocals as a class tend to require yttrium-aluminum-garnet capsulotomies at a greater rate and sooner than monofocal IOLs. This is due to multifocal IOLs being more sensitive to contrast loss and higher expectations of multifocal patients. Following implantation, be sure to aspirate all of the viscoelastic that may be behind the lens.

Centering of the 3-piece Tecnis multifocal is not necessary, because its design is self-centering by nature. The 1-piece Tecnis multifocal and ReSTOR aspheric 4.0/3.0 may benefit by nudging the optic nasally in the bag. This action helps align the optical axis with the visual axis. The Tecnis multifocal IOL is a little more forgiving, in that its central ring is 35% larger than the ReSTOR's, allowing for a slightly larger "sweet spot."

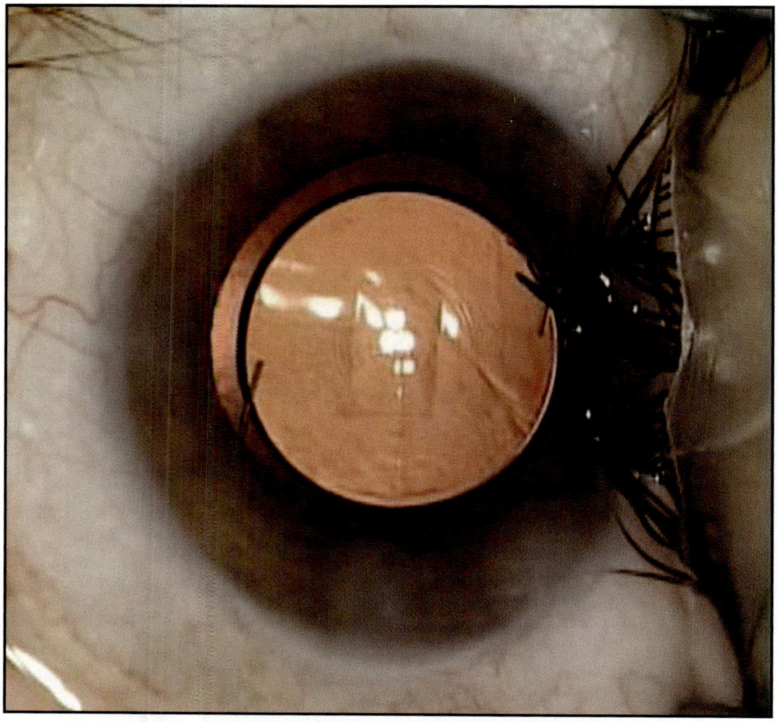

Figure 16-1. Tecnis ZMA00 multifocal with overlapping capsulorrhexis.

Postsurgical Patient Interactions

Once surgery is done, it is important to continue to engage patients. In the postoperative period, patients do not know what to expect, so they assume their vision should be perfect. It is important for both you and your staff to provide an encouraging environment. When patients come in for follow up, my staff always starts checking the visual acuity at the patient's preoperative uncorrected visual acuity level. This allows the patient to see the progress he or she has made in distance vision. I like to start with a binocular evaluation, because this is going to be better than the monocular values. I then show the patients his or her monocular vision so that he or she understands comparing one eye to the other is not a fair test of their vision. This shows that his or her eyes work better together than either one does by itself.

Near vision is then tested, with a near card in a normally lit room. I start with the near card at arm's length and then let the patient bring it in slowly until it comes into best focus. This allows the patient to understand there is a sweet spot for his or her near vision. After the patient has found his or her ideal reading position, I then use a pair of -3.00 D glasses for the patient to read through. The patient is quickly surprised that his or her near vision disappears. At this point, I explain that this is what his or her near vision would be like if he or she had chosen a standard monofocal IOL. It is important to show this to all of your multifocal patients to cement in what they truly have gained by having multifocal IOLs.

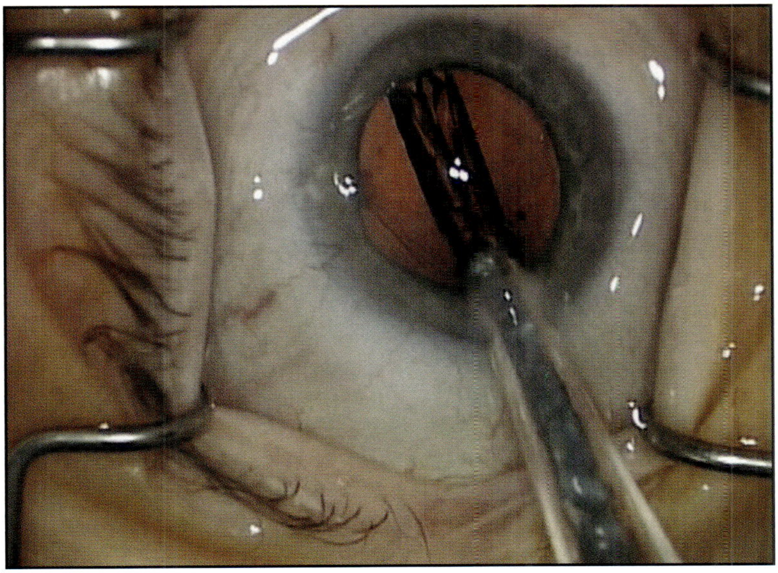

Figure 16-2. Tecnis ZMB00 being injected through a 2.2-mm incision.

On early postoperative visits, it is important to stress that the patient's vision will constantly be improving. This improvement makes the greatest leaps during the first 3 months but continues over the next year. The patient should be made aware that not only will the vision become clearer, but the glare and halos will diminish, and the depth of field will increase. This should be a time of encouragement and support.

Strategies for Enhancements

Though we plan for perfection, we often are left with suboptimal outcomes. One needs to be comfortable with some basic skills or have access to techniques such as corneal relaxing incisions, piggyback lenses, and LASIK/PRK. When dealing with enhancements, it is best to wait until at least 1 month postoperatively when the eye has stabilized. At this point, one needs to determine the cause of dissatisfaction. Is it astigmatism, sphere, or both, and how much?

If you are dealing with small amounts of cylinder, a corneal relaxing incision can be quite effective (Figure 16-2). The multifocal platform can tolerate a little bit of residual sphere, whether myopic or hyperopic. Always anticipate what your post-LRI spherical equivalent is going to be. If it is going to be more than 0.5 D hyperopic or more than 0.75 D myopic, a different form of enhancement may be warranted.

If you are correcting residual sphere, there are a couple of options at your disposal. IOL exchange may be an obvious solution but may be a little more challenging than the other options. A relatively easy and cost-effective solution is the use of a piggyback lens. The STAAR Surgical AQ5010 is an ideal platform for piggybacking, as it has a 6.2 mm optic, which will overlap the multifocal optic and not require precise centration. In addition, it has very long haptics that allow for secure placement in the ciliary sulcus. The lens is made out of silicone and is not prone to interface opacification when piggybacked on an acrylic multifocal IOL. Basic piggyback calculation can be done on several software programs, or you can multiply residual sphere by 1.7 to come up with the piggyback power needed. Piggyback lenses have also been shown to decrease temporal dysphotopsias and reduce glare and halos.

LASIK and PRK can be used to treat not only residual astigmatism and sphere but also a combination of the 2. This can be a very accurate but expensive way to enhance a patient. Concerns have been voiced about the possibility of inducing extra spherical aberration and dry eyes. Wavefront-optimized ablations or standard ablations would be preferred over wavefront guided ablations, as wavefront data from eyes with multifocals can be inaccurate.

Extended Depth of Focus Intraocular Lenses

Abbott's Symfony family of lenses has its roots in the Tecnis product lineup. It uses the same one-piece acrylic platform and A-constant as the Tecnis family of lenses. It is available in both spherical and toric versions. The Symfony IOLs use diffractive optics to minimize both spherical and chromatic aberrations. Unlike multifocal IOLs that use diffractive optics to split light to obtain 2 focal points, though, the Symfony diffractive optics uses constructive interference to maximize light transmission and results in a relatively flat defocus curve over 1.5 D and very usable vision over 2.5 D, with minimization of haloing and glare seen in multifocal designs.

These design elements allow for the use of the Symfony lens in patients with not only pristine eyes but also those with mild pathology and previous refractive surgery. The relatively flat defocus curve makes this lens a good choice in postrefractive patients when surgical planning and biometry are more variable. This family of lenses also lends itself to mini monovision and being used in the dominant eye in mix-and-match scenarios with a multifocal in the nondominant eye.

The benefits of the Symfony lens are negated by large corneal and macular pathology. In these scenarios, a monofocal IOL would be appropriate. Even in these situations, the platform could be considered unlikely to cause harm. Due to the spherical aberration reduction in the design, hyperopic LASIK patients may have a greater problem with haloing and reduced-contrast sensitivity.

References

1. Holladay JT, Piers PA, Koranyi G, van der Mooren M, Norrby NE. A new intraocular lens design to reduce spherical aberration of pseudophakic eyes. *J Refract Surg.* 2002;18(6):683-691.
2. Wang L, Dai E, Koch DD, Nathoo A. Optical aberrations of the human anterior cornea. *J Cataract Refract Surg.* 2003;29(8):1514-1521.
3. Prakash G, Prakash DR, Agarwal A, Kumar DA, Agarwal A, Jacob S. Predictive factor and kappa angle analysis for visual satisfaction in patients with multifocal IOL implantation. *Eye (Lond).* 2011;25:9:1187-1193.
4. Basmak H, Sahin A, Yildirim N, Papakostas TD, Kanellopoulos AJ. Measurement of angle kappa with synoptophore and Orbscan II in a normal population. *J Refract Surg.* 2007;23:456-460.

Chapter 17

Accommodating Implants
The Crystalens

Robert J. Weinstock, MD

Perhaps in the not-so-distant future we will be performing clear lens extractions on plano presbyopic patients and replacing the natural lens with a clear, soft, jelly-like material that can accommodate fully. However, until that time, the only implants available in the United States that can somewhat mimic the natural action of a physiologic prepresbyopic eye are the Crystalens and its sister toric version called the Trulign (Bausch & Lomb) accommodating implants. Many surgeons around the globe have turned to these lenses as their premium implant of choice because of their ability to provide high-quality vision at distance while also allowing the patient to maintain some spectacle independence in the middle and near zones as well. The Crystalens and Trulign are really just an early step in the evolution of a lens implant's ability to perform a more physiologic function and allow the eye to have a full natural range of vision without the need for glasses. The distinct advantage of the Crystalens and Trulign is that they do not use any multifocality to achieve middle and near vision and therefore do not suffer from the pitfalls of having refractive or diffractive optical rings that cause loss of contrast sensitivity that is well-documented in the use of multifocal implants. However, surgeons must be aware that the Crystalens accommodating implant also has its own drawbacks, such as the challenge of achieving precise refractive outcomes and the inability of the lens to fully accommodate so that all patients are completely spectacle independent and have a full range of accommodation. As the Crystalens design improves and other accommodating implants are brought to market in the future, surgeons will have the luxury of a variety of implants to choose from when trying to achieve spectacle independence for their patients. The Crystalens' modified plate haptics with flexible hinge design is the novel feature allowing reduced spectacle dependence compared with conventional monofocal implants (Figure 17-1).

Hovanesian JA.
Refractive Cataract Surgery: Best Practices and Advanced Technology, Second Edition (pp 199-212). © 2017 SLACK Incorporated.

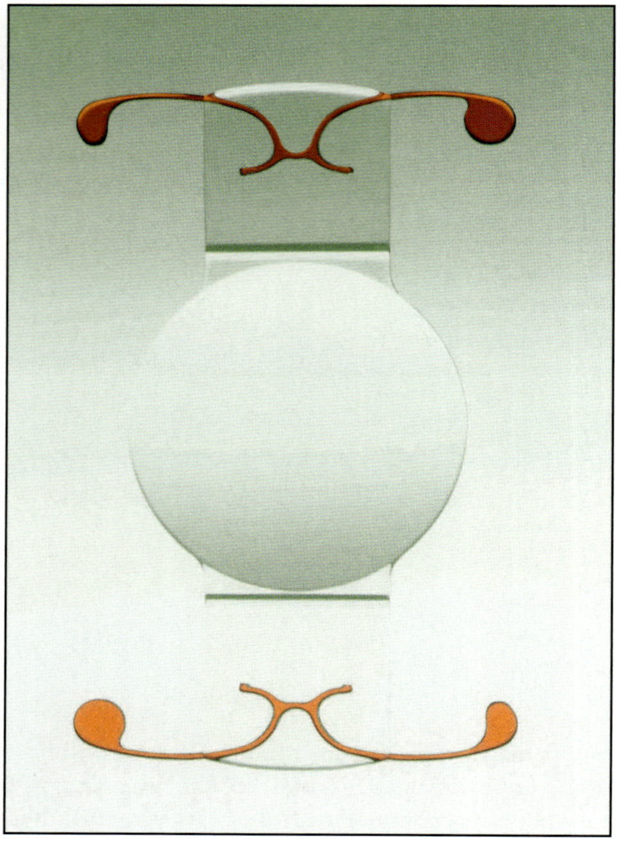

Figure 17-1. Image of the Crystalens AT50AO. It has a 5-mm optic, made of Biosil, and asymmetric polyimide loop haptics at the ends to aid in proper anterior posterior orientation.

Currently, there are 3 versions of the Crystalens that are available for the surgeon: the Crystalens AT50SE, Crystalens HD, and Crystalens AO. These 3 lenses were brought to market in that particular order, and currently most surgeons are using the Crystalens AO due to the aspheric optic that has been incorporated into the lens design. Some surgeons still prefer to use the Crystalens AT50SE, which does not have an aspheric optic design, and other surgeons also use the Crystalens HD, which has a small area of thickening in the central 1.5 mm of the optic, causing induced negative spherical aberration and increased depth of field. Crystalens HD tends to perform better at near than the other models; however, its refractive targeting outcome must be near plano to ensure proper functioning and high visual satisfaction. The Crystalens AO is a little bit more forgiving in terms of the exact refractive outcome that is necessary to have high-quality vision and a happy patient. Its aspheric design with no induced spherical aberration allows for a slightly positive amount of spherical aberration. All models have a square-edge design to inhibit posterior capsule opacification and are made of the proprietary copolymer, Biosil. The Crytalens comes in 0.5 diopter (D) power steps from 8 to 30 and 0.25 D steps from 18 to 22. The Trulign is built on the same exact platform as the Crystalens AO, except it incorporates a toricity power in addition to the spherical power (Figure 17-2). It comes in 3 different toric powers designed to cover a range of preoperative corneal astigmatism.

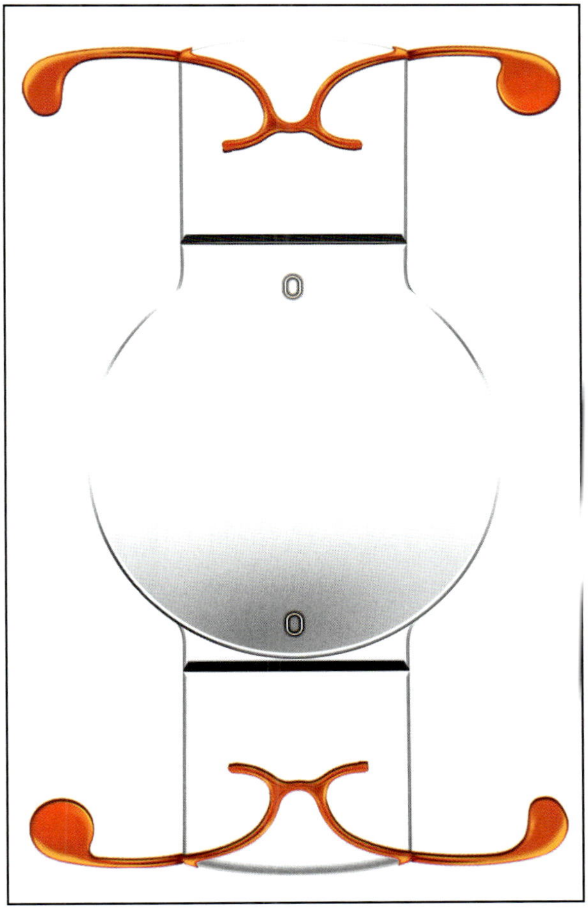

Figure 17-2. Image of the Trulign toric implant.

It comes in 1.25 D, 2.00 D, and 2.75 D correlating to 0.83 D, 1.33 D, and 1.83 D correction at the corneal plane. There are small marks in the peripheral optic adjacent to the hinge to guide axis placement.

Patient Selection

A critical aspect to successful Crystalens and Trulign usage is proper patient selection. When a surgeon is performing his or her initial cases, it is important to find patients with very reasonable expectations who can accept that there still may be a need for light reading glasses after the procedure. A patient who has a normal-shaped eye with average axial length and K-value readings will aid the surgeon in picking the correct implant power. The absence of any other ocular pathology or history of previous ocular surgery will also stack the cards in favor of the surgeon for achieving success with his or her initial cases. Patients who have had previous vitrectomies, glaucoma surgeries or lasers, pseudoexfoliation, history of ocular trauma, advanced significant epiretinal membrane pathology, or other vascular compromises to the retina or optic nerve should not be considered candidates when first starting to use the implant. It is possible to correct mild to moderate amounts of astigmatism with laser or manual limbal relaxing incisions (LRI), but ideally for the first few Crystalens patients, it is better to choose an eye that has less than 1 D of astigmatism present on the cornea. For over 1 D of astigmatism, a Trulign can be used. In addition, if a patient has had prior corneal refractive surgery such as photorefractive keratectomy, LASIK, radial keratotomy, or conductive keratoplasty, it will be very challenging to acquire accurate keratometric values and proper intraocular lens (IOL) power selection. A more advanced biometric approach is needed for the patients, and the use of intraoperative aberrometry is useful.

Another important consideration in patient selection is the general disposition and personality of the patient. Since there is an out-of-pocket expense, many patients have different levels of expectations with regard to how they think vision should be postoperatively. A consistent message coming from both the surgeon and the staff about realistic expectations is paramount for a good result and a happy patient postoperatively. The patient needs to understand that although this technology is advanced and has the ability for the lens to move/accommodate inside the eye, there is no guarantee that the patient is not going to need reading glasses or rely on corrective lenses after surgery. Additionally, the patient needs to understand that certain situations can arise in the operating room that would preclude the surgeon from using the Crystalens or Trulign, and a standard implant may be used in its place. It is best to inform patients that although the implant does an excellent job of providing a continuous range of vision from distance to near, in certain situations where the print is extremely small or there is not enough ambient light, there might likely be a need to use a low-power pair of over-the-counter reading glasses. Since, as with any procedure, there are unexpected outcomes and refractive surprises that can occur as the eye heals, patients must be informed that additional vision correction procedures may be needed to fine-tune or augment the visual outcome, including LRIs, laser corrective surgery, and possibly even an implant exchange in rare cases. Patients who accept these considerations and understand that they will occasionally need a light pair of reading glasses for fine print and are mostly seeking independence from glasses in the distance and middle range are the ideal candidates for the Crystalens and Trulign. It is wise for a surgeon to listen closely to the staff and surgical counselors, because often times these members of the team spend more time with the patient and may have more insight into the patient's expectations than the surgeon does. If the staff feels that the patient may not be a good candidate from a personality perspective and that the patient's expectations are too high, it would be prudent for the surgeon to discuss things further with the patient or even decide not to use a premium implant in that particular case. Many surgeons like to use a preoperative questionnaire in evaluating a patient for premium implants to help guide the decision process. The Dell questionnaire is a nice tool for evaluating personality type and visual demands (see Figure 3-3).

When setting up expectations for a Crystalens patient, it is important for the surgeon to realize that, unlike multifocal IOLs, the Crystalens and Trulign very rarely cause any nighttime visual disturbances and it is very unusual to have a patient complain of nighttime glare, halos, or reduced contrast sensitivity. However, the near vision, especially for very small print, is not as clear with the Crystalens/Trulign as it would be with a multifocal IOL with a strong near power. This distinction is very important for a potential premium implant patient to fully grasp in regard to the expectations and the pros and cons of different IOL technology. If a surgeon does desire to make a person completely spectacle independent with the Crystalens or Trulign, there is an opportunity to use them in a modified or full monovision arrangement. This is especially helpful if a patient has a history of successful monovision contact lens wear in the past.

Preoperative Measurements

As with any cataract surgery, accurate preoperative measurements are required to achieve an excellent refractive outcome. This is especially true with Crystalens/Trulign patients because the surgeon is required to deliver a precise refractive outcome in order for the patient to have reduced spectacle dependence and a high-quality visual result. In addition to a standard A-scan that is performed prior to cataract surgery, the surgeon would be wise to obtain additional refractive measurements to help guide the procedure. Many surgeons perform multiple axial length measurements as well as multiple corneal curvature measurements using different diagnostic technologies. It may be worthwhile to employ 2 forms of A-scan technology to help choose the proper IOL for the patient. A very common protocol is to perform both an IOLMaster (Carl Zeiss Meditec) or Lenstar (Haag-Streit) as well as an immersion A-scan on each patient. It is recommended that a surgeon also perform a very thorough evaluation of the corneal curvature and regularity of the corneal architecture. This can be performed with any topography machine, and some surgeons are even using wavefront imaging to obtain a reading of optical aberrations that are present in the optical system. It is important not to underestimate the value of manual keratometry in evaluating patients preoperatively for Crystalens/Trulign surgery, and once all of the preoperative measurements are taken, it is valuable to spend time evaluating and comparing all of the values to determine which are the most accurate readings. It is very helpful when different technologies result in the same or similar implant power readings, giving the surgeon a high degree of confidence in the lens power selection. If the readings from different machines do not corroborate each other, it is prudent to repeat the measurements and try to figure out what the most predictable readings are, especially with keratometric values in patients who have previously undergone refractive corneal surgery. These preoperative measurements not only help guide the surgeon in IOL power selection but also identify any unusual corneal pathology that may preclude a desired refractive outcome. The surgeon must also determine how much corneal cylinder exists and what mode of technology, if any, should be employed to correct the corneal astigmatism at the time of the cataract surgery or afterward. Occasionally, a surgeon will find a significantly higher amount of corneal astigmatism that was not present on manifest refraction because the lenticular astigmatism was counterbalancing it. The Trulign should be used in these situations, along with corneal arcuate incision if needed. Another important measurement that should be done preoperatively is an endothelial cell count to ensure that the patient has healthy corneal endothelium to prevent a situation in which there is prolonged corneal edema postoperatively and an undesirable refractive outcome. If the patient has a borderline endothelial cell count, it would be best to use a dispersive viscoelastic to coat and protect the cornea during the surgical procedure. If the endothelial cell count and clinical examination reveal that there is a high likelihood of prolonged corneal edema or the patient may have a diagnosis of Fuchs endothelial dystrophy, using the Crystalens would be contraindicated.

Intraocular Lens Selection and Targeting

Some surgeons prefer to do surgery on the dominant eye first with a plano target, while other surgeons prefer to do the nondominant eye first with a slightly myopic target. Regardless of this decision, it is important to check the patient postoperatively after the first eye has been completed to ensure that the eye is healing well and that the refractive target is where the surgeon intended. If it is not, then a slight adjustment can be made on the second eye to ensure a good refractive result. When selecting the IOL power in patients who have had previous corneal refractive surgeries, it is especially important to do an accurate assessment of the keratometric values and also to employ software, such as that available on the American Society of Cataract and Refractive Surgery website, to help determine the correct IOL power selection. An acceptable targeting strategy for an average patient would be to target somewhere between plano and -0.25 for the dominant eye and somewhere between -0.25 and -0.50 to the nondominant eye. This small amount of anisometropia is extremely well tolerated by the patient, and the slight difference allows the patient to have a good range of vision and often results in minimal need for reading glasses after the procedure is completed. To ensure good outcomes, some surgeons are now using intraoperative aberrometry. These machines can do aphakic autorefractions and recommend a lens power while the patient is on the operating table. They can also provide a refraction once the implant is placed in the eye to help guide the correct axis placement for the Trulign and determine whether the implant is sitting in the proper position (Figure 17-3). For average eyes, the SRK-T formula works well. For eyes with axial lengths under 22 mm, Ks flatter than 42, steeper than 47, and postrefractive surgery cornea, the Holladay 2 formula is better suited.

Surgical Considerations

As with any cataract surgery, an efficient atraumatic surgical procedure is paramount for ensuring a good refractive outcome. Some important features that are specific to a good refractive outcome with a Crystalens/Trulign include creating a well-constructed corneoscleral wound and a 5- to 6-mm centralized capsulorrhexis. If too small of a capsulorrhexis is made, it can lead to capsular contraction and fibrosis of the anterior capsule. The fibrosis can then cause a shift in the lens position within the eye. Conversely, if too large of a capsulorrhexis is created, it can lead to an unstable platform for the Crystalens implant and prevent optimal performance of the lens (Figure 17-4).

When removing the nucleus and cortical material, it is extremely important for the surgeon to be as gentle as possible with the capsular bag. If there is excessive manipulation of the capsule, it can cause zonular dialysis or tearing of the capsule. If this occurs, the implant will not sit properly inside the eye and will not perform properly postoperatively. If there is unexpected damage to the capsule during surgery, it may be best to abandon the Crystalens/Trulign and use a standard monofocal implant. Another important

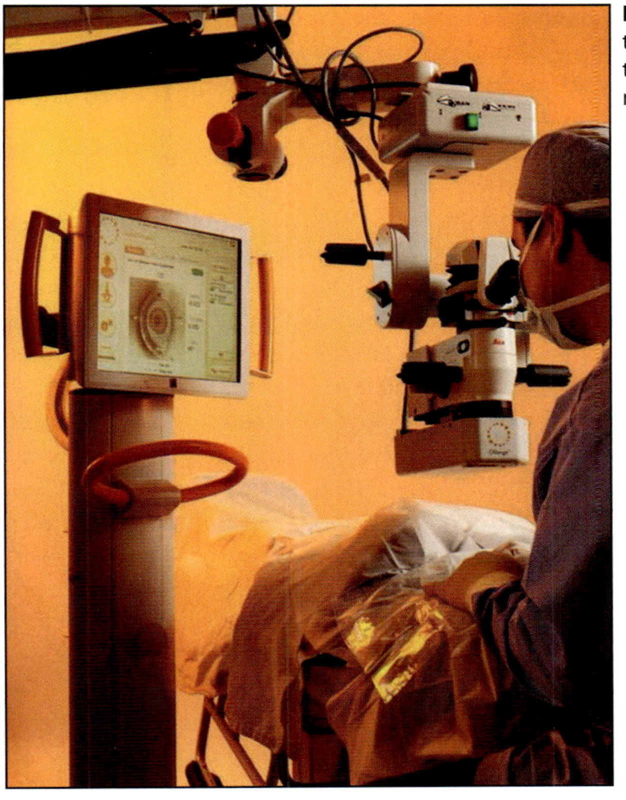

Figure 17-3. The ORange intraoperative aberrometer (WaveTec Vision Systems) can be helpful in achieving optimal refractive outcomes.

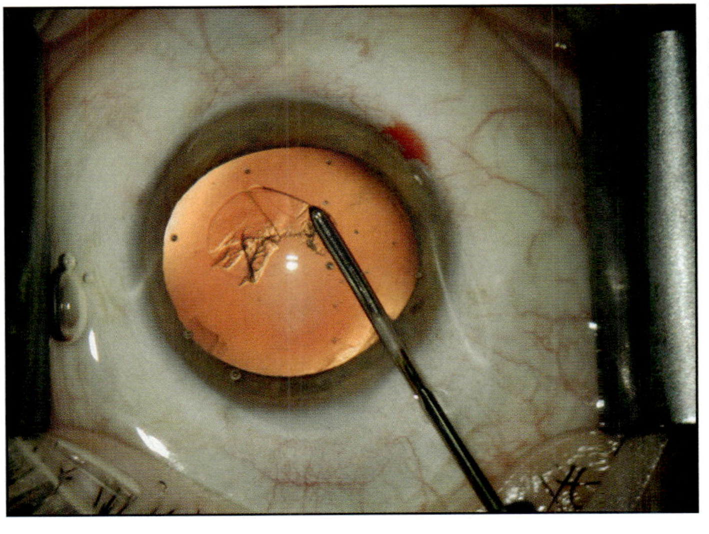

Figure 17-4. A well-centered 6- to 7-mm capsulorrhexis is an important feature of a successful procedure and outcome. Here a microcapsular forceps is used to have precise control of the tear.

strategy in the cataract surgery is to ensure a complete and thorough cortical clean-up. Many surgeons gently polish the capsule to ensure all endothelial cells are removed from the capsular bag; this can be a double-edged sword, because overzealous polishing of the capsule can lead to zonular tearing and damage. If cortical material or endothelial cells are left behind in any significant amount, it can affect the patient's vision postoperatively and also cause excessive scarring, fibrosis, and irregular contraction of the capsule, leading to a displacement in the IOL position. Some surgeons even like to polish the undersurface of the anterior capsular rim.

Crystalens/Trulign insertion can be accomplished with a variety of injector systems, but most commonly employed is the Crystalsert (Bausch & Lomb) injector. This device works with any of the implant models and allows for a smooth, controlled delivery. It is best to place the injector well into the eye and deep into the capsular bag prior to injecting the lens. This ensures that the lens will be delivered into the bag and not into the sulcus or anterior chamber. Filling the bag and chamber completely with a dispersive viscoelastic is helpful to ensure a safe delivery. A good goal is to at least deliver the leading haptics into the capsule, and often the entire lens can be placed in the bag with a single action. If the trailing haptics do not go in the bag, a Sinskey or Kuglen hook can be used to push posteriorly on the edge of the optic. The trailing plate and haptics generally follow the optic and can then be delivered into the capsule. Care should be taken not to let the lens haptic enter the sulcus space, as it can embed into and get stuck in the anterior zonules. If this happens, usually the only solution is to forcefully push it out with a Kuglen hook, which may tear a few anterior zonules. It is also important to see that the leading haptic has the round, orange polyimide loop on the right and the oval loop on the left. If that is not able to be visualized, you can also look at the trailing haptic where the round one should be on the left and the oval one on the right (Figures 17-5 through 17-10).

In most cases, it is good to use a hook or the irrigation/aspiration handpiece to rotate the implant inside the bag to help it center and take a posterior vaulted position against the posterior capsule. For Trulign cases, the lens must be placed in correct axis to ensure astigmatism reduction. Following implantation of the Crystalens/Trulign, it is important to remove the viscoelastic from behind the implant and from all the fornices of the capsule so that the implant sits centrally and vaulted posteriorly within the capsular bag (Figures 17-11 and 17-12). If the anterior chamber is not stable and deep, the Crystalens has the propensity to bow or vault forward at the end of the procedure; therefore, it is critical to create a well-sealed wound and make sure the lens is vaulted posteriorly and pressed against the posterior capsule. It is easy to rotate the lens inside the capsular bag. This can help with centration as well as freeing up any hidden cortex. If the eye is not sealed postoperatively and the chamber is unstable, there is risk of the IOL prolapsing anteriorly. Sometimes it is wise to place an astigmatically neutral suture across the primary wound at the end of the case to ensure there is no leakage. If striae are seen in the posterior capsule, the implant should be rotated or manipulated, and the wound should be checked for leakage. Once the lens is seated and vaulted posterior with the eye sealed and under normal intraocular pressure, there should not be any striae in the posterior capsule. The surgeon must also not forget to perform LRIs on patients who have greater than 0.75 D of preoperative measured corneal astigmatism or use a Trulign for greater amounts of astigmatism (Figure 17-13).

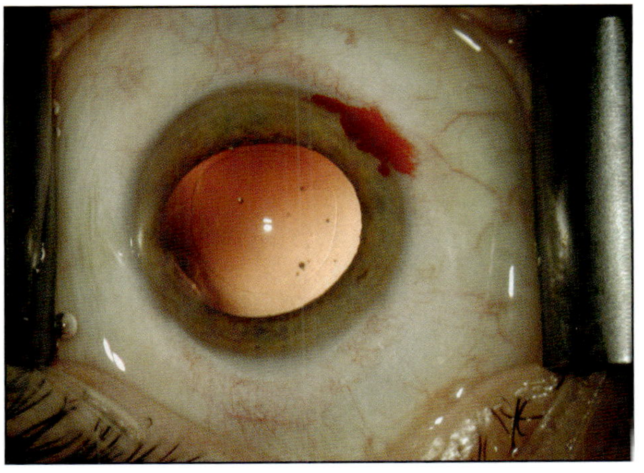

Figure 17-5. The entire capsule and anterior chamber are filled with a cohesive viscoelastic prior to lens insertion. Notice how clean the capsule is, with no residual cortex.

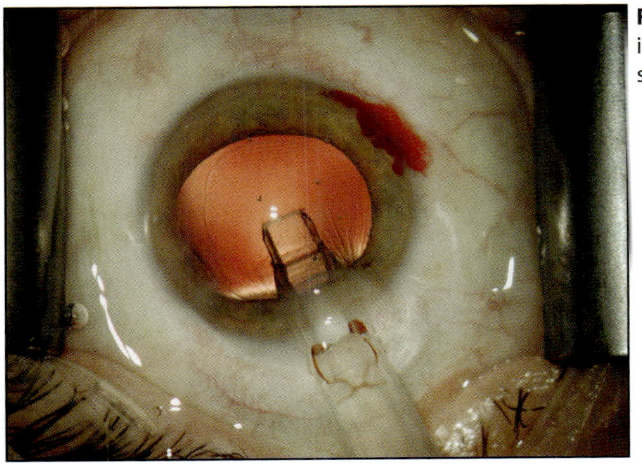

Figure 17-6. The injector is placed well inside the wound and deep in the capsule prior to lens release.

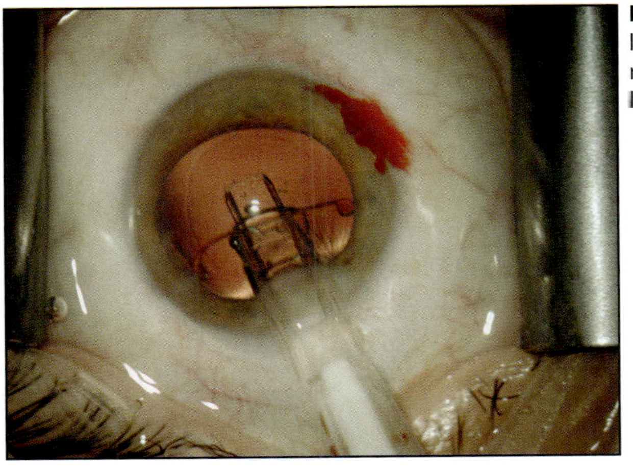

Figure 17-7. The leading haptic is delivered into the capsule. Notice how the round loop is on the right and the oval loop is on the left.

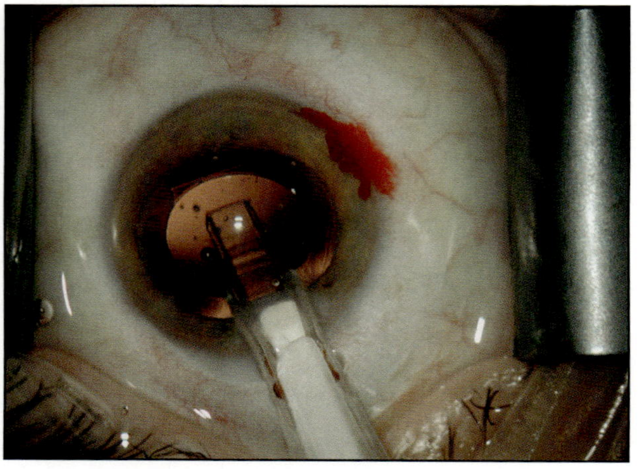

Figure 17-8. The optic is delivered into the capsular bag, and the leading haptics disappear from the surgeon's view.

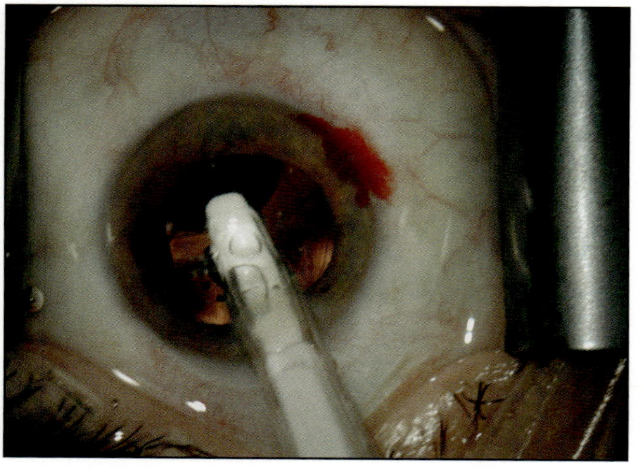

Figure 17-9. The trailing haptics can be delivered into the bag if the injector is kept in the center of the eye and just below the level of the capsulorrhexis.

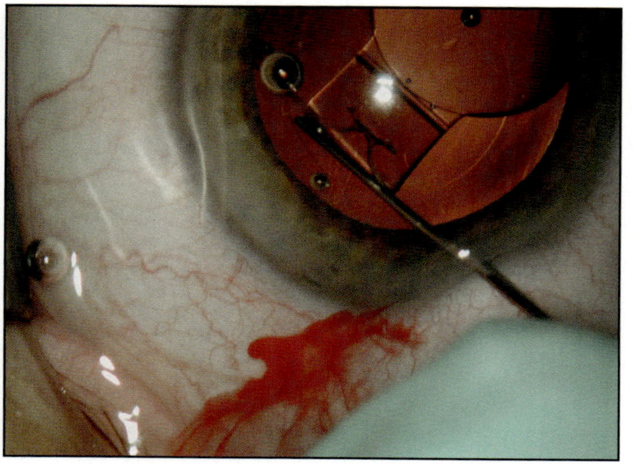

Figure 17-10. A Kuglen hook can be used to tuck the trailing haptics into the capsule.

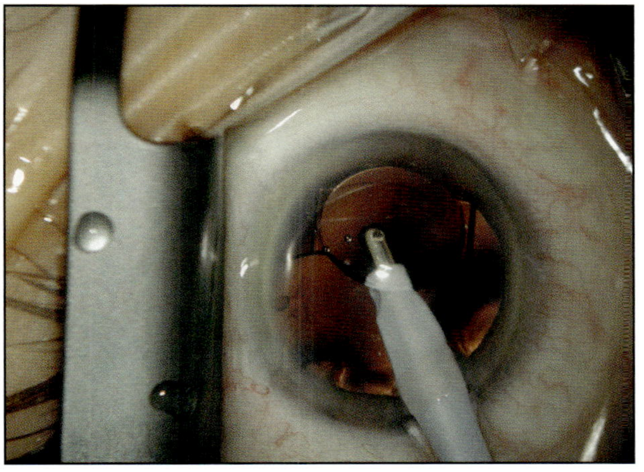

Figure 17-11. The irrigation/aspiration handpiece can be placed under the optic to remove all the viscoelastic.

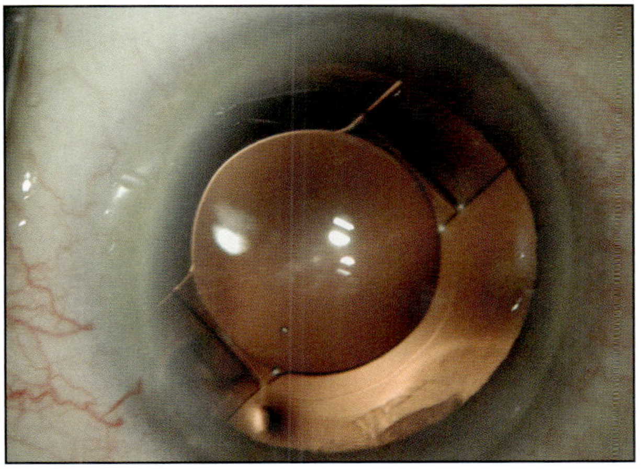

Figure 17-12. The Crystalens should take a well-centered position against the posterior capsule at the completion of the case. Notice the absence of striae in the posterior capsule.

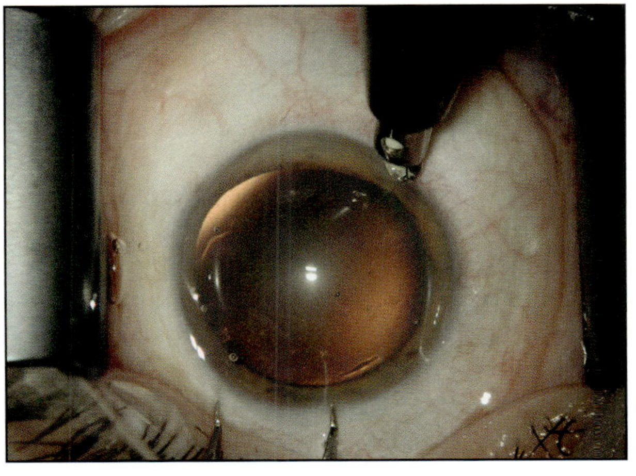

Figure 17-13. An LRI is placed to reduce corneal cylinder.

Postoperative Considerations

In providing successful cataract surgery with implantation via a Crystalens/Trulign implant, postoperative follow up and management become the next crucial event. In the early days of Crystalens surgeries, it was recommended that surgeons atropinize patients postoperatively to prevent ciliary muscle movement and accommodation so that the Crystalens would remain in a posterior vaulted position until it had settled in and started to fibrose to the capsule. This was partially due to the fact that the earlier designs of the Crystalens had smaller plate haptics and a propensity to move anteriorly perioperatively, with some surgeons seeing myopic shifts in the early postoperative period. However, since modifications were made several years ago to the optic and haptic design, and since the release of the Crystalens AO, some surgeons are no longer atropinizing patients postoperatively and are using a traditional postoperative cataract pharmaceutical regimen of antibiotics, steroids, and nonsteroidal medication. On the postoperative day 1 visit, it is important to check uncorrected visual acuity and examine the anterior segment to make sure that the Crystalens/Trulign is in a good position, vaulted posteriorly, and the eye is healing well. Many surgeons bring the patient back sometime within the first week to recheck the vision and ensure that the refractive targeting is as intended. It is appropriate to wait at least 1 week between doing surgery on the first and second eye to allow the eye to heal and vision to improve and to ensure that the eye is healing as planned in regard to its refractive outcome. Depending on the refraction of the eye at 1 week, the surgeon can make slight modifications to the targeting of the second eye. For example, if the first eye is emmetropic and the patient has a good uncorrected distance visual acuity, the surgeon may choose to slightly increase the power of the IOL in the second eye to ensure good middle and near functioning in the second eye. Conversely, if the patient is experiencing good near vision after the 1-week-postoperative visit and the distance vision is not adequate, then the surgeon may choose an implant power closer to plano targeting or even potentially a +0.25 D hyperopic target in the second eye to ensure at least one eye achieves a good uncorrected distance visual acuity. Fortunately, the small amount of anisometropia that is seen postoperatively in patients is well tolerated and most of the time the surgeon will not need to do any further refractive procedures. If a hyperopic result is found early in the postoperative period, the first thing to do is to make sure that there is no corneal or retinal edema and that the lens is in its posterior position. If the lens seems to be seated posteriorly and the eye is healing well with a clear cornea, then it must be assumed that the IOL power selection was not accurate for that particular eye, and that needs to be taken into account in performing surgery on the second eye. Therefore, if the patient has similar axial length and keratometric values in the second eye, the surgeon would be advised to select a slightly stronger IOL power in the second eye to compensate for the possible hyperopic outcome that was seen in the first eye. Occasionally, unexplained mild hyperopic or myopic results will be seen, and some feel this may be due to how the lens sits in different-sized capsular bags. In a small hyperopic capsular bag, the implant may vault more posteriorly than anticipated, and the opposite is true for larger myopic capsular bags where the implant can take a more planar anterior position. In these cases, it is often best to let the eye heal, perform a yttrium-aluminum-garnet (YAG) capsulotomy around 90 days postoperatively, and then consider corneal refractive surgery if indicated. Small to moderate amounts of residual astigmatism can be addressed with an

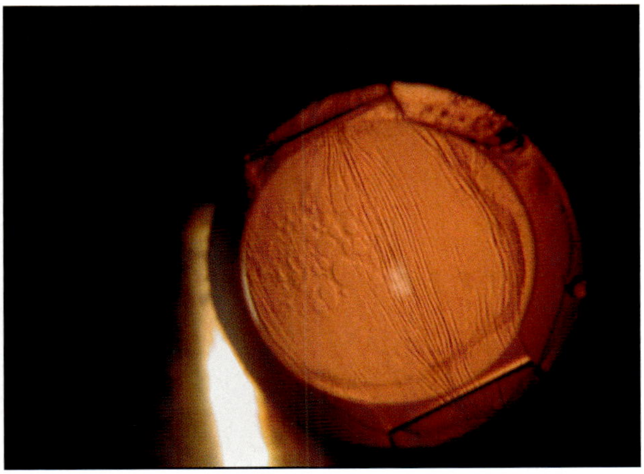

Figure 17-14. An example of posterior capsule opacification behind the implant, which can be treated easily with a YAG capsulotomy.

LRI at the slit lamp or minor procedure room. Cycloplegic postoperative refractions are also helpful in determining the refractive status of the eye.

YAG capsulotomies are very safe to perform in Crystalens/Trulign patients and can be performed as soon as 1-month postoperatively if needed. However, it is generally recommended to wait 90 days. When performing a YAG capsulotomy, it is best to use a lower than average power setting and make a smaller than usual central opening in the posterior capsule (Figure 17-14). If too large of an opening is created, it can lead to vitreous prolapse around the optic and into the anterior chamber. This can even lead to a slight malposition of the implant. Very rarely, a surgeon will encounter the so-called *z syndrome*. In this situation, asymmetric capsular fibrosis causes a localized contraction of the capsule that squeezes the haptics, bowing it anterior. This causes lens tilt, the patients complain of a change in vision, and manifest refraction/topography reveals noncorneal astigmatism. This can usually be remedied by treating the fibrosed/contracted area of the capsule with the YAG laser. This laser treatment is usually done right behind the haptic that is bowed forward, and sometimes the surgeon can actually watch the lens move back into normal position as the YAG treatment is being performed. If significant anterior capsular phimosis occurs, the YAG laser can also be used to make small nicks in the anterior capsule, releasing the tension and enlarging the opening (Figure 17-15).

Pearls for Success With Your First Few Crystalens Patients

- ▲ Find a hyperope who wears glasses full-time.
- ▲ Make sure there is less than 0.75 D of corneal cylinder and the keratometry readings are between 41 and 44 D. The axial length should be between 22 and 24 mm.
- ▲ Make sure the patient understands that he or she may need a light pair of reading glasses for reading very small print.
- ▲ Use an IOLMaster with SRK/T formula and target the dominant eye near plano and the nondominant eye near -0.37 D. Use recommended A-constant or surgeon factor.

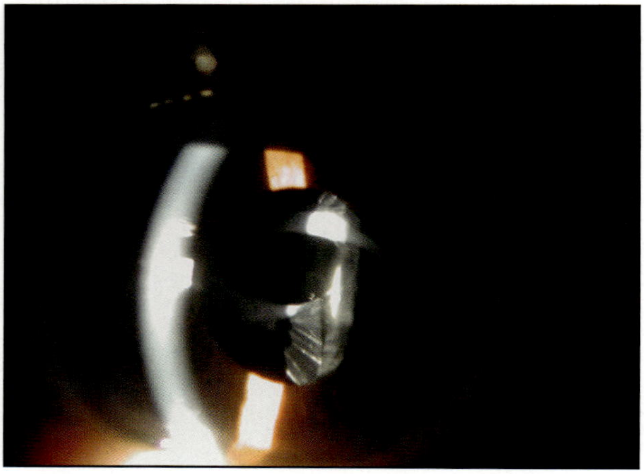

Figure 17-15. Anterior capsule phimosis can cause a shift in optic position. It can be treated with the YAG laser.

- Create a 5- to 6-mm capsulorrhexis. Do not stress the zonules during the case, and do a thorough capsular cortex removal.
- Fill the entire capsule and chamber with a cohesive viscoelastic prior to lens insertion.
- Deliver the Crystalens directly into the capsule and tuck the trailing haptic into the capsule with a Kuglen hook if needed. Spin the implant to ensure a central position and a posterior vault with the optic pressed against the posterior capsule.
- Remove all the viscoelastic from the eye with irrigation/aspiration. Tilt, rock, or go behind the implant with the aspirator to make sure all is removed.
- Hydrate the wound and place a 10-0 suture if needed to ensure wound closure and no leakage. Ensure that the lens is vaulted posterior at the completion of the case.
- Check the refraction of the first eye prior to doing the second eye, and adjust IOL power selection if needed.

Conclusion

The Crystalens and Trulign accommodating implants are a vital component to providing premium cataract surgery. The advanced design of these implants has led to less spectacle dependence than other monofocal lenses can deliver. With careful patient selection, preoperative testing, and intraoperative technique, a surgeon can deliver high-quality visual results to the patient and achieve personal satisfaction in a job well done.

Bibliography

Agarwal A. *Bimanual Phaco.* Thorofare, NJ: SLACK Incorporated; 2005.

Agarwal A. *Refractive Surgery Nightmares.* Thorofare, NJ: SLACK Incorporated; 2007.

Chang DF. *Mastering Refractive IOLs: The Art and the Science.* Thorofare, NJ: SLACK Incorporated; 2008.

Garg A. *Mastering the Techniques of Advanced Phaco Surgery.* New Delhi, India: Jaypee Brothers Medical Publishers; 2008.

Garg A. *Surgical Techniques in Ophthalmic Surgery: Cataract Surgery.* New Delhi, India: Jaypee Brothers Medical Publishers; 2010.

Section III

Postoperative Considerations and Enhancements

Chapter 18

Refractive Intraocular Lenses

Managing Unhappy Patients

Eric Donnenfeld, MD;
Alanna Nattis, DO; Eric Rosenberg, DO;
and Allon Barsam, MD, MA, MRCOphth

Preoperative Education

There are several important steps that dramatically increase postoperative success with refractive intraocular lens (IOL) cataract surgery. In general, cataract surgery, and more specifically premium IOL cataract surgery, requires careful patient selection and counseling, along with precise surgical technique. Recent design advances in IOLs have resulted in excellent visual outcomes after cataract surgery.[1] As a result, many patients now have higher expectations for vision following surgery, including complete spectacle independence.[1] The use of diffractive multifocal IOLs is an effective way to satisfy the desire for excellent distance and near vision.[1] The principle by which diffractive IOLs work is to provide a focused image with zero order diffraction for distance vision, and first order diffraction for near vision.[1] However, with this optical setup, the focused retinal image will always be overlaid by an out-of-focus image from another diffractive portion of the lens, and also by background light, or light scattering due to diffraction inefficiency.[1] This phenomenon often results in unintended adverse effects after implantation of diffractive multifocal/accommodative IOLs, including decreased contrast sensitivity and unwanted dysphotopsias, such as glare and halos.[1]

For the less experienced surgeon, the best candidates for multifocal or accommodative IOLs are hyperopes or higher myopes who are motivated to reduce their dependence on spectacles, and who have more significant cataracts with minimal astigmatism. Both emmetropes and low myopes may feel that their distance or near vision was better prior to surgery than with a presbyopic IOL and should be counseled accordingly. Multiple options of add power allow physicians and patients to make individualized choices, in terms of target diopters, to customize patients' lenses to their lifestyle.[1] For example,

Hovanesian JA.
Refractive Cataract Surgery: Best Practices and Advanced Technology, Second Edition (pp 215-224). © 2017 SLACK Incorporated.

lower add power provides better intermediate vision for using computers and electronic devices.[1] Patients often perform best with bilateral multifocal or accommodative IOL implantation and usually have the second cataract surgery completed within 1 month of the first surgery.

Multifocal IOL implantation requires the same surgical technique as conventional monofocal cataract surgery. However, optic insertion of these presbyopic lenses requires precise centration, necessitating a well-centered capsulorrhexis and good zonular integrity in order to achieve optimal visual results. Control of astigmatism alongside accurate biometry with advanced technology, such as the IOLMaster or Lenstar, is essential in maximizing outcomes. The lens constant must be carefully personalized to the individual surgeon. For this reason, tracking postoperative results is imperative to refine surgical outcomes. Postoperative astigmatism should be reduced to 0.5 diopter (D) or less. Refractive errors in general, and notably in patients with astigmatism, have a greater effect on quality of vision in multifocal IOL patients than in monofocal IOL patients. For patients with astigmatism greater than 0.5 D, limbal relaxing incisions (LRI), LASIK, or photorefractive keratectomy (PRK) may be required, and the patient should be informed about this prior to surgery.

In patients who are seeking spectacle independence but have significant preoperative astigmatism, a multifocal IOL may not be the best option. Toric multifocal IOLs, such as the AcrySof ReSTOR (Alcon) and other lenses on the horizon, combine diffractive optics with a toric component, thus offering astigmatic patients the option of having a multifocal IOL.[2] Toric multifocal IOLs have been found to result in increased spectacle independence and improved ability to perform near, intermediate, and distance tasks.[2] Despite the ability to produce spectacle independence, toric multifocal IOLs are not without drawbacks, such as diminished contrast sensitivity, halos, and/or glare.[2] Monofocal toric, or accommodating toric IOLs (Trulign [Bausch & Lomb]) offer excellent quality of vision and may be preferable options to discuss with the patient. Toric monofocal IOLs are also better options for patients with other coexisting ocular pathology. Patients with dry eye, macular pathology, glaucoma, or optic nerve disease may be relative or absolute contraindications to multifocal IOLs but do very well with toric monofocal IOLs. The only patient who should not be considered for a toric IOL is the patient who wishes to wear a gas permeable contact lens following surgery, such as those individuals with keratoconus.

The first step in any refractive procedure is to determine the patient's visual requirements. Clinicians should fully educate their patients about possible postoperative symptoms and carefully interview them about lifestyle and postoperative expectations before selecting an IOL.[1] Asking the patients to complete a questionnaire like the one shown in Figure 18-1 (originally described by Steven Dell) is very helpful for this purpose. It is important to understand the differences between the various presbyopic IOLs in order to tailor the IOL choice to the needs of the individual patient.

Patient understanding of acceptable and expected surgical outcomes is imperative for the achievement of optimal results. Patients with unrealistic expectations for visual improvement and patients with excessive complaints about spectacles or contact lenses may not be optimal candidates for multifocal IOLs. This may also be true for patients whose occupation requires significant night driving and those who experience excessive glare and halo at night. There are many different multifocal IOLs currently available,

Date___________

Name______________________________

Cataract and Refractive Lens Exchange Questionnaire

The term "cataract" refers to a cloudy lens within the eye. When a cataract is removed, an artificial lens is placed inside the eye to take the place of the human lens that has become the cataract. Occasionally, clear lenses that have not yet developed cataracts are also removed to reduce or eliminate the need for glasses or contacts. This questionnaire will assist us in providing the treatment best suited for your visual needs if it is determined that surgery is appropriate for you. It is important that you understand that many patients still need to wear glasses for some activities after surgery. Please fill this form out completely and give it to the doctor. If you have questions, please let us know and we will assist you with this form.

1. Are you interested in seeing well **at distance** without glasses after surgery?
___Prefer no distance glasses. **___Not important to me. I wouldn't mind wearing distance glasses.**

2. Are you interested in seeing well **at near** without glasses after surgery?
___Prefer no reading glasses. **___Not important to me. I wouldn't mind wearing reading glasses.**

3. Zones of Vision.

We divide vision into 5 "Zones of Vision"

Near ⟷ **Far**

Zone 1	**Zone 2**	**Zone 3**	**Zone 4**	**Zone 5**
(12-20 in)	**(2-4 ft.)**	**(6-20 ft.)**	**(20-100 ft.)**	**(100 ft.+)**
Newsprint	Headlines	Indoors	Day-far	Night-far
Phone book	Computer	TV	Driving	Night driving
Maps	Menus	Cooking	Golf	Movies
Sewing	Price tags	Cleaning	Road signs	Star gazing

Which group of "Zones of Vision" is the **most** important group to you? Please choose **only one** of the following three options of Group A, B or C:

Figure 18-1. Questionnaire. *(continued)*

____**Group A: Zones 1, 2 and 3.** ____**Group B: Zones 2, 3 and 4.**
____**Group C: Zones 3, 4 and 5.**

4. If you **had** to wear glasses after surgery for one activity, for which activity would you be **most** willing to use glasses? ____**Reading fine print.**
____**Computer.** ____**Driving**

5. If you could have good **distance vision during the day** without glasses, and good **near** vision for reading without glasses, but the compromise was that you might see some **halos** around lights at night, would you like that option?
____**Yes** ____**No**

6. If you could have good **distance vision during the day and night** without glasses, and good **computer-distance (Zone 2)** vision without glasses, but the compromise was that you might need glasses for reading the finest print at near, would you like that option? ____**Yes**
____**No**

7. Please place an "X" on the following scale to describe your personality as best you can:

[---I------------------------------
--------------------------------]
Easy going
Perfectionist

Please Sign Here________________________________

Figure 18-1 (continued). Questionnaire.

with different adds that range from 2.5 to 4.0 D. Patients who wish to perform fine near tasks such as threading a needle may prefer the high add IOLs, and patients who spend more time at a computer or using a smart phone will appreciate the lower add multifocal IOLs. In general the risk of visual disturbance, such as glare and halo, is greatest with the higher add IOLs, while quality of vision is better with the lower adds. The size of halo experienced is proportional to the size of the out-of-focus retinal image produced by the IOL, which depends on the add power.[1] However, even though the halo may be smaller with lower add powers, the intensity of halo may be greater, and therefore it will impact how a patient experiences his or her visual symptoms.[1] In addition, topical nonsteroidal anti-inflammatory drugs (NSAID) should be used perioperatively to decrease the risk of subclinical cystoid macular edema (CME) and thereby improve retinal and visual function.[3]

Preoperative Expectations

The next step in dealing with presbyopic IOL patients is to set realistic expectations preoperatively. Always talk to patients before surgery about common concerns such as glare, halo, quality of vision, residual refractive error, and the need for enhancements. Preoperative glare testing may be useful as well.[1] Chair time spent with these patients before surgery pays dividends later on. For example, when informing a patient that he or she may experience postoperative dysphotopsias, he or she will be prepared for the problem should it result. However, if they are not adequately informed preoperatively, it will be perceived as a complication.

Management of the Unhappy Postoperative Patient: The Seven Cs

When a patient is unhappy following cataract surgery, our technicians are instructed to perform a refraction, topography, and optical coherence tomography (OCT) prior to the surgeon evaluating the patient. Residual refractive error is the most common reason patients are unhappy. Residual error is evaluated with refraction, while the residual cylinder that could be missed with refraction is diagnosed with topography. In addition, the topography will show dropout, as evidenced by white areas where the tear film has been disrupted. Topography can be extremely valuable in diagnosing dry eye and ocular surface disease. OCT will help diagnose CME, in addition to any other macular pathology that might have been overlooked. By following these steps and the 7 Cs that follow, the most common problems leading to postoperative visual complaints will be identified. The primed ophthalmologist may now walk into the patient's room, give an informed expert opinion as to why the patient might be dissatisfied, and suggest solutions immediately. Our patients who are unhappy know that we are working with them to try to resolve their problems.

There are 7 different causes of unhappy patients after refractive IOL implantation, which should be looked for in any patient who is not completely satisfied following presbyopic IOL cataract surgery.

Consecutive Treatment

When implanting presbyopic IOLs, it is important to tell patients that they will likely be dissatisfied with their vision after only one eye has been operated on. It is expected that patients will not be fully functional until the second IOL is placed, and they should be informed about this preoperatively. The importance of having both eyes completed is critical for the success of the procedure, along with providing for an adequate neuroadaptation period. However, in the rare circumstance that the patient is extremely unhappy following surgery on the first eye, we do not recommend operating on the second eye until the first surgical result has been optimized. The second IOL choice may be predicated on the patient's response to the first surgery.

Cylinder and Residual Refractive Error

Presbyopic IOL patients are incredibly sensitive to small refractive errors, and the surgeon must be willing and able to treat these errors. Any astigmatism greater than 0.50 D in a symptomatic patient should be evaluated for treatment. LRIs can be useful in up to 1.50 D of cylinder, while surface ablation or LASIK provides more accurate results in patients with more than 1.50 D of cylinder. For patients with high cylinder, it is reasonable to debulk the refractive error with an LRI, followed by fine-tuning with the excimer laser. In patients with toric IOLs, it is important that the IOL be placed at the correct axis. For every 1 degree the IOL is off axis, there is a 3% loss of astigmatic correction. Newer technology such as intraoperative aberrometry and devices like the Verion (Alcon) and Callisto (Carl Zeiss Meditec) that display the axis of astigmatism intraoperatively can help refine cylinder outcomes. For patients with residual cylinder following toric IOL implantation, the website www.astigmatismfix.com is helpful in determining the correct axis for the physician to rotate the IOL.

Capsular Opacification

Multifocal IOL patients in particular are extremely sensitive to any opacification of the posterior capsule. The loss of contrast sensitivity and the glare created by the multifocal IOL is made worse by any capsular opacity. Depending on the patient's complaint and mesopic/scotopic pupil size, multifocal IOL patients may require a larger capsulotomy than normal. An important consideration is that once the posterior capsule is opened, it makes a safe IOL exchange increasingly more difficult. Therefore, it is important to be sure that the capsule is the problem before proceeding. We commonly communicate to patients that when we "break" the posterior capsule, they "buy" the IOL.

Cystoid Macular Edema

The best way to look for CME after cataract surgery is with OCT. In addition, OCT is a very effective screening tool preoperatively for epiretinal membranes and lamellar macular holes. Patients who have undergone conventional cataract surgery without capsular breakage and have no risk factors have up to a 70% chance of developing macular thickening on OCT.[3] Without the use of a topical NSAID, these same patients also have a 12% chance of developing visually significant CME.[4] In addition, the loss of contrast sensitivity associated with a multifocal IOL is made much worse by CME.[5] Once the normal architecture of the retina is lost, that visual quality is degraded for life. Snellen visual acuity will improve, but the contrast sensitivity will be permanently reduced. Multifocal IOL patients will not tolerate the lenses if they have significant maculopathy.[6] We recommend using a topical NSAID for 3 days preoperatively and continuing it for 4 to 6 weeks postoperatively to help prevent CME.

Cornea and Ocular Surface Disease

Vision starts with the tear film, as the tear film is the most important refracting surface of the eye. The concept of stressing the visual system also applies to ocular surface disease, which is a common problem in presbyopic patients. Even mild disruption of the

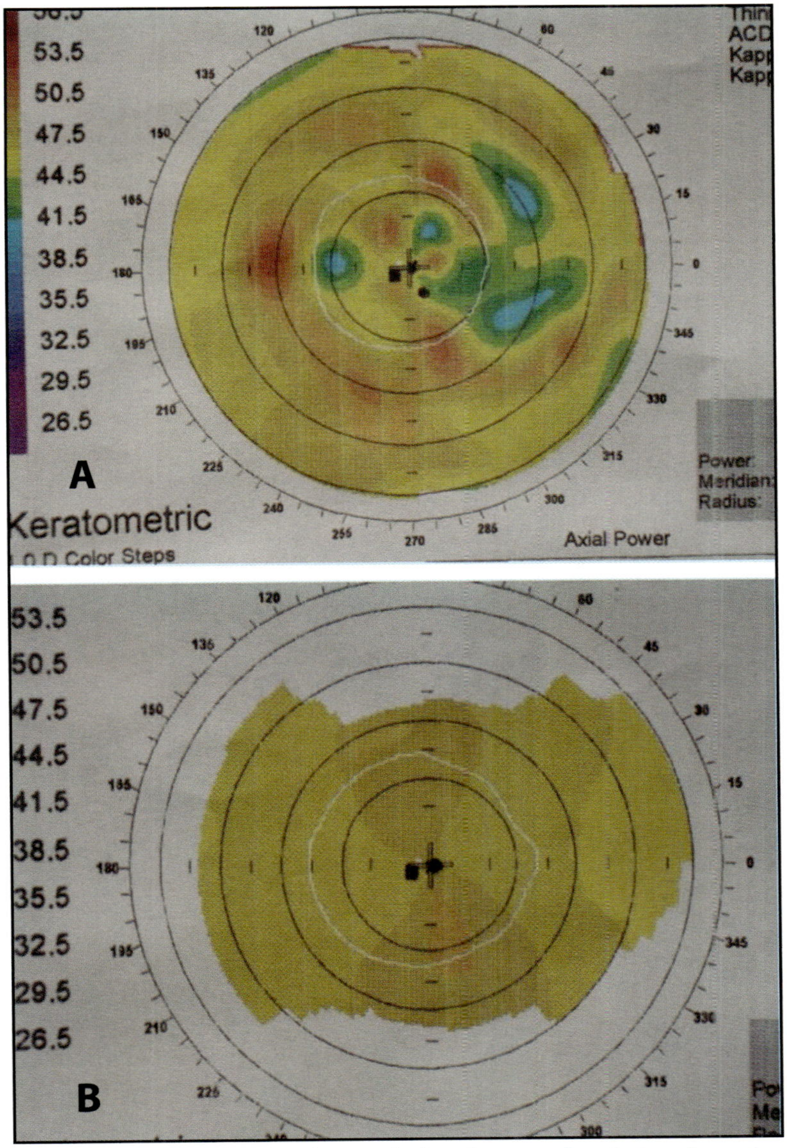

Figure 18-2. Topography before and after the use of topical cyclosporine 0.05%.

tear film greatly impacts the quality of vision. Patients without dry eye receiving bilateral multifocal IOL implantation had significantly improved mesopic and scotopic contrast sensitivity in the eye that received topical cyclosporine compared with eyes that received only an artificial tear[7] (Figure 18-2). In addition, these patients were more satisfied with the eye that received the topical cyclosporine.[7] When assessing the tear film, the meibomian glands must be evaluated. New treatments with re-esterified oral omega-3 nutritional supplements, hot compresses, and topical azithromycin have been shown to dramatically improve lid function.[8] A more regular tear film and ocular surface will also help to improve the quality of vision.

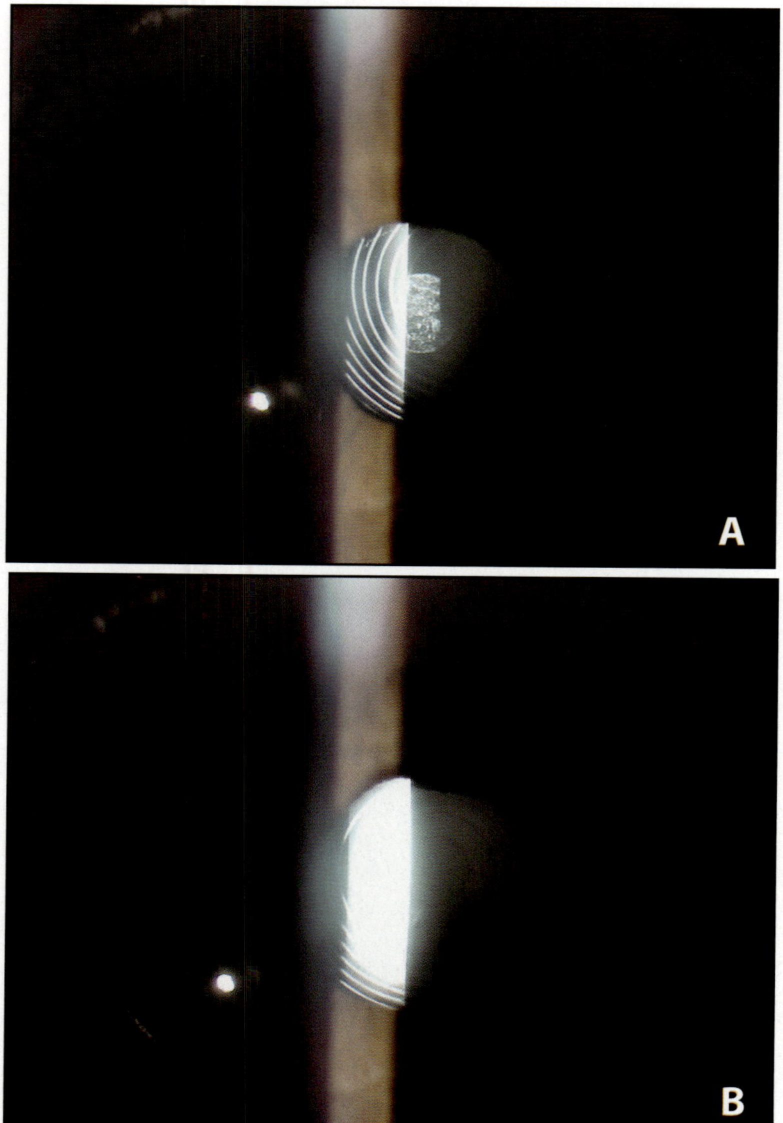

Figure 18-3. IOL not centered under pupil (A) before and (B) after argon laser iridoplasty.

Centration of the Intraocular Lens Relative to the Pupil

It is important to look for the centration of the IOL behind the pupil. If the pupil and the center of the capsular bag do not coincide, then the lens will appear decentered (Figure 18-3). In a symptomatic patient, an argon laser iridoplasty may be performed.[9] In this procedure, 4 spots are positioned in the iris midperiphery in the direction that the clinician would want the pupil pulled. The laser parameters frequently used are a power setting of 500 mW and a 500-μm diameter spot size for half a second.[9] In certain circumstances, an anterior capsulotomy may be performed as well, to help manage negative dysphotopsias.[10] An iridoplasty may also be elected prior to an excimer laser enhancement. The goal is to center the IOL on the pupil so that ablation is not performed off the visual axis or off the center of the lens. It is important to remember that although considered interventional, these procedures may spare a symptomatic patient the need for an IOL exchange.

Circumference of the Pupil Relative to the Intraocular Lens

Circumference of the pupil relative to the ICL becomes an important variable in patients who have had a ReSTOR IOL. If a patient has poor reading vision with this lens, he or she requires constriction of the pupil to increase the proportion of light being handled by the +3.00 or +4.00 central reading add. This can be achieved by prescribing topical brimonidine or pilocarpine. On the other hand, if the patient has poor distance vision, he or she may benefit from dilation of the pupil to increase the proportion of light being transmitted through the distance-dominated periphery of the lens. This may be accomplished either pharmacologically or with 360 degrees of midperipheral argon laser iridoplasty.

Patient Management

Patients who are unhappy following presbyopic IOL implantation require attention to detail from a surgical, pharmacological, and psychological perspective. Although visual outcomes with multifocal IOLs may be excellent, many surgeons have concerns about their use, partly due to the notion that even the latest generation of multifocal IOLs has been associated with photic phenomena such as glare, halos, or difficulty functioning in certain lighting conditions.[11] This can negatively affect daily life activities, limiting the patient's ability to perform and thus affecting quality of life.[11] Most importantly, dissatisfied patients should never feel abandoned, and it should be emphasized that the clinician will always work with them to solve their problems, although this process may take time. An unhappy patient should never be told, "You should be happy." The unhappy patient deserves a thorough evaluation of all possible reasons for his or her complaint. Patients may also be reminded that in a worst-case scenario, an IOL exchange for a monofocal IOL is almost always an alternative.

Attempts at expediting treatment as soon as it becomes safe for the unhappy or unsatisfied patient are frequently met with gratitude and positive feedback. Commonly, LRIs can be performed as early as 2 weeks following surgery. Patients who require LASIK or PRK are treated as soon as 1 month following multifocal IOL surgery and as early as 4 months following Crystalens implantation. It should be noted that our group always performs a posterior capsulotomy prior to an excimer laser enhancement in Crystalens patients, as the capsulotomy may change the refractive error if done afterward. Additionally, we have found that eliminating the additional financial burden on those patients who need additional procedures following IOL implantation yields a happier patient and, more importantly, a patient for life. This step also goes a long way to preserve the doctor-patient relationship.

In conclusion, there are multiple ways of improving visual outcomes in patients with refractive IOLs. Multifocal technology has already improved the quality of life for many pseudophakic patients by reducing or eliminating their dependence on spectacles, while new technologies are constantly evolving. Quality of vision with good near and far foci may make these lenses superior to excimer laser photoablation for some refractive errors in presbyopic patients. Accommodating IOLs preserve quality of vision and increase depth of focus for many patients. As physician comfort with these lenses improves over the coming years and decades, it is probable that multifocal and accommodative IOLs will dramatically increase in popularity with both cataract and refractive surgeons and their patients. When multifocal IOLs are not an option, toric IOLs are low-risk, high-reward options that should be offered to all patients with astigmatism who are interested in reducing spectacle dependence. When refractive IOL patients are unhappy following surgery, it is important to investigate and treat organic problems first before assuming that neuroadaptation will resolve all of the issues. With attention to residual refractive error, the ocular surface, CME, the posterior capsule, pupil centration, and pupil size, the unhappy refractive IOL patient can be converted to the happy postoperative patient.

References

1. Kim JS, Jung JW, Lee JM, Seo KY, Kim EK, Kim TI. Clinical outcomes following implantation of diffractive multifocal intraocular lenses with varying add powers. *Am J Ophthalmol.* 2015;160(4):702-709.
2. Knorz M, Rincon J, Suarez E, et al. Subjective outcomes after bilateral implantation of an apodized diffractive +3.0d multifocal toric IOL in a prospective clinical study. *J Refract Surg.* 2013;29(11):762-767.
3. Donnenfeld E. The effect of NSAIDS on quality of vision with multifocal IOLs. Paper presented at: American Society of Cataract and Refractive Surgery Symposium on Cataract, IOL, and Refractive Surgery; March 17-22, 2006; San Francisco, CA.
4. Rossetti L, Autelitano A. Cystoid macular edema following cataract surgery. *Curr Opin Ophthalmol.* 2000;11:65-72.
5. Donnenfeld E, Perry H, Wittpenn J, et al. Preoperative ketorolac tromethamine 0.4% in phacoemulsification outcomes: pharmacokinetic-response curve. *J Cataract Refract Surg.* 2006;32(9):1474-1482.
6. Donnenfeld E, Solomon K, Chu R. The effect of a topical NSAID on quality of vision with a multifocal IOL. *Invest Ophthalmol Vis Sci.* 2006;47:617.
7. Donnenfeld E, Solomon R, Roberts CW, Wittpenn JR, McDonald MB, Perry HD. Cyclosporine 0.05% to improve visual outcomes after multifocal intraocular lens implantation. *J Cataract Refract Surg.* 2010;36:1095-1100.
8. Malhotra C, Singh S, Chakma P, Jain AK. Effect of oral omega-3 fatty acid supplementation on contrast sensitivity in patients with moderate meibomian gland dysfunction: A prospective placebo-controlled study. *Cornea.* 2015;34(6):637-643.
9. Solomon R, Barsam A, Voldman A. Argon laser iridoplasty to improve visual function following multifocal intraocular lens implantation. *J Refract Surg.* 2012;28(4):281-283.
10. Hood C, Sugar A. Subjective complaints after cataract surgery: common causes and management strategies. *Curr Opin Ophthalmol.* 2015;26(1):45-49.
11. Cillino G, Casuccio A, Pasti M, Bono V, Mencucci R, Cillino S. Working-age cataract patients: Visual results, reading performance, and quality of life with three diffractive multifocal intraocular lenses. *Ophthalmology.* 2014;121(1):34-44.

Chapter 19

Enhancement With Piggyback or Intraocular Lens Exchanges

Adi Abulafia, MD and Warren E. Hill, MD

Although less frequent today than in years past, even with significant advances in measurement technology and formula accuracy, refractive surprises following all forms of lens-based surgery still occur. With patient expectations steadily increasing, surgeons should have in place a well-developed strategy for enhancing an unanticipated refractive outcome that includes the placement of a piggyback intraocular lens (IOL) or a lens exchange.

Situations in which refractive surprises occur most commonly are seen in the setting of high myopia and hyperopia, unusual anterior segments with exceptionally deep or shallow anterior chambers, small or large corneal diameters, the extremes of central corneal power, or any combination of these.

When faced with a refractive surprise, 5 basic management options are available: spectacle correction within the limits of tolerated anisometropia, the placement of a contact lens, corneal refractive surgery by LASIK or photorefractive keratectomy (PRK), a secondary piggyback IOL, or an IOL exchange.

Piggyback Intraocular Lens

There are several requirements for a successful piggyback IOL. First, the primary IOL should be contained completely within the capsular bag and preferably have 360 degrees of anterior capsule overlap. There should also be satisfactory space for another IOL between the posterior surface of the iris and the anterior surface of the primary IOL. This can usually be determined at the slit lamp. In addition, the capsular bag IOL should not have a strongly positive shape factor in the form of a steep anterior

Hovanesian JA.
Refractive Cataract Surgery: Best Practices and Advanced Technology, Second Edition (pp 225-232).

radius, as is sometimes seen with very high plus (+) power lenses. A steep anterior radius for the capsular bag IOL may displace the ciliary sulcus IOL forward or cause it to shift to one side of the visual axis.

The first advantage of a piggyback IOL is that the power of the capsular bag IOL does not need to be known. When using a piggyback IOL, optical power is simply being added to, or subtracted from, an existing optical system. A second advantage is that visual rehabilitation is usually rapid and the procedure carries a relatively low risk when compared with that of a lens exchange. And most importantly, determining the power of a piggyback IOL is an axial length–independent exercise. If the spherical equivalent (SphEq) of the refractive error is within ±7.00 diopters (D), and the Ks are in normal range, only the manifest refraction need be known if the intended refractive outcome is plano.[1]

Calculating the Power of a Piggyback Intraocular Lens

To calculate the power of a piggyback IOL, a simple rule of thumb is the following:

- ▲ For hyperopic refractive errors with a SphEq equivalent of less than +7.00 D, the SphEq is multiplied by 1.50 for a plano result. For example, for a refractive surprise of +3.75 +0.50 x 180, with Ks in a normal range, the piggyback IOL power for a plano result would be +4.00 D x 1.50 = +6.00 D.
- ▲ For myopic refractive errors of less than -7.00 D, the SphEq is multiplied by 1.30 for a plano result. For example, for a refractive surprise of -1.75 +0.50 x 180, with Ks in a normal range, the piggyback IOL power for a plano result would be -1.50 D x 1.30 = -1.95 D. Here, a -2.00 piggyback IOL would be used.
- ▲ For hyperopic and myopic refractive errors of greater than ±7.00 D, for unusual Ks, as are seen with refractive surgery, or if the refractive target is something other than plano, more accurate results are obtained using the refractive vergence formula or the Barrett Rx formula.

Working with the refractive vergence formula requires knowing the SphEq of the manifest refraction, current Ks, and the effective lens position of the IOL to be implanted. Once again, the great advantage here is that this is an axial length–independent exercise. Repeating the calculation using the same measurements but a different theoretical formula may lead to disappointments. For most cases, it was an incorrect assumption by a theoretical formula that resulted in the original refractive surprise.

As a general rule of thumb, the effective lens position of the piggyback IOL is simply the optimized effective lens position for the capsular bag lens that has been reduced by 0.65 mm. An optimized lens constant for the piggyback IOL would not be appropriate, as this second IOL will be sitting on top of the capsular bag IOL. See Table 19-1 for a method of approximating the effective lens position based on an optimized SRK/T A-constant.

For example, a Crystalens (Bausch & Lomb) patient undergoes scleral buckling more than a year after cataract surgery. A capsulotomy has already been completed. Due to axial length elongation by the scleral buckle, the refractive error has now shifted myopic and stabilizes at -2.50 + 0.50 x 180 for a SphEq of -2.25 D. The Ks are 42.25 x 42.75, and the capsular bag IOL has an optimized effective lens position of 5.61 mm. The adjusted piggyback effective lens position would therefore be 4.96 mm. The refractive target is plano.

Table 19-1
Approximation of Effective Lens Position Based on an Optimized SRK/T A-Constant

A-constant	*ELP*	*A-constant*	*ELP*	*A-constant*	*ELP*
118.0	4.97	118.5	5.26	119.0	5.55
118.1	5.02	118.6	5.32	119.1	5.61
118.2	5.02	118.7	5.37	119.2	5.67
118.3	5.14	118.8	5.43	119.3	5.72
118.4	5.20	118.9	5.49	119.4	5.78

Abbreviation: ELP, effective lens position.

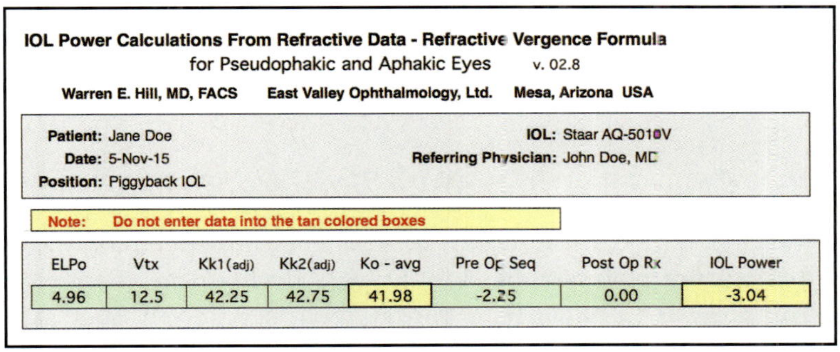

Figure 19-1. Piggyback IOL power calculation using the refractive vergence formula as described by Holladay in the form of a simple Microsoft Excel spreadsheet.

For this scenario, 3.04 D less power would be needed, added in the form of a minus (-) power secondary piggyback IOL at the plane of the ciliary sulcus in order to achieve the intended refractive outcome. The surgeon selects a -3.00 D AQ-5010V (Staar Surgical) piggyback IOL. See Figure 19-1 for the calculation carried out using the refractive vergence formula.

An explanation of how the refractive vergence formula works, along with examples, can be found on the Internet at www.doctor-hill.com/iol-main/piggyback.htm. A free, downloadable refractive vergence formula calculator in a Microsoft Excel format based on a description by Holladay[2,3] can be downloaded at www.doctor-hill.com/physicians/download.htm.

The Holladay R formula contained within the Holladay IOL Consultant (Holladay Consulting) software is a more sophisticated, commercially available version of the refractive vergence formula.

The Rx formula, recently introduced by Graham Barrett (available at www.apacrs.org), provides a solution for 3 scenarios: piggyback IOL, IOL exchange, and the optimal rotation of an existing toric IOL to a new meridian of alignment.

The Barrett Rx formula is derived from the Barrett Universal II formula. It first determines the actual ELP for the postoperative refractive error and uses this as the basis for the calculation. For this reason, the results may be somewhat different than for the Holladay R formula, or the refractive vergence formula, which use an IOL-specific value as the basis for the ELP. A shortcoming of this method is that the predicted outcome remains unchanged when different IOL powers are implanted for a particular refractive outcome.

The Barrett Rx formula also allows surgeons to select an alternative IOL option when the calculation assumes the predicted ELP is correct. This option should be chosen for eyes with prior refractive surgery, or if the error is thought to be due to a mislabelled or unknown IOL power. In this case, the piggyback IOL prediction will be similar to that of the Holladay R and the refractive vergence formulas.

The Barrett Rx formula requires axial length, postoperative Ks, optical anterior chamber depth, power of the implanted IOL, and 2 lens constants: 1 for the actual IOL implanted and 1 for the IOL selected for an IOL exchange. The constant for the IOL can be adjusted if the IOL exchange is planned for the sulcus, and this is indicated in a popup window.

The Barrett Rx formula will predict the resultant spherical equivalent, the IOL power, and also the recommended toric cylinder for an IOL exchange or a piggyback IOL.

Choosing a Piggyback Intraocular Lens

When choosing a piggyback IOL, it is generally best to select a 3-piece silicone lens with rounded edges. For powers from -4.00 D to +4.00 D, many consider the STAAR AQ-5010V (Figure 19-2) to be an ideal choice, with its relatively large 6.3-mm optic with smooth, rounded edges and a 14.0-mm haptic length. For higher plus (+) powers, the STAAR AQ-2010V is frequently used. In the United States, placing an IOL in the ciliary sulcus remains an off-label use. However, in other countries, there are available IOLs that are approved for sulcus implantation, such as the popular Sulcoflex (Rayner Intraocular Lenses Limited).

Important Caveat

In general, when selecting a piggyback IOL, it is best to avoid the use of 3-piece acrylic IOLs. Unless there is a large amount of space between the anterior surface of the capsular bag IOL and the posterior iris, the combination of square, truncated edges and a semi-tacky nature of the acrylic material may result in interaction with the posterior iris. This may lead to any combination of transillumination defects, pigment dispersion, secondary glaucoma, and intermittent uveitis. A single-piece acrylic IOL would never be placed in the ciliary sulcus.[4]

Piggyback Intraocular Lens Surgical Technique

Placing a piggyback IOL differs from primary lens implantation in that there is generally less room in which to work and the intended location is always the ciliary sulcus. When implanting silicone optic piggyback IOLs, it is often helpful to work under a

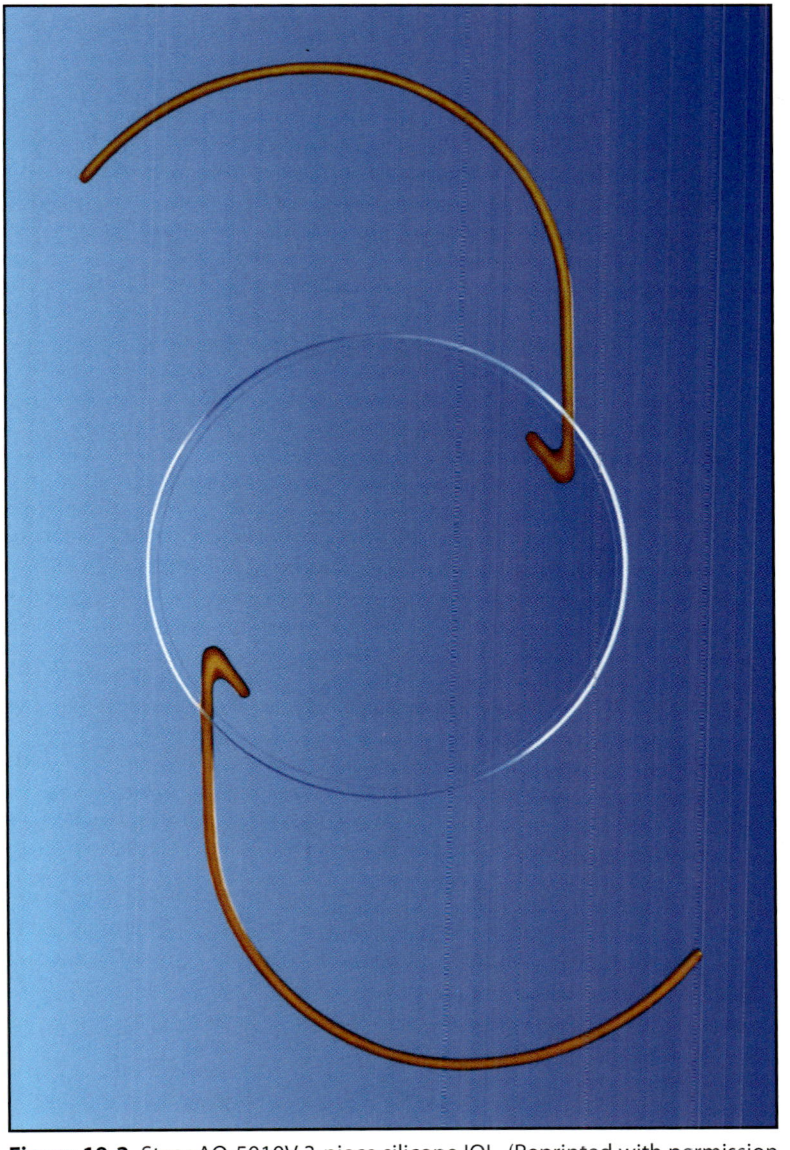

Figure 19-2. Staar AQ-5010V 3-piece silicone IOL. (Reprinted with permission from STAAR Surgical.)

highly retentive viscoelastic, such as Healon GV (Abbott Medical Optics) and have the optic exit the insertion cartridge nozzle as slowly as possible to avoid the lens rapidly and forcefully unfolding in the anterior chamber. There is no particular alignment necessary for the haptics. Following the removal of viscoelastic, a quick check confirms that adequate space exists between the posterior iris and the anterior surface of the IOL.

Residual Astigmatism

If less than 1.50 D, residual refractive astigmatism following the placement of a piggyback IOL can be managed by limbal relaxing incisions. For higher amounts, LASIK or PRK would be the better option within the effective treatment range of the procedure. For small amounts of preoperative refractive astigmatism, the corneal incision for the piggyback IOL can be made on axis. For surgeons outside the United States, the Sulcoflex IOL (Rayner) is also available in a toric model.

Intraocular Lens Exchange

An IOL exchange is the preferred option for a refractive surprise early in the postoperative course, when the power of the existing IOL is known with certainty and/or when a piggyback IOL would not be a workable option.

The 4 most common reasons for a lens exchange are formula inaccuracy, difficulties with preoperative measurements, an unhappy multifocal patient, or the unsettling occurrence of dysphotopsia. In addition to the use of older 2-variable, third-generation formulas, preoperative keratometry remains one of the weakest links in the process of IOL power calculation.[5]

Calculating the Power of an Exchange Intraocular Lens

As with a piggyback IOL, when calculating the power for a lens exchange, we are simply adding power to or subtracting power from an existing optical system. For a lens exchange, using the refractive vergence formula, the Holladay R formula, or the Barrett Rx formula is recommended.

Working with the refractive vergence formula requires knowing the SphEq of the manifest refraction, current Ks, and the effective lens position of the IOL to be implanted. Once again, this is an axial length–independent exercise. The effective lens position of the exchange IOL can be approximated using Table 19-1.

For example, a patient undergoes uncomplicated surgery with a +18.50 D SN6AD1 ReSTOR (Alcon) multifocal IOL, and it is later discovered that the wrong Ks were entered into the IOL power calculation formula. As a result, there is a hyperopic postoperative refractive error of +1.50 +0.25 x 180 (SphEq = +1.68 D). The Ks are 42.25 x 42.50, the capsular bag IOL has an optimized effective lens position of 5.55 mm, and the refractive target is plano. For this scenario, 2.53 D more power would be needed for the exchange IOL at the plane of the capsular bag in order to achieve the intended refractive outcome. The power of the exchange IOL would be 18.50 D + 2.50 D = +21.00 D (Figure 19-3).

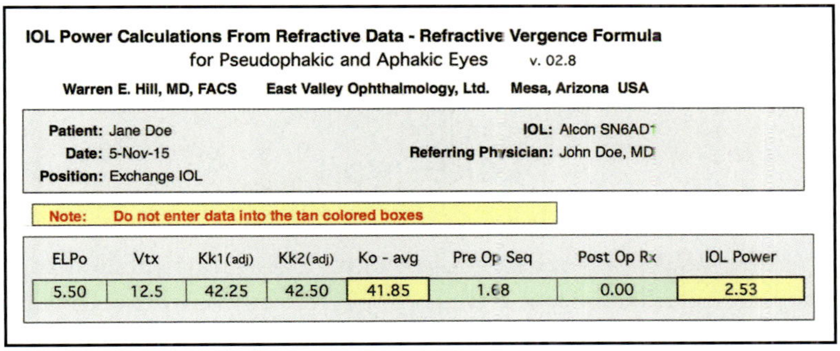

IOL Power Calculations From Refractive Data - Refractive Vergence Formula
for Pseudophakic and Aphakic Eyes v. 02.8
Warren E. Hill, MD, FACS **East Valley Ophthalmology, Ltd.** **Mesa, Arizona USA**

Patient: Jane Doe
Date: 5-Nov-15
Position: Exchange IOL
IOL: Alcon SN6AD1
Referring Physician: John Doe, MD

Note: **Do not enter data into the tan colored boxes**

ELPo	Vtx	Kk1 (adj)	Kk2 (adj)	Ko - avg	Pre Op Seq	Post Op Rx	IOL Power
5.50	12.5	42.25	42.50	41.85	1.68	0.00	2.53

Figure 19-3. Exchange IOL power calculation using the refractive vergence formula as described by Holladay in the form of a simple Microsoft Excel spreadsheet.

Intraocular Lens Exchange Surgical Technique

Removing an existing IOL from the capsular bag is relatively easy when carried out early in the postoperative course. The technique is generally as follows:

- ▲ Via multiple paracentesis sites, the capsulorrhexis edge is first dissected off the anterior surface of the existing IOL in all quadrants with a dispersive viscoelastic, often by using a bevel-up 30-gauge needle on the end of the viscoelastic syringe.
- ▲ Viscoelastic is next injected between the leaflets of the anterior and posterior capsules using a 30-gauge cannula at the location of both optic-haptic junctions where the anterior and posterior aspects of the capsular bag are being held apart. It is not uncommon to witness a "wave" of viscoelastic dissecting the capsular bag around the edge of the optic during this process. The dispersive viscoelastic Viscoat (Alcon) is ideal for this purpose.
- ▲ The bulbous terminations of single-piece acrylic haptics may require additional viscodissection in order to free up that portion of the haptic from its location in the equator of the capsular bag. The haptics are then gently rotated out of the capsular bag. If the haptics cannot be safely removed, they can be amputated and left in place without problems.
- ▲ Occasionally, additional viscoelastic is injected between the posterior capsule and the back surface of the IOL to completely mobilize the optic of the IOL.
- ▲ With the IOL now completely mobile, the optic can either be cut in half or folded using the combination of IOL folding forceps aided by the use of a cyclodialysis spatula placed under the IOL from a location 180 degrees from the entry of the folding forceps. There are many instruments available for cutting the optic of a foldable IOL prior to explantation. The Mackool Foldable Lens Removal System (Ambler Surgical) and the Packer/Change IOL Cutters (MicroSurgical Technology) are especially good for cutting both silicone and acrylic IOLs.

With few exceptions, it is generally possible to preserve the capsular bag and place the new IOL in the same location as the one explanted. Maintaining the effective lens position of the new IOL allows for accurate refractive outcomes. If the posterior capsule is compromised, a 3-piece IOL implanted in the ciliary sulcus or stabilized by optic capture, with the necessary power adjustment, are effective alternatives.

Conclusion

The placement of a piggyback IOL offers the advantage of a relatively low-risk procedure that combines rapid visual rehabilitation with a calculation methodology that does not involve the same pitfalls that lead to the original refractive surprise. Disadvantages are that most low power, silicone IOLs only come in 1.00 D steps, and there may not always be adequate space between the posterior iris and the anterior surface of the capsular bag IOL for this option.

An IOL exchange is typically carried out early in the postoperative course and is best accomplished when it is anticipated that the capsular bag can be preserved and the power of the implanted IOL is known with certainty. Similar to a piggyback IOL, calculating the power of the exchange lens does not involve needing to know the axial length, as power is simply being added to an existing optical system.

Fortunately, calculating the power of a piggyback IOL and an exchange IOL can be carried out with great accuracy.

References

1. Hill WE, Byrne SF. Complex axial length measurements and unusual IOL power calculations. *Focal Points—Clinical Modules for Ophthalmologists*. Module 9. San Francisco, CA: American Academy of Ophthalmology; September 2004.
2. Holladay JT. Refractive power calculations for intraocular lenses in the phakic eye. *Am J Ophthalmol.* 1993;116(1):63-66.
3. Chang DF, Masket S, Miller KM, et al; ASCRS Cinical Cataract Committee. Complications of sulcus placement of single-piece acrylic intraocular lenses: recommendations for backup IOL implantation following posterior capsule rupture. *J Cataract Refract Surg.* 2009;35:1445-1458.
4. Holladay JT. Standardizing constants for ultrasonic biometry, keratometry and intraocular lens power calculations. *J Cataract Refract Surg.* 1997;23(9):1356-1370.
5. Jin, GJ, Crandal AS, Jones JJ. Intraocular lens exchange due to incorrect lens power. *Ophthalmology.* 2007;114(3):417-424.

Chapter 20

Excimer Laser Enhancements After Intraocular Lens Surgery

Jay Bansal, MD and Arun C. Gulani, MD, MS

New technologies and heightened expectations are forging pathways for premium cataract surgery and, more importantly, raising the bar on outcomes.

The demographic of patients who are opting to pay for an upgrade to a premium lens means increasing expectations, clinically as well as emotionally. The ever-elusive fountain of youth is not their actual goal, but the baby boomers who are transitioning from being prime LASIK candidates and becoming cataract patients have new sets of expectations and demands. They expect to have the vision of their youth and may become a surgeon's loudest advocate for happiness or chagrin depending on how well a surgeon navigates the process. For "20/happy" all around, it is essential that the entire team is involved in negotiating patients' expectations, providing information that gives them choices, and preparing them for options in enhancement scenarios.

Setting the Stage

While many surgeons may have a preferred lens, the patient's visual needs dictate the lens choice. Considering the many choices of premium IOLs available, counseling is a critical component of helping patients understand what the technology can give them, what tradeoffs they should expect when they choose a premium lens, and what may be necessary to achieve optimum visual function postsurgery. Many practices have taken counselors from their LASIK team and utilized them in helping patients walk through their options. Sending materials and having a point of contact before the initial examination is proving successful in preparing patients for their choices. Privacy and an office

Hovanesian JA.
Refractive Cataract Surgery: Best Practices and Advanced Technology, Second Edition (pp 233-244). © 2017 SLACK Incorporated.

space where discussions on their choices in the lane and with the surgical scheduler are often appreciated.

Achieving maximum visual function after premium IOL implantation may take several months, and the more patients understand this and have a contact in the practice who is empathetic, patient, and available, the better the period of their neuroadaptation will be. It is critical that the patient be comforted ahead of time regarding this and also be educated about the possible need for additional treatments preoperatively, including optimization of the ocular surface, neodymium-doped yttrium aluminum garnet (Nd:YAG) laser posterior capsulotomy, and keratorefractive surgery.

Ophthalmologists have various options available when it comes to premium IOLs. These include the AcrySof ReSTOR IOL +3.0 D, +4.0 D and Toric (Alcon), the ReZoom and Tecnis IOLs (Abbott Medical Optics), and the Crystalens 5.0, HD, and AO (Bausch & Lomb).

To produce optimal visual outcomes and excellent patient satisfaction after premium IOL surgery, laser vision correction enhancement procedures such as LASIK or photorefractive keratectomy (PRK) are necessary additional skills for a successful cataract surgeon. The enhancement element is creating several trends as surgeons consider the best-case scenario for their patients. Some cataract surgeons are outsourcing enhancements to LASIK surgeons whom they are partnering with, while others are investing in equipment and training to do their own enhancements, and/or they are using open access centers and doing the enhancements themselves there.

Enhancements are a necessary and important part of achieving the optimal outcomes for patients who have a presbyopia-correcting IOL. For some patients, correcting even small amounts of residual refractive error—sometimes as small as 0.5 D of myopia, hyperopia, or astigmatism—can really change the patient's perception of the outcome. Cataract surgeons who provide premium IOLs (toric, accommodating, and multifocal) must be able to offer enhancement procedures to achieve excellent outcomes and thus satisfy their patients' expectations. Ultimately, until optimal vision is obtained, the patient's care is not complete.

Laser vision correction enhancements to premium IOL cases can be classified as follows[1]:

- Planned laser combination surgeries
- Laser enhancement for unexpected, visually significant refractive errors
- Laser surgery to correct complications

Enhancement Options: Photorefractive Keratectomy, LASIK, Conductive Keratoplasty, and Radial Keratotomy

Most surgeons employ LASIK or PRK to correct residual refractive error in these premium IOL patients. Laser vision correction gives surgeons the confidence to achieve emmetropia even with a refractive surprise or significant preoperative astigmatism. While an IOL exchange is certainly an option for treating residual spherical refractive errors (especially large errors), a strong argument can be made for treating smaller residual refractive errors and/or astigmatism with laser vision correction after cataract surgery.

Any additional intraocular surgical procedure for an IOL exchange is stressful for both the patient and surgeon, along with the significant additional expense of returning to an operating room. While the prospect of performing LASIK surgery may be daunting even to seasoned cataract surgeons, surface ablation with PRK is a simple and powerful means by which to adjust residual refractive errors that remain after cataract surgery. PRK is a simpler technique with equivalent efficacy for the majority of patients.

Performing topographic mapping and corneal pachymetry for IOL patients, as well as a complete eye evaluation and IOL calculations, is wise in the event that refractive surgery is necessary postoperatively. External disease is treated and the ocular surface optimized before the cataract surgery. As it has been observed that minor postoperative fluctuations in vision are frequently related to dry eyes, an aggressive pretreatment may be in order to achieve a healthy ocular surface.

Additionally, if there are concerns or doubt about the topography or pachymetry of the cornea, proceeding with PRK instead of LASIK for the enhancement may be the better course of treatment.

Some patients may ask about having LASIK instead of PRK. LASIK is an outstanding first choice, but for many older patients, their poorly adherent corneal epithelium will be a red flag. Furthermore, PRK is less likely to induce extreme ocular dryness, and dryness is a frequent (albeit usually temporary) byproduct of even cataract surgery alone. Also, older patients are more prone to vascular disease, increasing the (still unlikely) possibility that the prolonged suction required during LASIK could precipitate a retinal vascular event. Surface ablation for elderly patients who require laser vision correction after cataract surgery is often a procedure of choice.

TIMING

It is important to allow the refractive error and best corrected visual acuity to stabilize after surgery and to resist the urge to jump right in. A period of observation is especially important if the patient has had prior refractive surgery, because fluctuations in corneal shape, and hence refractive error, may continue. Under- or overcorrection is readily evident 1 to 2 weeks postoperatively in an eye that has never undergone refractive surgery. Eyes that had prior LASIK, PRK, or radial keratotomy (RK) may take longer to stabilize. If the patient has more than 2.5 D of unintended refractive error, an IOL exchange within the first postoperative month may be a better option, depending on the surgeon's comfort with the exchange vs laser vision correction. For a PRK enhancement after IOL surgery, it is not necessary to wait 3 to 6 months before enhancing the result of prior PRK or LASIK; 6 to 8 weeks is usually sufficient. Surgeons should prescribe spectacles if patients need them postoperatively. If the unintended refractive error is less than 2.00 D, anisometropia should be tolerable. If the patient does not achieve the expected correction, surgeons should look for and treat other causes of decreased best corrected visual acuity that may distort the refraction (eg, cystoid macular edema).

The following are some things to consider prior to any enhancement:

- ▲ Has the ocular surface been optimized?
- ▲ Is there another issue that needs to be resolved first (eg, cystoid macular edema, posterior capsular opacification)?

Open the Capsule?

Consider performing an Nd:YAG laser capsulotomy before PRK. If the subjective visual acuity endpoint is not distinct with manifest refraction, an Nd:YAG capsulotomy often allows for the determination of a consistent refraction with which to plan a PRK enhancement. If the patient has received the Crystalens (Bausch & Lomb), it is advisable to perform the capsulotomy before any refractive surgery, because the effective IOL position may shift.

Laser or Incisions?

An excimer laser rather than limbal relaxing incisions (LRI) to enhance premium IOL recipients' outcomes is preferred due to the control over the astigmatic correction. LRIs may be fairly unpredictable for patients who have more than 1.00 D of astigmatism. The advanced IOL calculations for premium cataract surgery leave most patients' postoperative spherical equivalent close to plano. Consequently, the amount of postoperative correction these patients need is generally very small (less than 3.00 D). With the predictability and stability of laser vision correction available today, there are very few cases in which either conductive keratoplasty or RK may be of greater benefit than the excimer laser.

Wavefront-Guided Versus Optimized Versus Conventional

For optimal results, regardless of attention to detail during biometry and meticulous surgery, a refractive correction may be necessary after IOL surgery regardless of the lens selected. This can occur secondarily to other factors also: incision related refractive change, over- or undersized capsulorrhexis, effective lens position, biometry error, etc. The refractive surgery enhancement choices include PRK, LASIK, conductive keratoplasty, RK, astigmatic keratotomy, and IOL exchange. There is greater refractive predictability using LASIK to correct hyperopic refractive errors post-IOL surgery. With laser vision correction, however, the decision must be made between wavefront guided vs optimized vs conventional treatment.

It is advisable to obtain wavefront measurements on everyone; however, for simple myopia and myopic astigmatism, a treatment of choice is often conventional PRK using a transepithelial approach. This method is engaged primarily because of the rapid re-epithelialization, minimal ablation depth, and less induced dry eye postoperatively.

Multifocal IOLs can affect the accuracy of the wavefront aberrometer, and thus wavefront-guided treatments are not appropriate. Wavefront-optimized treatments are also an excellent treatment option in all cases, and even more pronounced in higher refractive errors.

Nomograms, Special Considerations for Patients

The laser vision correction procedures (LASIK and PRK) are performed exactly the same way for primary and secondary treatments, utilizing the same nomogram adjustments.

Counseling

When planning premium IOL surgery in which a primary goal is clear, uncorrected vision, it must be determined ahead of time whether the patient is a candidate for an enhancement with PRK. If so, this is the time to share with the patient that laser vision correction may be an option to enhance less-than-perfect results. The fees for this may be separated or included, depending on the practice's preference. Patients need to know that an IOL exchange may be the only surgical option if residual spherical error remains. Most patients are not overly worried about the risks of intraocular manipulation during cataract surgery, but it may be comforting that this can be accomplished without another operating room procedure.

Further discussion with patients about their visual recovery after PRK is usually a good idea. Individuals undergoing PRK often have the misguided idea that they will see well immediately, as they are likely to know someone who has undergone LASIK. Letting them know that their vision will fluctuate significantly for the first 4 to 6 days until the bandage contact lens is removed is essential, along with emphasizing that full recovery may take 8 weeks or longer. Most patients achieve functional vision in the 20/30-to-20/50 range within days of the bandage contact lens removal. If they are aware that visual recovery is a process, patients tend to be more accepting of the time it involves. Again, the time and investment in developing meaningful patient information packets with timelines, answers to frequently asked questions, and having a counselor who is able to communicate swiftly and reassuringly can make all the difference in the world.

Preoperative Evaluation

The Ocular Surface

Ocular surface instability from dry eye and/or lipid tear deficiency from meibomitis frequently causes refractive changes after cataract surgery. Patients with multifocal IOLs will be especially sensitive to this. Eyelid hygiene, Restasis (cyclosporine), artificial tear supplements, and punctal occlusion are all valuable treatments in this situation and should be used aggressively to optimize lubrication before any decisions about a PRK enhancement. Ocular rosacea is common; consideration should be given to the use of adjunctive topical azithromycin and/or oral tetracycline, doxycycline, or minocycline to improve meibomian gland function before surgery in such patients. Sufficient lubrication of the ocular surface is essential during the post-PRK healing process. Consider prescribing preservative-free artificial tears 4 times daily postoperatively, placement of permanent punctal plugs, and initiation of Restasis therapy (Allergan, Inc). If the patient was using

Restasis before surgery, it is recommended that usage stop until topical antibiotics are discontinued.

A large group of patients who are having cataract surgery have pre-existing dry eye or blepharitis and have compromised ocular surfaces. A healthy ocular surface ensures accurate measurements of the cornea and is essential to a successful outcome with all cataract surgery. Optimizing the ocular surface dramatically improves patient satisfaction, quality of vision, and may potentially reduce the need for postoperative enhancements. Based on the clinical evaluation, there are a variety of methods to optimize the ocular surface, varying from topical medications to therapeutic treatments and/or nutritional supplements.

Intraoperative Steps

Verify that topography correlates with the refractive error. Although most patients have some degree of orthogonal, regular corneal astigmatism before and after surgery, those who experience epithelial sloughing during cataract surgery can develop irregularities in the epithelial surface that manifest as increased refractive astigmatism, as can patients with keratoconus.

To correct astigmatism in eyes with intraoperative epithelial sloughing, superficial keratectomy (epithelial debridement) is preferable to PRK or LRIs. If the corneal topography appears to be normal and unexplained astigmatism is still present, the surgeon should examine the IOL for evidence of tilt or decentration. If the position of the IOL is in doubt based on the slit-lamp examination, imaging with a device such as the Pentacam Comprehensive Eye Scanner (Oculus, Inc) or anterior segment optical coherence tomography can be helpful.

The laser vision correction procedures (LASIK and PRK) are performed exactly the same way for primary and secondary treatments utilizing the same nomogram adjustments. PRK and LASIK enhancements 8 to 12 weeks after the original lenticular surgery are our standard timetable, and we usually prefer PRK to LASIK for these secondary procedures, because the former will not compromise the integrity of the capsular bag or zonules and is less likely to induce dry eyes. If it seems likely preoperatively that the patient will need a re-treatment (for example, a very high-cylinder patient), a LASIK flap will be created before performing the cataract surgery, and then 8 to 12 weeks later the flap is able to be lifted and the enhancement completed. This is possible using the femtosecond laser to cut all LASIK flaps, because it places much less pressure on the post-surgical eye than do mechanical microkeratomes. For PRK, it is important for surgeons to be comfortable with the techniques for gently removing the corneal epithelium during surgery (a rotary brush or transepithelial approach are preferable) and with the strategies to optimize the management of pain postoperatively.

For wavefront-optimized PRK treatment with the Allegretto Wave excimer laser (Alcon): first use a rotary brush to remove the corneal epithelium and verify all epithelium is removed with a dry Merocel sponge. After ablation, apply chilled balanced saline solution for 45 seconds, followed by a bandage contact lens.

For conventional PRK with the VISX Star excimer laser (Abbott Medical Optics): the transepithelial no-touch approach is preferred. The laser is preprogrammed in the epithelial mode (-0.75 D spherical and 45 microns plano) to remove the epithelium followed by the actual correction. This allows for very smooth epithelial edges and quite rapid recovery. Again, after ablation, apply chilled balanced saline solution for 45 seconds, followed by a bandage contact lens.

An extended-wear lens with high oxygen permeability, such as the O2Optix (CIBA Vision) with a base curve of 8.6 mm and a diameter of 14.2 mm, or the Oasys lens (Acuvue) with a base curve of 8.4 mm, seems to work well. For patients who have steeper corneas (46.00 D and up), the Soflens 66 steep/medium lens (Bausch & Lomb) is the bandage contact lens of choice. The lens should fit snugly but not be overly tight. On the day after PRK, an optimally fit bandage contact lens should move slightly (0.25 mm) with blinking or be movable with gentle upward digital pressure on the lower eyelid.

Many refractive surgeons now use a single dose of intraoperative dilute mitomycin C (MMC; usually 0.02%) routinely during PRK surgery for 12 to 20 seconds, especially for eyes that have undergone prior LASIK or RK. MMC is not necessary for eyes undergoing treatment for small corrections, as discussed earlier, but surgeons will need to be comfortable using this agent if they plan to treat eyes that have had prior corneal surgery. The best method by which to deliver MMC to the central cornea (where it needs to be applied) seems to be incubation with a saturated corneal light shield. Once the light shield is removed, it is important to irrigate the corneal surface generously with chilled, balanced salt solution. The use of MMC during PRK is considered off-label, and it is prudent to obtain a separate, informed consent for this practice.

Postoperative Care

Proper postoperative medical therapy after PRK is key to success. Fitting a bandage contact lens after PRK enhances the patient's comfort and helps to ensure prompt healing of the corneal epithelium. A collagen punctal plug in the eyes of all PRK patients to enhance lubrication of the ocular surface and maintain hydration of the bandage contact lens performs well.

Medical therapy after PRK consists of topical antibiotic prophylaxis as well as anti-inflammatory treatment with topical steroids and nonsteroidal anti-inflammatory drugs (NSAIDs). In practice, patients may use a fourth-generation fluoroquinolone solution and prednisolone acetate 1% suspension 4 times daily for 1 week, at which time the epithelium has healed and the bandage contact lens has been removed (generally on postoperative day 4 for myopes and day 5 for hyperopes). Additionally, for pain relief, patients take a topical NSAID, Xibrom (bromfenac ophthalmic solution), twice daily until the bandage contact lens is removed.

After 1 week, antibiotics are discontinued, and topical steroids are tapered by 1 drop/day every 1 week during a 4-week period. While a topical NSAID is very helpful for controlling pain, it can impede epithelial healing and incite sterile corneal stromal inflammation in some patients if continued for too long. Thus it is discontinued when the bandage lens is removed. Oral analgesia after PRK is also important for patients' comfort. If there are no medical contraindications, oral NSAID therapy with higher doses of ibuprofen (600 to 800 mg twice daily) or naproxen sodium (440 mg twice daily) is helpful and can minimize the need for stronger medications.

Turning Back the Clock

Laser Advanced Surface Ablation: Premium Lens Implant Combinations in Previous Refractive Surgery Cases

With millions of people who have had previous refractive surgeries seeking 20/20 again, we need to be well prepared to face an inevitable epidemic in the world of ophthalmology—an evolving population of previous refractive surgery patients who are now in their cataract age. Most of these patients can be corrected back to enjoy the excellent vision that they had once appreciated by using premium lens implants; in a way, turning back the clock!

Once we understand this concept of laser advanced surface ablation (ASA) surgery combination with premium lens implants as a required and mandatory skill of a premium cataract surgeon, you shall see how every patient deserves an opportunity for premium lens implants.

With this vision-oriented approach, we first manipulate the intraocular optical elements of such cases using specific lens implants to be followed by using the cornea as a vision rehabilitative platform (with the excimer laser) in turning back the clock and once again aiming for unaided emmetropia with the technologies and expectations of the present times.[2,3]

What Functions Does the Excimer Laser Achieve in Previous Refractive Cases?

The need for staged laser combination following premium lens implants in previous refractive surgeries using the PRK mode (ASA) is a conceptual shift from thinking in terms of just *refractive enhancement* to *optimizing vision.* The excimer laser ASA can additionally be used to correct all of the following:

- Residual refractive error
- Irregular astigmatism
- Superficial irregularity/scars
- Increasing the effective optical zone
- Optimizing/reversing corneal optics to compensate for previous keratorefractive surgery

This concept of looking at the excimer laser ASA surgery as an essential component of premium lens implant surgery in previous refractive cases (Figure 20-1) will enable millions of suitable candidates to enjoy the technology and vision of the 21st century.

It will also extend the indications to include patients with conditions like Fuchs dystrophy (Figure 20-2) and keratoconus (Figure 20-3) as premium lens candidates and provide patients with inadequate or complicated premium lens outcomes a second chance for vision (Figure 20-4).

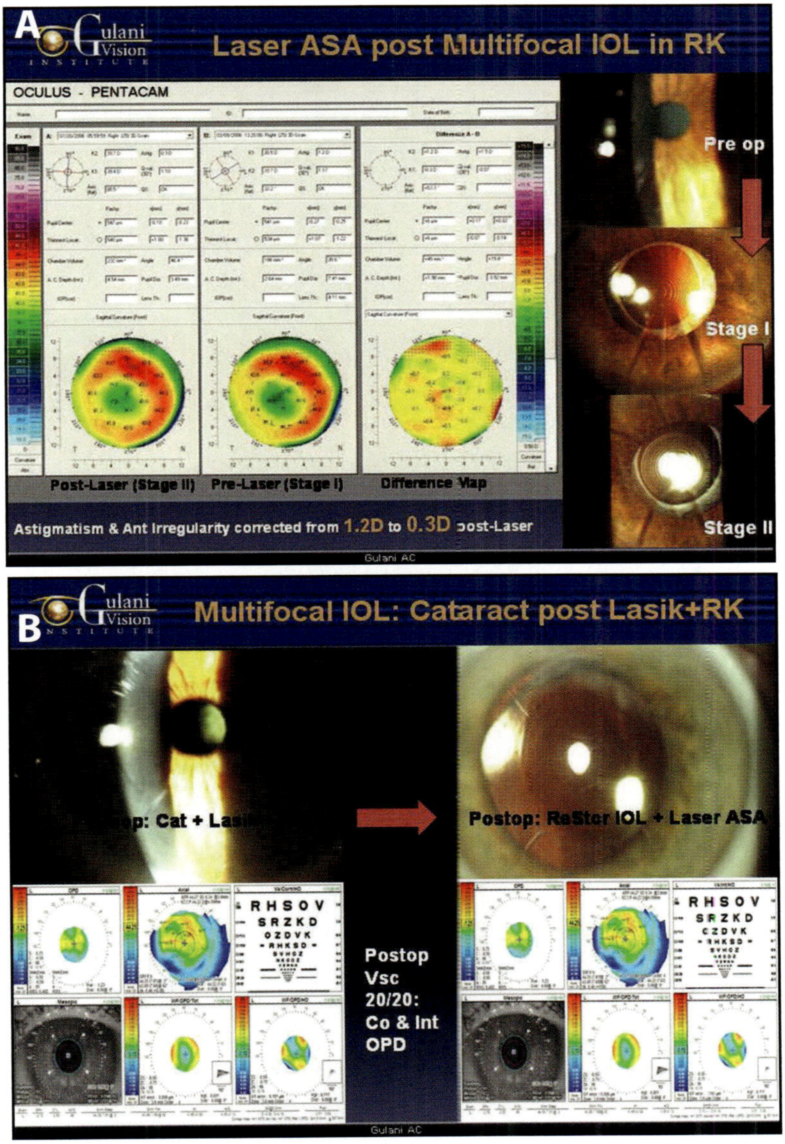

Figure 20-1. (A) Laser ASA following multifocal lens implant in an RK case; (B) ASA-based selection of premium IOL in case of LASIK and RK cataract to 20/20 outcomes.

Converting "Not a Candidate" Into "Candidate"

Many cases of previous RK, PRK, or LASIK, including those with keratoconus or corneal scars, can be converted to premium cataract surgery both in applications and expectations by planning for a staged laser surgery following lens implantation.

For example, a case of keratoconus can first be prepared with asymmetric INTACS (Addition Technology) to be followed by toric IOL to result in myopic astigmatism, to

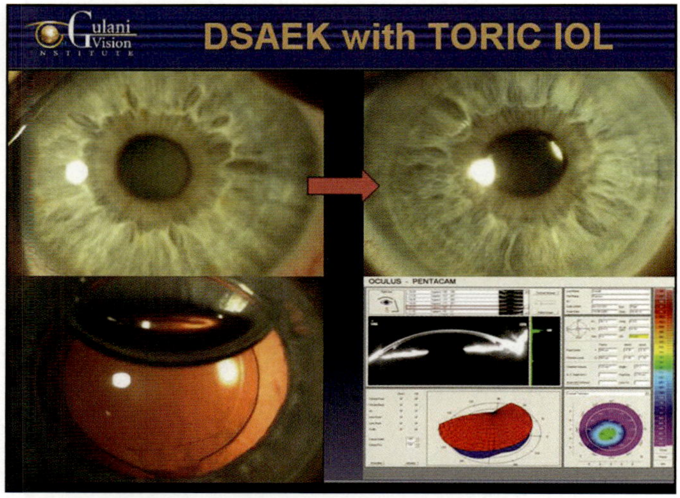

Figure 20-2. Toric lens implant in Descemet stripping automated endothelial keratoplasty.

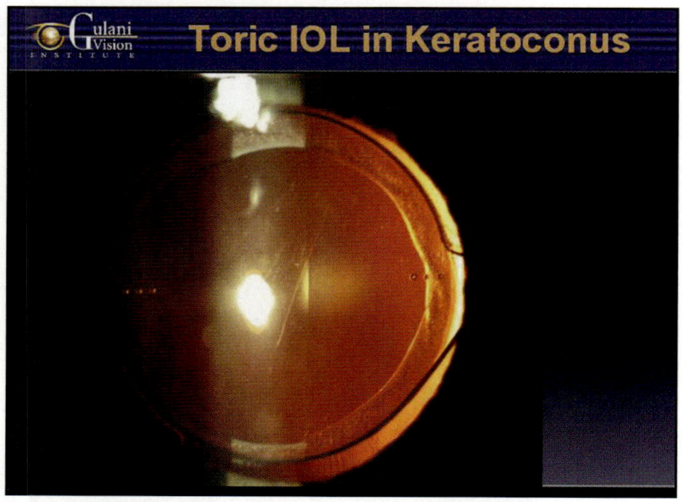

Figure 20-3. Toric lens implant in a keratoconus case.

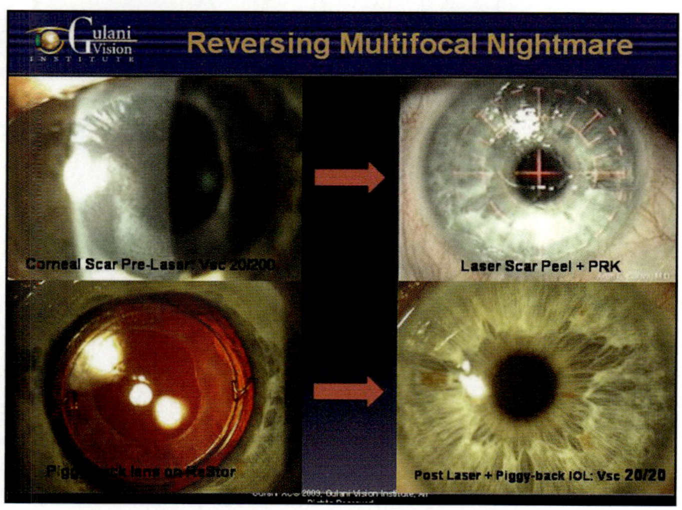

Figure 20-4. Reversing complication of a multifocal lens implant with laser ASA.

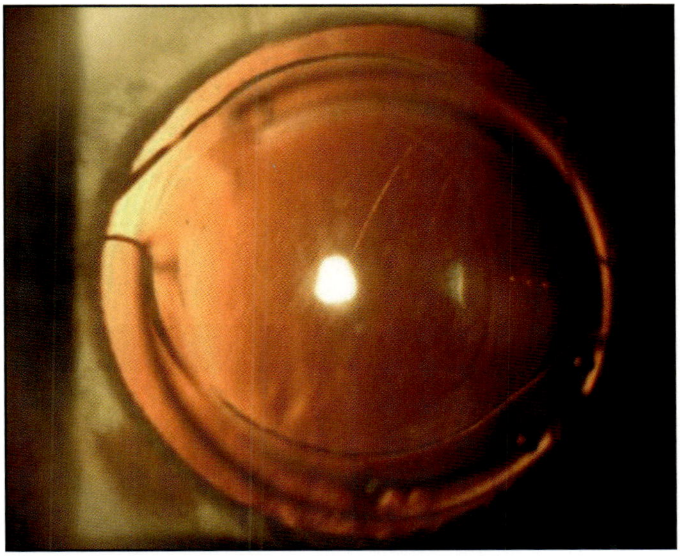

Figure 20-5. Preparatory INTACS before premium toric IOL followed by laser PRK enhancement.

then be followed by excimer laser PRK in a myopic mode to increase optical zone, flatten keratometry, and correct residual refractive error (this can then be cross-linked) (Figure 20-5).

Cases of RK can be corrected with combined laser PRK in a planned staged manner 3 to 4 weeks apart to emmetropia (Figure 20-6).

Femtosecond lasers can help turn cases of white mature cataracts into successful outcomes (due to consistent capsulorrhexis) and then, given possible poor IOL calculation, one can apply LASIK surgery to emmetropia.[4-6]

Even in complex cases with compromised anatomy we can manipulate the optics using technology to the patient's advantage like in this case which allowed this active patient to have premium IOL /Cataract surgery (Figure 20-7).

Conclusion

Cataract surgeons offering premium IOLs have a good array of enhancement options at hand to fine-tune residual refractive errors and optimize the final visual outcome after IOL procedures. Patients will appreciate receiving all of their care from their treating cataract surgeon, which makes it well worth these ophthalmologists' efforts to acquire the requisite skills for successful excimer laser enhancements after IOL surgery.

Additionally, patients who were deemed "not a candidate" can now become candidates for premium IOL surgery with a planned preparatory stage or conclusive staged laser surgery.

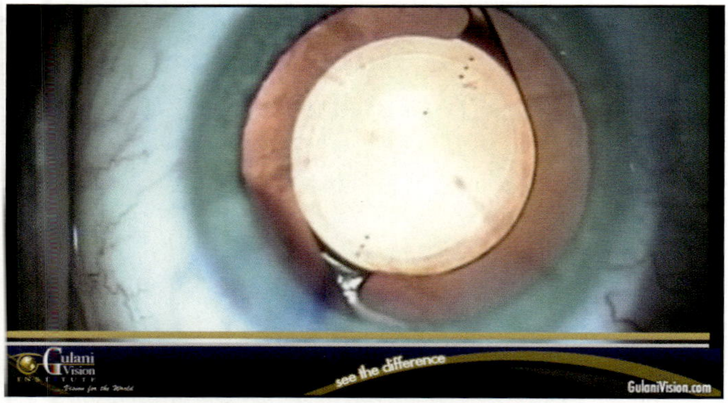

Figure 20-6. Premium toric IOL in RK case followed by planned laser PRK.

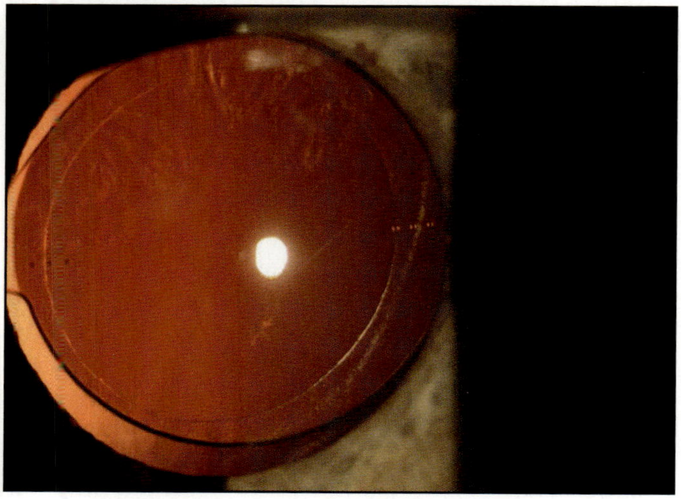

Figure 20-7. Femtosecond laser capsulorrhexis in a mature white cataract enabled good placement of a premium IOL, to be followed by LASIK surgery to emmetropia.

References

1. Gulani AC. Refractive surgery to the rescue. Presented at XXXII World Congress of Ophthalmology; June 5-9, 2010; Berlin, Germany.
2. Gulani AC. Corneoplastique. *Tech Ophthalmol.* 2007;5(1):11-20.
3. Gulani AC. Art of vision surgery. *Video Journal of Cataract and Refractive Surgery.* 2006;XXII(3).
4. Gulani AC. Femtosecond lasers in complex cataract surgery. *Cataract and Refractive Surgery Today.* 2015;15(4):92.
5. Gulani AC. Femtosecond lasers: are they becoming a necessity in cataract surgery? *Cataract and Refractive Surgery Today.* 2013;13(11):25-26.
6. Gulani AC. Sharpen your LASIK technique. *Rev Ophthalmol.* 2015;2:68-69.

Bibliography

Hardten D. Surgeon offers advice for optimum vision after premium IOL surgery. *Refractive Surgery News.* June 24, 2010.

Manrique C. Laser enhancements after premium cataract surgery: my experience compared with limbal relaxing incisions. *Cataract and Refractive Surgery Today.* February 2010.

Talamo JH. How to perform excimer laser enhancements after premium IOL implantation: making a good thing even better: a primer for cataract surgeons. *Cataract and Refractive Surgery Today.* February 2010.

Chapter 21

Enhancements With Micro-Radial Keratotomy/ Astigmatic Keratotomy

Frank A. Bucci Jr, MD

The efficient and accurate correction of residual refractive errors following the implantation of presbyopic-correcting intraocular lenses (IOL) is critical for achieving high levels of both spectacle independence and patient satisfaction. One diopter (D) of astigmatism corresponds to an uncorrected distance vision of 20/30. Almost all patients receiving presbyopic-correcting IOLs, but especially those paying additional fees for these premium IOLs, will experience 20/30 uncorrected distance acuity as unacceptable. They will frequently even perceive a significant difference between 20/25 and 20/20 uncorrected distance visual acuity. Limiting your patient selection to those patients with low amounts of preoperative cornea cylinder will not eliminate your need to acquire skills for correcting residual refractive errors. Wound dynamics and other unpredictable factors inherent in IOL placement will frequently result in residual astigmatism of at least 0.75 D, even though preoperative keratotomy readings predicted that this would not occur.

My general guideline is that 0.50 D or less of spherical error and 0.50 D or less of astigmatism are consistent with acceptable uncorrected visual outcomes by the post–presbyopic-correcting IOL patient. When spherical and cylindrical postoperative refractive errors reach 0.75 D or greater, patients will perceive a meaningful benefit with surgical treatment of their residual refractive error.

The most frequently performed procedures for correcting residual refractive errors following use of posterior chamber IOLs include 1) limbal relaxing incisions (LRIs) at the time of implantation, 2) LASIK at least a few months postoperatively, and 3) postoperative surface laser ablation, such as photorefractive keratectomy (PRK), at least 1 month following implantation. In the majority of cases, I use an alternative technique that I call micro-RK/AK (radial keratotomy/astigmatic keratotomy).

Hovanesian JA.
Refractive Cataract Surgery: Best Practices and Advanced Technology, Second Edition (pp 245-256). © 2017 SLACK Incorporated.

What is micro-RK/AK? This technique is performed no sooner than 3-weeks postoperatively. It includes arcuate incisions in the peripheral cornea that are identical to those used in any other LRI or AK procedure. The surgeon can use his or her nomogram of choice for correcting astigmatism. The second component of the micro-RK/AK technique is the micro-RK. When the implant power is selected preoperatively, the target for the spherical outcome is plano to -0.50. So, in more than 90% of cases, the spherical outcome is either plano or slightly myopic. Micro-RK is used to correct the small degrees of myopia in a relatively noninvasive manner.[1]

It should be noted that LRIs or AK incisions performed at the time of surgery can now be performed in the traditional manner, with handheld diamond blades or with femtosecond lasers. The femto-AK procedure and incision have distinct advantages and disadvantages when compared with the alternative procedures mentioned above, including micro-RK/AK.

The capacity of femtosecond lasers to correct corneal astigmatism is in its developmental stages. In the future, I believe this emerging technology will compete with or surpass competing techniques for correcting corneal astigmatism at the time of cataract surgery or as an independent procedure. Currently, the character of the femto-AK incision and the procedure performed by the femtosecond laser does not compare favorably with the incision created by an experienced diamond blade incisional AK or LRI surgeon.

The term *micro-RK*[2] is used to distinguish this technique from both mini-RK[3] and traditional RK, in which optical zones as small as 3.00 mm are frequently used. In micro-RK, the optical zone is never smaller than 5.00 mm. Since only a very small amount of myopia is being corrected usually, only 1 or 2 micro-radial incisions are necessary. The length of these incisions is always less than 2.50 mm. This is less than the thickness of 2 dimes (2.75 mm). A small portion of the Lindstrom 2-incision mini-RK nomogram (Figure 21-1) is used to select the surgical optical zone. I have been using this nomogram for 25 years, and it is extremely accurate. Fluctuating vision and hyperopic shifts do not occur with radial incisions this small.

Advantages of Micro-Radial Keratotomy/Astigmatic Keratotomy

The advantages of using this technique compared with the alternative techniques are numerous. The advantages of micro-RK/AK vs LRI are mostly related to accuracy, and accuracy is even more critical when dealing with demanding elective presbyopic patients. Since the micro-RK/AK is performed 3 or more weeks postoperatively, the surgeon has the advantage of knowing the exact amount of cylinder, the exact axis of the cylinder, and the exact amount of spherical error. The micro-RK component then provides you with an opportunity to fix small amounts of residual myopia with excellent precision. There is greater ease and precision when this procedure is performed on a nonphaco day, because 1) the pupil is not dilated, 2) it is easier to mark the axis, 3) it is easier to perform pachymetry at each incision site and custom set your diamond blade, and 4) the temporal and paracentesis wounds are more stable.

The advantages of micro-RK/AK over conventional LASIK are also significant. The typical premium IOL patient is usually older than 45 years and at an increased risk for

2 INCISION MRK NOMOGRAM

	SURGICAL OPTION										
AGE	**2 x 3.0**	**2 x 3.25**	**2 x 3.5**	**2 x 3.75**	**2 x 4.0**	**2 x 4.25**	**2 x 4.5**	**2 x 4.75**	**2 x 5.0**	**2 x 5.25**	**2 x 5.5**
20	1.60	1.40	1.20	1.08	0.96	0.84	0.72	0.60	0.48	0.36	0.24
21	1.64	1.44	1.23	1.11	0.98	0.86	0.74	0.62	0.49	0.37	0.25
22	1.68	1.47	1.26	1.13	1.01	0.88	0.76	0.63	0.50	0.38	0.25
23	1.72	1.51	1.29	1.16	1.03	0.90	0.77	0.65	0.52	0.39	0.26
24	1.76	1.54	1.32	1.19	1.06	0.92	0.79	0.66	0.53	0.40	0.26
25	1.80	1.58	1.35	1.22	1.08	0.95	0.81	0.68	0.54	0.41	0.27
26	1.84	1.61	1.38	1.24	1.10	0.97	0.83	0.69	0.55	0.41	0.28
27	1.88	1.65	1.41	1.27	1.13	0.99	0.85	0.71	0.56	0.42	0.28
28	1.92	1.68	1.44	1.30	1.15	1.01	0.86	0.72	0.58	0.43	0.29
29	1.96	1.72	1.47	1.32	1.18	1.03	0.88	0.74	0.59	0.44	0.29
30	2.00	1.75	1.50	1.35	1.20	1.05	0.90	0.75	0.60	0.45	0.30
31	2.04	1.79	1.53	1.38	1.22	1.07	0.92	0.77	0.61	0.46	0.31
32	2.08	1.82	1.56	1.40	1.25	1.09	0.94	0.78	0.62	0.47	0.31
33	2.12	1.86	1.59	1.43	1.27	1.11	0.95	0.80	0.64	0.48	0.32
34	2.16	1.89	1.62	1.46	1.30	1.13	0.97	0.81	0.65	0.49	0.32
35	2.20	1.93	1.65	1.49	1.32	1.16	0.99	0.83	0.66	0.50	0.33
36	2.24	1.96	1.68	1.51	1.34	1.18	1.01	0.84	0.67	0.50	0.34
37	2.28	2.00	1.71	1.54	1.37	1.20	1.03	0.86	0.68	0.51	0.34
38	2.32	2.03	1.74	1.57	1.39	1.22	1.04	0.87	0.70	0.52	0.35
39	2.36	2.07	1.77	1.59	1.42	1.24	1.06	0.89	0.71	0.53	0.35
40	2.40	2.10	1.80	1.62	1.44	1.26	1.08	0.90	0.72	0.54	0.36
41	2.44	2.14	1.83	1.65	1.46	1.28	1.10	0.92	0.73	0.55	0.37
42	2.48	2.17	1.86	1.67	1.49	1.30	1.12	0.93	0.74	0.56	0.37
43	2.52	2.21	1.89	1.70	1.51	1.32	1.13	0.95	0.76	0.57	0.38
44	2.56	2.24	1.92	1.73	1.54	1.34	1.15	0.96	0.77	0.58	0.38
45	2.60	2.28	1.95	1.76	1.56	1.37	1.17	0.98	0.78	0.59	0.39
46	2.64	2.31	1.98	1.78	1.58	1.39	1.19	0.99	0.79	0.59	0.40
47	2.68	2.35	2.01	1.81	1.61	1.41	1.21	1.01	0.80	0.60	0.40
48	2.72	2.38	2.04	1.84	1.63	1.43	1.22	1.02	0.82	0.61	0.41
49	2.76	2.42	2.07	1.86	1.66	1.45	1.24	1.04	0.83	0.62	0.41
50	2.80	2.45	2.10	1.89	1.68	1.47	1.26	1.05	0.84	0.63	0.42
51	2.84	2.49	2.13	1.92	1.70	1.49	1.28	1.07	0.85	0.64	0.43
52	2.88	2.52	2.16	1.94	1.73	1.51	1.30	1.08	0.86	0.65	0.43
53	2.92	2.56	2.19	1.97	1.75	1.53	1.31	1.10	0.88	0.66	0.44
54	2.96	2.59	2.22	2.00	1.78	1.55	1.33	1.11	0.89	0.67	0.44
55	3.00	2.63	2.25	2.03	1.80	1.58	1.35	1.13	0.90	0.68	0.45
56	3.04	2.66	2.28	2.05	1.82	1.60	1.37	1.14	0.91	0.68	0.46
57	3.08	2.70	2.31	2.08	1.85	1.62	1.39	1.16	0.92	0.69	0.46
58	3.12	2.73	2.34	2.11	1.87	1.64	1.40	1.17	0.94	0.70	0.47
59	3.16	2.77	2.37	2.13	1.90	1.66	1.42	1.19	0.95	0.71	0.47
60	3.20	2.80	2.40	2.16	1.92	1.68	1.44	1.20	0.96	0.72	0.48
61	3.24	2.84	2.43	2.19	1.94	1.70	1.46	1.22	0.97	0.73	0.49
62	3.28	2.87	2.46	2.21	1.97	1.72	1.48	1.23	0.98	0.74	0.49
63	3.32	2.91	2.49	2.24	1.99	1.74	1.49	1.25	1.00	0.75	0.50
64	3.36	2.94	2.52	2.27	2.02	1.76	1.51	1.26	1.01	0.76	0.50
65	3.40	2.98	2.55	2.30	2.04	1.79	1.53	1.28	1.02	0.77	0.51
66	3.44	3.01	2.58	2.32	2.06	1.81	1.55	1.29	1.03	0.77	0.52
67	3.48	3.05	2.61	2.35	2.09	1.83	1.57	1.31	1.04	0.78	0.52
68	3.52	3.08	2.64	2.38	2.11	1.85	1.58	1.32	1.06	0.79	0.53
69	3.56	3.12	2.67	2.40	2.14	1.87	1.60	1.34	1.07	0.80	0.53
70	3.60	3.15	2.70	2.43	2.16	1.89	1.62	1.35	1.08	0.81	0.54
71	3.64	3.19	2.73	2.46	2.18	1.91	1.64	1.37	1.09	0.82	0.55
72	3.68	3.22	2.76	2.48	2.21	1.93	1.66	1.38	1.10	0.83	0.55
73	3.72	3.26	2.79	2.51	2.23	1.95	1.67	1.40	1.12	0.84	0.56
74	3.76	3.29	2.82	2.54	2.26	1.97	1.69	1.41	1.13	0.85	0.56
75	3.80	3.33	2.85	2.57	2.28	2.00	1.71	1.43	1.14	0.86	0.57
76	3.84	3.36	2.88	2.59	2.30	2.02	1.73	1.44	1.15	0.86	0.58
77	3.88	3.40	2.91	2.62	2.33	2.04	1.75	1.46	1.16	0.87	0.58
78	3.92	3.43	2.94	2.65	2.35	2.06	1.76	1.47	1.18	0.88	0.59
79	3.96	3.47	2.97	2.67	2.38	2.08	1.78	1.49	1.19	0.89	0.59
80	4.00	3.50	3.00	2.70	2.40	2.10	1.80	1.50	1.20	0.90	0.60
AGE	**2 x 3.0**	**2 x 3.25**	**2 x 3.5**	**2 x 3.75**	**2 x 4.0**	**2 x 4.25**	**2 x 4.5**	**2 x 4.75**	**2 x 5.0**	**2 x 5.25**	**2 x 5.5**

Find patient age, then move right to find result closest to refractive myopia without going over

Figure 21-1. Lindstrom 2-incision mini-RK nomogram. Highlighted area designates the part of the nomogram used for micro-RK. Note that optical zones less than 5.00 mm are never used with micro-RK.

dry eye (especially women). Even lesser degrees of aqueous or evaporative dry eye can compromise the visual outcomes of these already demanding patients. Micro-RK/AK does not create a neurotropic cornea, as does the cutting of a flap with LASIK. The central 5.00 mm of the cornea is untouched. There will be no flap complications, no diffuse lamellar keratitis, and no central epithelial defects.

Some surgeons wait up to 3 to 6 months before performing LASIK following an implant, because of concern about wound stability during creation of the flap. Micro-RK/AK can be performed with confidence much sooner. The cost of laser access (purchase or facility fee) and the procedure (procedure card and microkeratome blade) will almost always be significantly greater than this incisional technique. Since the optics of multifocal IOLs are not compatible with custom LASIK, the advantage of a custom ablation cannot be realized when performing LASIK following the implantation of diffractive and refractive IOLs. LASIK enhancements further complicate the patient's neurotropic dry eye, and cost again becomes a factor. The small incisions of this technique produce no greater postoperative symptoms than LASIK. LASIK becomes my preferred technique when the residual cylinder or sphere increases significantly. As the residual refractive error increases, there is a relative increase in precision with laser vision correction compared with an incisional technique.

The advantages of micro-RK/AK compared with traditional PRK are also substantial. The central 5 mm of the cornea remains untouched. There is less postoperative discomfort. Bilateral surgery is possible, and the visual recovery is quicker for these demanding patients. No bandage contact lens is required, there are fewer postoperative visits, and again this incisional technique is much less costly. There is much less stress on healing of the ocular surface, especially for patients with pre-existing ocular surface disorders, such as aqueous dry eye, meibomian gland dysfunction, anterior blepharitis, or delayed epithelial healing secondary to diabetes. There is frequently a subtle subepithelial haze following PRK that is usually tolerated by the typical PRK patient. In the multifocal implant patient who has already lost contrast sensitivity, the visual consequences of the subepithelial haze may be poorly tolerated.

The advantages of micro RK/AK over femto-AK begin with the architecture of the incisions. The vertical incisions of femto-AK are much less effective and efficient for correcting astigmatism than diamond blade incisions that are constructed perpendicular to the corneal surface. The effectiveness of the incisions is highly dependent on the achieved depth. Limitations in the visualization technology of many femtosecond lasers require a large margin of error when calculating the depth of the AK incision, and effectiveness is sacrificed. Larger arcuate incisions with smaller optical zones are required to correct equal amounts of astigmatism. Many femtosecond incisions require a secondary manual true opening of the incision, because of the "postage stamp" microcorrections of tissue characteristic of femtosecond tissue separation, as observed with femtosecond LASIK flaps.

In general, AK incisions with larger optical zones are less sensitive to small errors in axis alignment. Femto-AK is currently limited to smaller optical zones, because femtosecond incisions cannot be constructed in the peripheral cornea because of the arcus senilis frequently observed in patients undergoing cataract surgery. Axis alignment can also be challenging with the current femtosecond technology. Although companies are developing *iris registration* to manage torsional rotation, which will eventually improve outcomes, the process is in its early stages of evolution. As with LRI or AK performed at the time of surgery, femto-AK cannot correct small amounts of residual myopia, and the cost is also much greater than micro RK/AK.

I have used micro-RK/AK to correct residual refractive error following implant surgery in more than 2500 cases during the past 25 years. Figures 21-2 and 21-3 summarize the results of this technique in 320 eyes after receiving multifocal IOLs.[4] Note that the final uncorrected visual acuity in the Array (Abbott Medical Optics) eyes (n = 111) is slightly better, because this group is exclusively lensectomy patients vs the ReZoom (Abbott Medical Optics) and ReSTOR (Alcon) eyes (n = 209), which are a mix of lensectomy and older cataract patients with less healthy maculas.

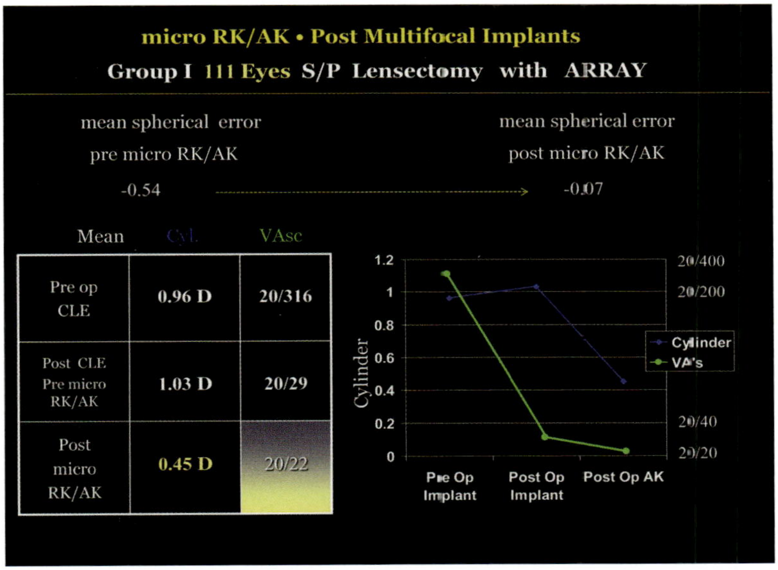

Figure 21-2. Postoperative results following micro-RK/AK in 111 eyes status post–refractive lensectomy with a multifocal IOL.

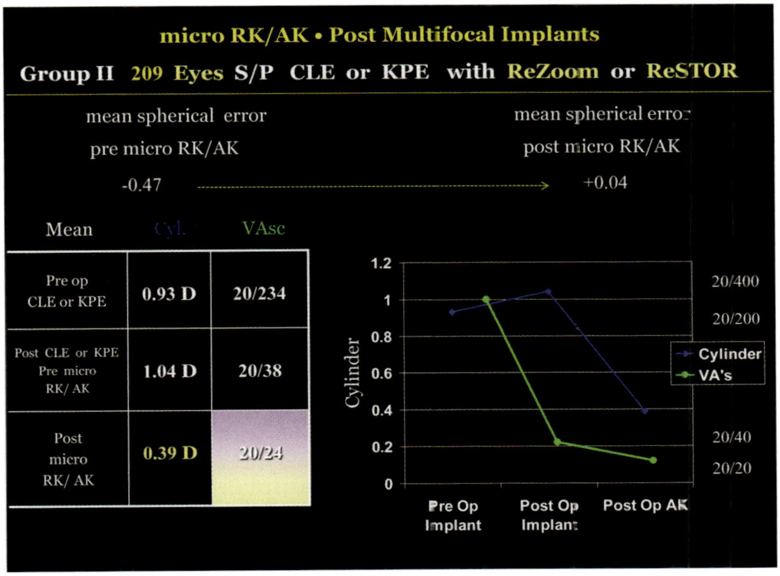

Figure 21-3. Postoperative results following micro-RK/AK in 209 eyes status post–cataract extraction or refractive lensectomy with a multifocal IOL.

Preoperative Pearls

Although the stress on the ocular surface is frequently much less than experienced with PRK and LASIK, the principle of optimizing the ocular surface health prior to a refractive surgery still strongly applies. A healthy preoperative ocular surface obviously enhances postoperative visual outcomes. In addition, an optimized ocular surface

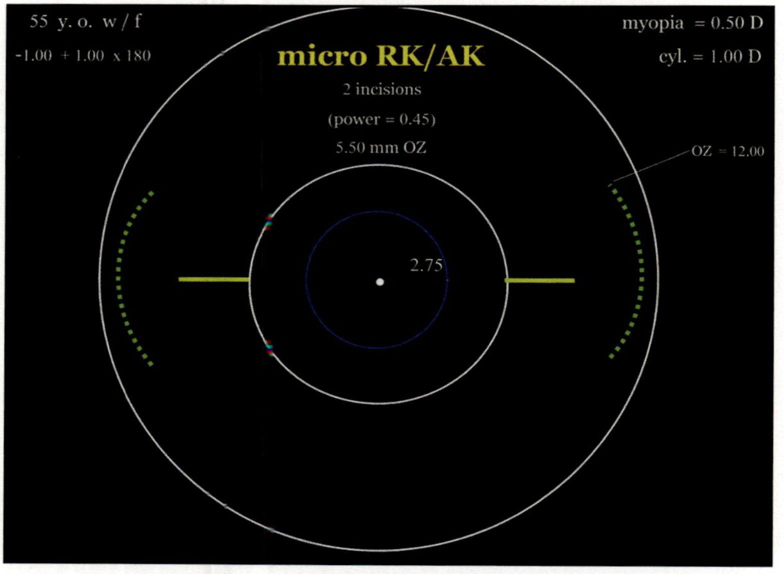

Figure 21-4. An example of a 2-incision micro-RK with 2 arcuate keratotomies corresponding to the steep axis of astigmatism. Note that the optical zone of 5.50 mm for the micro-RK incisions in a 55-year-old patient is taken from the Lindstrom 2-incision mini-RK nomogram and is expected to achieve 0.45 D of myopic correction.

promotes a more accurate detection of the true preoperative residual refractive error. We always perform a manifest refraction, WaveScan (VISX), and corneal topography on the day of surgery to help detect any last-minute changes in the residual refractive error after aggressively pursuing an optimized ocular surface in the days and weeks prior to the procedure. Tears, gels, plugs, Restasis (cyclosporine), omega-3 fish oils (pure triglyceride omega-3s, not ethyl ester omega-3s), tetracyclines, lid hygiene, Azasite (azithromycin), and TobraDex ST (tobramycin/dexamethasone) are all used proactively to treat aqueous dry eye, evaporative dry eye, and various forms of meibomian gland dysfunction or meibomitis.

As previously alluded to, the presence of 1) irregular astigmatism from conditions such as anterior basement membrane dystrophy, 2) a history of advanced dry eye, and 3) relative amounts of myopia, hyperopia, or astigmatism greatly influence the procedure of choice when correcting residual refractive errors. If there is no irregular astigmatism, micro-RK/AK is the treatment of choice for relatively small amounts of residual myopia with low and moderate amounts of astigmatism. Since great care is given to preoperative testing related to IOL power selections, residual myopia greater than 1.00 D is relatively rare. However, since we cheat toward plano to slight myopia when selecting IOL powers, a residual myopia of -0.25 to -0.62 D is not uncommon. Correcting these commonly observed small amounts of residual myopia along with astigmatism from 0.50 to 2.00 D would define the typical case in which micro-RK/AK would be employed (Figure 21-4). Higher amounts of astigmatism can also be corrected in atypical cases when laser vision correction is contraindicated (ie, history of severe dry eye). The AK component of the

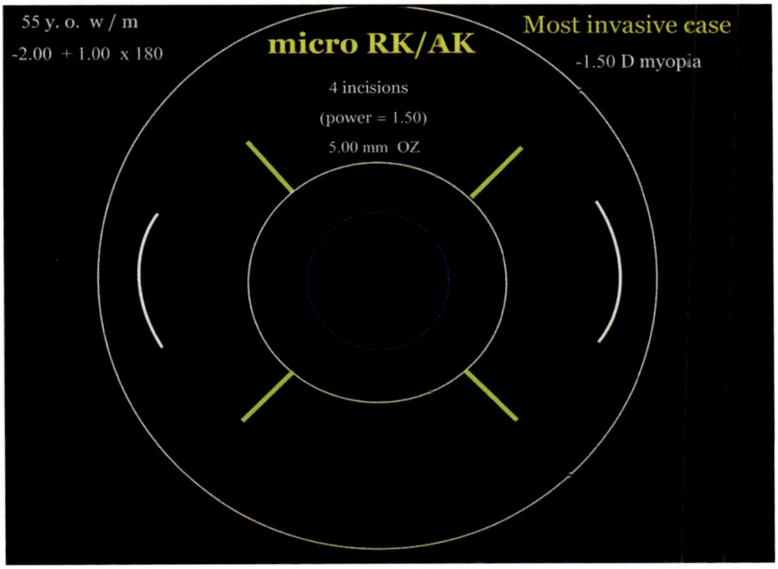

Figure 21-5. This is an example of a 4-incision micro-RK/AK with the smallest optical zone allowed (5.00 mm) and demonstrates that up to 1.50 D of myopia can be corrected in a 55-year-old patient.

technique can be made more aggressive by using larger arcuate incisions and/or by moving the incisions closer to the center of the cornea (smaller optical zone).

Pushing the upper limits of myopic correction for micro-RK to replace laser vision correction is only considered with a history of advanced dry eye or a history of a poor outcome in the opposite eye secondary to an ocular surface disease. The upper limits of myopic correction are guided by the age-dependent nomogram and the rule of thumb that the optical zone should never be smaller than 5.00 mm. Thus, as per the nomogram 1.50 D of myopia in a 55-year-old patient (Figure 21-5) and 2.00 D of myopia in an 80-year-old patient could safely be corrected with a 4-incision micro-RK procedure with an optical zone of 5.00 mm. There are both a 2-incision (see Figure 21-1) and a 4-incision micro-RK nomogram, which are adapted from Dr. Lindstrom's original mini-RK nomograms.

If significantly greater amounts of hyperopia are encountered beyond the refractive target, we choose laser vision correction to treat the residual hyperopia or hyperopic astigmatism. The choice between LASIK and PRK is beyond the scope of this chapter, but in general a greater degree of irregular astigmatism, corneal scarring, or a history of advanced dry eye would favor surface ablation over LASIK.

For those patients seeking multifocal technology, the increasing availability of multifocal toric IOLs offers an alternative treatment for patients with higher amounts of corneal astigmatism. Multifocal toric IOLs may eliminate the need for postoperative enhancements of residual astigmatism. If, however, they reduce the astigmatism from very high preoperatively to moderately low postoperatively, the micro RK/AK technique is an ideal enhancement procedure for optimizing their visual outcome by eliminating the residual astigmatism and/or low myopia.

The refractive target for astigmatism is obviously always zero. However, the target for the spherical outcome can be dependent on the type of premium IOL and the existing postoperative or target outcome of the opposite eye. For example, a diffractive multifocal IOL such as the Tecnis (Abbott Medical Optics) multifocal would have a spherical target between +0.25 D and plano, while the target refraction for a ReZoom or a ReSTOR 3.0 would be from plano to -0.25 D.

The spherical targets for the Crystalens (Bausch & Lomb) could be even more myopic but are very patient dependent. The target refraction for any given patient, as previously stated, should also be chosen in light of existing or intended refractive outcomes in the opposite eye. This is especially true when using the Crystalens bilaterally, when at least a minimonovision is frequently necessary to achieve acceptable levels of patient satisfaction.

Do not perform incisional or laser refractive procedures for residual refractive errors prior to an anticipated yttrium-aluminum-garnet (YAG) laser capsulotomy after implantation with a Crystalens. We have reported[5] frequent and significant shifts in the spherical refractive error following YAG laser capsulotomies. More than 54% of eyes had a shift of greater than or equal to 0.50 D. Hyperopic shifts occurred almost 4 times as often as myopic shifts. Hyperopic shifts of 0.75 D occurred 23% of the time, while 1.00-D hyperopic shifts occurred in 14% of cases. The capsulotomy probably alters the physical relationship and interactive forces between the Crystalens and the remaining capsular bag. Micro-RK/AK can be performed with confidence in the presence of other premium IOLs prior to anticipated YAG laser capsulotomies.

Perioperative Pearls

All patients are instructed to use artificial tears 4 times daily for 7 days prior to their micro-RK/AK, even if there are no deficiencies in the health of their ocular surface. This increases the probability of obtaining a more accurate immediate preoperative manifest refraction and enhances the integrity of the epithelium when performing the surgery. A fourth-generation fluoroquinolone antibiotic is used 4 times daily 2 days preoperatively and 7 days postoperatively or until the epithelium over the incision is completely healed. There is also pulsing of the antibiotic immediately following the procedure. Patients are also instructed to perform lid hygiene at bedtime for 2 nights prior to surgery.

A nonpreserved nonsteroidal anti-inflammatory drug (NSAID) is used immediately following the procedure and for 7 days postoperatively. The NSAID given immediately after the surgery is administered to decrease symptoms of pain and discomfort. However, the small micro-RK/AK incisions usually heal very quickly, so discomfort is actually a minor issue. Continued use of the NSAIDs for 1 week or more is prescribed as a prophylactic against subclinical cystoid macular edema in these recently implanted lensectomy or cataract patients. A topical steroid is also given immediately postoperatively and 4 times daily for 7 days thereafter. Artificial tears are used every hour while awake for 3 days, with a tapering dose as determined by the needs of the patient.

Collagen plugs are placed in the punctum of both the upper and lower lids on the day of surgery to accelerate healing of the epithelium and to enhance the short-term postoperative visual outcomes. For patients who already have a silicone plug in the lower

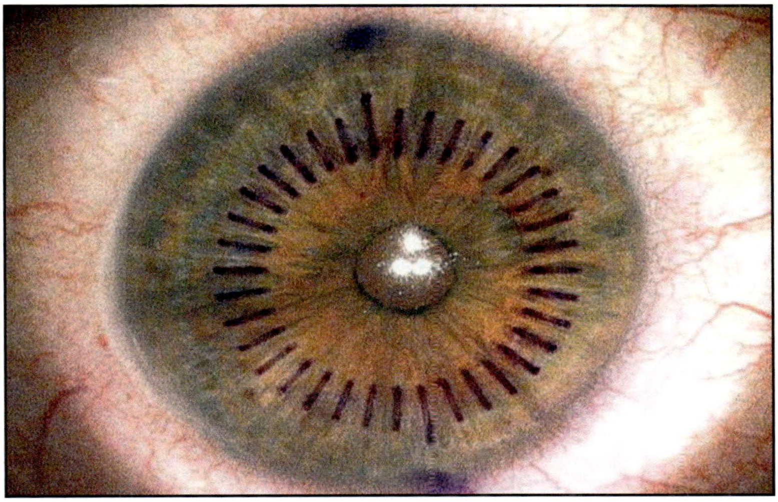

Figure 21-6. Gentian violet markings created by a Thornton corneal marker for locating the correct axis when placing either arcuate incisions or on-axis (plus cylinder) micro-RK incisions.

lid from previous treatment, a collagen plug is added to the upper lid. More aggressive treatment for ocular surface issues as previously discussed is added, as indicated by the needs of each individual patient.

Nonpreserved artificial tears are administered upon arrival on the day of surgery prior to taking the uncorrected vision and performing a manifest refraction, corneal topography, and WaveScan. WaveScans are very useful for accurately determining the axis of astigmatism regardless of which premium IOL has been implanted. WaveScans are extremely unreliable in detecting residual spherical error in eyes containing multifocal implants. Corneal topography and indices such as the surface regulatory index can aid in assessing the health of the ocular surface.

All corneas are marked at the slit lamp prior to taking the patient to the operating room. A gentian violet marker is used to place a small limbal mark at the 12 and 6 o'clock positions. Subsequently, under the surgical microscope, a Thornton corneal marker is properly aligned using the previous limbal markings at 12- and 6-o'clock. The Thornton marker contains 36 small markings placed every 10 degrees for 360 degrees at an optical zone of approximately 7.00 mm (Figure 21-6). The 12- and 6-o'clock marks represent the axis of 90 degrees. All surgical axes can be located by counting away from the 90-degree axis in 10-degree increments until the surgical axis is identified.

There are surgeons who advocate performing LRIs or AKs at the slit lamp. Even without the added challenge of the micro-RK incisions, I am not a supporter of this approach. If an ambulatory surgery center or treatment room with a surgical microscope is available, I highly recommend taking the patient to this setting to perform the procedure. The slit-lamp approach is even more strongly discouraged during the learning curve. The comfort and stability of both the patient and the surgeon will be greatly enhanced if the patient is horizontal and the surgeon is using a microscope.

Patients receive 5 to 10 mg of oral Valium (diazepam) approximately 20 minutes before surgery. Proparacaine 0.5% drops are used to anesthetize the cornea prior to

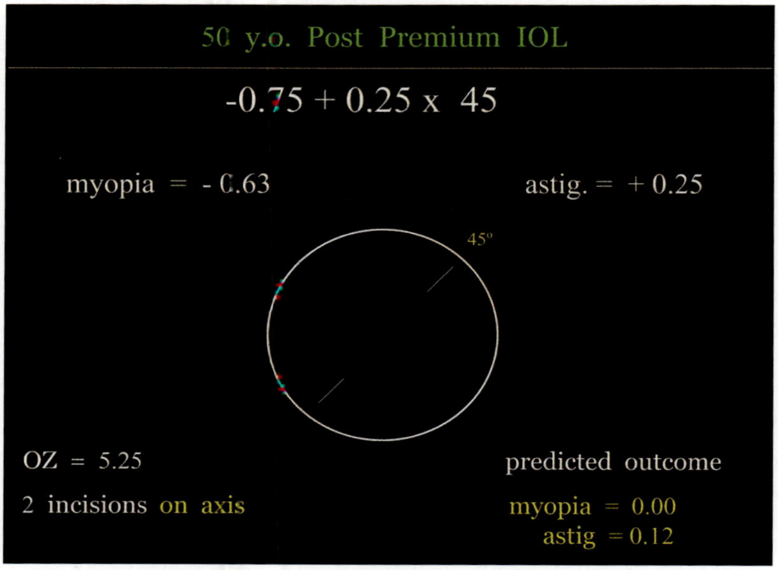

Figure 21-7. An example of a 2-incision on-axis micro-RK. Note that the 5.25-mm optical zone corresponds with the Lindstrom 2-incision nomogram recommendation for correcting 0.63 D of myopia in a 50-year-old patient.

placement of the lid speculum. The axis of all astigmatic procedures is determined by the Thornton maker as previously outlined. Optical zone markers (usually 5.00, 5.25, or 5.50 mm) are placed over the center of the pupil to define the placement of micro-RK incisions. The optical zone of the micro-RK incisions is derived from the patient's age and the amount of myopia to be corrected, as determined by the Lindstrom nomogram.

The typical 1 or 2 micro-RK/AK incisions are always placed on axis (plus cylinder) (Figure 21-7). Four micro-RK incisions would straddle the arcuate incisions used to correct astigmatism (see Figure 21-5).

It is important to understand the concept of radial incisions contributing to the correction of astigmatism. Two on-axis radial incisions are placed primarily to flatten the cornea and correct a small amount of myopia. However, it should be appreciated that, on average, twice as much flattening takes place in the axis of the incisions compared with the meridian 90 degrees away. The original 2-incision mini-RK with smaller optical zones (and longer incisions) developed by Dr. Lindstrom could contribute greatly to flattening the plus cylinder axis as an independent treatment for astigmatism or in conjunction with additional arcuate incisions, depending on the amount of astigmatism correction needed. The anticipated result of a classic 2-incision on-axis mini-RK would be complete elimination of the myopia and a 50% reduction in the astigmatism (see Figure 21-7).

If the surgeon is electing to correct a small amount of myopia (less than 1.0 D) when only 0.25 D of astigmatism is present, he or she would place the 2 micro-RK incisions on axis (plus) and elect not to use any arcuate incisions. As previously stated, the optical zone of the 2-incision micro-RK would be determined by the patient's age and amount of myopia to be corrected. The on-axis placement of the incisions further reduces the residual refractive error by making a small but meaningful reduction in the residual astigmatism.

Since the radial incisions of a typical 2-incision micro-RK/AK are placed on axis, the peripheral aspect of the incisions is frequently approaching an AK incision. Arcuate AK incisions are always placed first. The subsequent RK incision should never cross the AK incisions. The corners resulting from these crossed incisions will elevate and not heal with proper orientation.

Reports from various surgeons have revealed relatively inconsistent outcomes when performing LRI or AK incisions. Substantial differences in nomograms and other aspects of the surgical technique have been observed. I recommend that each surgeon use his or her nomogram and techniques of choice when planning and executing surgery to correct astigmatism. However, a few basic principles should be kept in mind. A greater surgical effect will obviously be observed with 1) incisions closer to the center of the cornea, 2) deeper incisions, and 3) incisions with increasing degrees of arc. Arcuate incisions are more efficient and effective than straight t-cuts. Although incisions closer to the center of the cornea yield greater effect, they are associated with a greater risk of inducing irregular astigmatism. Larger arcuate incisions located further from the center of the cornea (but of equal degree) are more forgiving and less likely to create significant variations from the ideal intended axis of correction.

Individual ultrasonic pachymetry is performed at the exact location of all micro-RK and AK incisions. The pachymetry for RK incisions is located over the optical zone mark on the cornea, corresponding to the most central and thinnest aspect of the incision. Pachymetry for AK incisions is located directly over the central part of the proposed arcuate incision. When very large arcuate incisions (greater than 60 degrees) are necessary, it is suggested that pachymetry readings should be taken at each end of the arc to check for large variations in corneal thickness.

A microscope (SIS Magnum Diamond) is used to set the blade depth for all incisions. RK blades are set at 99% to 100% of the pachymetry. AK blades are set at 90% to 96% of pachymetry. AK diamond blades traditionally have a squared-off rudder-type configuration. My RK blade of choice is a duotrak 35-degree pointed diamond with a full cutting surface on the angled edge with only 225 µm of cutting surface at the tip of the front straight edge of the blade.

Micro-RK incisions are constructed with a double motion after placing the blade into the cornea adjacent to the outer aspect of the indentation made from the optical zone marker. A classic *American pull motion* is then performed, moving from the central to peripheral cornea, stopping 1 to 2 mm before the limbus. Once the outer aspect of the incision is reached, and without raising the blade, a push motion is performed back to the central cornea with the leading front edge tip of the blade doing the cutting. This classic *Russian stroke* uses the 225 µm of sharp cutting surface at the tip of the front straight edge to square off the inner aspect of the incision. The noncutting surface above the tip of the straight edge stops the blade at the optical zone mark and prevents cutting across the visual axis of the central cornea. A proper squared-off incision is not created with the angled side of the blade during the downhill American stroke of this technique, so the uphill stroke is necessary to achieve the appropriate wound architecture.

The relatively noninvasive nature of micro-RK/AK compared with keratorefractive laser procedures and its favorable cost profile make it an attractive surgical alternative for many subtypes of patients who have received IOLs. Young postlensectomy patients in their 50s, young postcataract patients in their 60s, and older post–premium IOL cataract patients in their 70s or 80s can greatly benefit from this technique. In principle, any postcataract surgery patient with lower degrees of residual myopic astigmatism seeking improved uncorrected visual acuity is a candidate for this technique, even years following his or her initial implantation.

Micro-RK has also been very useful for correcting small amounts of residual myopic astigmatism following LASIK, PRK, and penetrating keratoplasties. When more than 2 years have passed since performing the initial LASIK procedure, raising the flap for an enhancement may be difficult. I have found that performing a micro-RK/AK over a well-healed LASIK flap to be more efficient and less invasive than performing PRK or cutting a new LASIK flap. If the patient has excessive amounts of higher-order aberrations, a custom PRK may be chosen over a micro-RK/AK procedure.

Some post-PRK patients continue to regress to small amounts of myopia after one or repeated PRK enhancements. This may be due to epithelial modulation of the ablated cornea. I have successfully corrected this persistent residual low myopia very accurately with micro-RK/AK. Micro-RK has also been used effectively in post–penetrating keratoplasty patients when LASIK is contraindicated because of ocular surface issues.

Performing AK or LRIs is a function of the new femtosecond cataract lasers. Research to develop the capacity for creating micro-radial incisions for the correction of low myopia has already begun.

Conclusion

Micro-RK/AK is an excellent alternative for correcting residual refractive errors following the use of presbyopia-correcting IOLs. In general, it is less costly, puts less stress on the ocular surface, is less invasive then laser vision correction, and is more accurate than intraoperative LRI.

References

1. Bucci FA Jr. Mini-RK: indications and technique. In Chang DF, ed. *Mastering Refractive IOLs: The Art and Science.* Thorofare, NJ: SLACK Incorporated; 2008:786-788.
2. Bucci FA Jr. Micro RK/AK for correcting residual refractive errors following presbyopic IOLs. Presented at: XXV Congress of the European Society of Cataract and Refractive Surgeons; September 2007; Stockholm, Sweden.
3. Lindstrom RL. Minimally invasive radial keratotomy: mini-RK. *J Cataract Refract Surg.* 1995;21:27-34.
4. Bucci FA Jr. "Micro RK/AK" for correcting residual refractive errors following presbyopic IOLs. Poster presented at: American Academy of Ophthalmology annual meeting; November 11, 2007; New Orleans, LA.
5. Bucci FA Jr. Do YAG capsulotomies in eyes with a Crystalens significantly impact spherical refraction and near visual function? Presented at: International Society of Refractive Surgery/American Academy of Ophthalmology Refractive Surgery Subspecialty Day; October 2009; San Francisco, CA.

Financial Disclosures

Dr. Adi Abulafia is a consultant for Haag-Streit, PhysIOL, and Hoya.

Dr. Jay Bansal has no financial or proprietary interest in the materials presented herein.

Dr. Allon Barsam has no financial or proprietary interest in the materials presented herein.

Dr. John P. Berdahl is a consultant for Alcon.

Dr. Frank A. Bucci Jr has no financial or proprietary interest in the materials presented herein.

Dr. David F. Chang is a consultant for AMO, PowerVision, Clarity, Calhoun Vision, and Zeiss.

Dr. Kevin J. Corcoran is president of the Corcoran Consulting Group.

Dr. Kendall E. Donaldson has financial interest in Alcon, Abbot, and Bausch & Lomb.

Dr. Eric Donnenfeld is a consultant and performs research for Allergan, Alcon, Advanced Medical Optics, and Bausch & Lomb.

Dr. Arun C. Gulani has no financial or proprietary interest in the materials presented herein.

Dr. Warren E. Hill is a consultant for Alcon and Haag-Streit.

Dr. John A. Hovanesian is a consultant for Alcon, Allergan, AMO, Bausch & Lomb, Glaukos, Ivantis, Ocular Therapeutix, Omeros, Shire, and Sight Sciences.

Dr. Kevin Jwo has no financial or proprietary interest in the materials presented herein.

Dr. Ji Won Kwon has no financial or proprietary interest in the materials presented herein.

Dr. Bryan S. Lee has no financial or proprietary interest in the materials presented herein.

Dr. Jimmy Lee has no financial or proprietary interest in the materials presented herein.

Dr. Jodi Luchs is a consultant for Allergan, Bausch & Lomb, Tear Lab, Shire, Omeros, and Sun Ophthalmics; is a clinical researcher for Allergan, Alcon, Bausch & Lomb, Shire, Auven, Aerie, and Inotek; and has ownership interest in CXLO, Insightful Solutions, Omega Ophthalmics, RPS Diagnostics, Calhoun Vision, and Trefoil Therapeutics.

Dr. Robert K. Maloney is a consultant for Advanced Medical Optics, Calhoun Vision, and Presbia; and an equity holder in Calhoun Vision and Stroma Medical.

Dr. J. E. "Jay" McDonald II has no financial or proprietary interest in the materials presented herein.

Dr. Alanna Nattis is a consultant for Alcon.

Dr. Jay S. Pepose is a consultant for Abbot Medical Optics, Bausch & Lomb, and Visiometrics.

Dr. Mujtaba A. Qazi is affiliated with Oasis.

Dr. R. Luke Rebenitsch receives speaking honoraria from Acufocus, Zeimer, and Staar Surgical.

Dr. Eric Rosenberg has no financial or proprietary interest in the materials presented herein.

Garth Rotramel has financial interest in Alcon, Abbot, and Bausch & Lomb.

Dr. Joel M. Solano has no financial or proprietary interest in the materials presented herein.

Dr. Jason E. Stahl has no financial or proprietary interest in the materials presented herein.

Paul Stubenbordt is a practice consultant.

Dr. Savak "Sev" Teymoorian is a consultant for Aerie, Alcon, Allergan, Bausch & Lomb, Ellex, MDbackline.com, and Glaukos; and does research for Bausch & Lomb, Aerie, and Allergan.

Dr. Farrell (Toby) Tyson is a consultant for AMO and Bausch & Lomb.

Dr. R. Bruce Wallace III is on the noncompensated physicians advisory board for LensAR.

Dr. George O. Waring IV has financial interest in AMO, Alcon, Bausch & Lomb, Visiometrics, and AcuFocus.

Dr. Robert J. Weinstock is a consultant for Bausch & Lomb, Alcon, and AMO.

Dr. William F. Wiley is a consultant for Alcon, AMO, Bausch & Lomb, Zeiss, Clarity Medical, Imprimis, Acufocus, Revision Optics, and LensAR.

Dr. Abu-Bakar Zafar has no financial or proprietary interest in the materials presented herein.

Index

advertising, 13–14, 75–86
  astigmatism surgery, 83–84
  budget, 76–77
  contact information, 77
  counselors, preparing, 85
  discussions, scheduling, 82
  elements of, 77
  hiring staff, 80–81
  honesty, 77
  internal marketing, 76
  laser-assisted cataract surgery, 84–85
  marketing medical practice, 76
  marketing plan, 76–77
    message, 76–77
    placement, 76–77
  media placement, 77–79
    newsprint, 79
    radio, 78
    social media, 79
    television, 78–79
  message, 76–77
  patient evaluation, 82–83
  placement, 76–77
    radio, 78
    social media, 79
    television, 78–79
  professional agency, 79–80
  reinforming patients, 77
  staff, preparing, 85
  telephone, 81–82
    rapport, 81–82
    role playing, 81
    scripting, 81
    trust, 81–82
  value, 77
allergy, unstable tear film, 29
astigmatic keratotomy, enhancement, 245–256
astigmatism correction, 17
astigmatism surgery, 83–84
axial length, preoperative testing, 44

Barrett toric calculator, toric intraocular lens, 162–163
bimanual microincisional cataract surgery, 129

blepharitis, unstable tear film, 28–29
budget, marketing, 76–77

calculations, 52–54
  formulas, 49–52
  solutions, 53–54
  sources of error, 52–53
capsular opacification, 220
capsulorrhexis, microincisional cataract surgery, 128–129
capsulotomy, 100–101
CME. *See* Cystoid macular edema
co-management, 67–71
communication with patient, 6–8
  cost of astigmatism, 181
  cost of monovision, 181–182
  counseling, 173
  educating patients, 87–92
  scheduling, 82
  scripting message, 186–187
  unsatisfied patients, 215–224
complications
  communication with patient, 13, 215–224
  patient communication, 13
conductive keratoplasty, excimer laser enhancement, 234–235
confidence, surgical, 3
conjunctival impression cytology, 33–34
contacting prospective patients telephone, 81–82
  rapport, 81–82
  role playing, 81
  scripting, 81
  trust issue, 81–82
contraindications, 23
corneal incisions, 102
corneal power, preoperative testing, 45–49
counselors, preparing, 85
covered services vs noncovered services, 62
Crystalens, 199–212
  intraocular lens selection, 204
  patient selection, 201–203
  preoperative measurements, 203–204
  surgical considerations, 204–209
CyPass, micro-invasive glaucoma surgery, 146
cystoid macular edema, 218, 220

data display, Optiwave Refractive Analysis system, 120
defining refractive intraocular lenses, 1–8
deluxe items, 64
discussions with patient, scheduling, 82
disease of ocular surface, 30–31
  allergy, unstable tear film, 29
  blepharitis, unstable tear film, 28–29
  conjunctival impression cytology, 33–34
  dry eye, unstable tear film, 28
  history, 31
  immunoglobulin E analysis, 33
  intraoperative considerations, 37
  lactoferrin analysis, 33
  matrix metalloproteinase-9 detectors, 32
  meibomography, 33
  point-of-care diagnosis, 31
  postoperative, 31, 37
  preoperative diagnosis, 31–36
    patient history, 31
    postoperative considerations, 31
  preparation, 27–39
  preparative measurements, 30
  risks, 29–30
  slit-lamp examination, 34–36
  tear film
    interferometry, 33
    osmolarity, 32
  treatment, 36–37
  unstable tear film, 28–29
dry eye, 22–23
  unstable tear film, 28
dysfunctional lens syndrome, 18–19

education of patient, 87–92
  family members, discussion with, 88
  follow-up, 91–92
  by physician, 89–90
  technology, 87–88
    upcoming, 10–11
endothelial cell loss, microincisional cataract surgery, 132–135

- equipment, office, 4–6
- error message, Optiwave Refractive Analysis system, 120
- error sources, intraocular lens calculation, 52–53
- estimated lens position, preoperative testing, 49–52
- ethical issues, 9–14
  - advertising for femtosecond laser, 13–14
  - complications, patient communication, 13
  - insurance company billing, 12
  - LASIK promotion, 11
  - noncovered service, pricing, 12–13
  - options, informing patient of, 10
  - residual postoperative refractive error, 13
  - upcoming technology, 10–11
- excimer laser enhancements, 233–244
  - conductive keratoplasty, 234–235
  - counseling, 237
  - intraoperative steps, 238–239
  - laser advanced surface ablation, 240
  - LASIK, 234–235
  - Nd:YAG laser capsulotomy, 236
  - nomograms, 237
  - ocular surface, 237–238
  - photorefractive keratectomy, 234–235
  - postoperative care, 239
  - radial keratotomy, 234–235
  - refractive lens implant, 240
- expectations of patient, 20–22

- family members, discussion with, 88
  - education of patient, 88
- femtosecond laser-assisted cataract surgery, 95–60
  - capsulotomy, 100–101
  - complicated cases, 106–110
  - complication rates, 105
  - corneal incisions, 102
    - clear corneal incisions, 102
  - ethical dilemmas, 110–111
  - laser platforms, 96–100
    - imaging, 99
    - patient interface, 96–99
  - lens fragmentation, 101–102
  - limbal relaxing incisions, 102–104
  - logistics, 104–105
  - outcomes, 105–111
  - procedure, 100–104
  - pupillary miosis, 110
  - refractive outcomes, 105
  - safety, 105
- financial waivers, 64–66
- FLACS. *See* Femtosecond laser-assisted cataract surgery
- follow-up education of patient, 91–92
- formulas, calculations, 49–52

- hiring staff, 80–81
- Hydrus, micro-invasive glaucoma surgery, 144
- hydrodissection, microincisional cataract surgery, 128–129

- image capture, Optiwave Refractive Analysis system, 117–121
- immunoglobulin E analysis, 33
- InnFocus Micro-Shunt, micro-invasive glaucoma surgery, 149
- insurance company billing, 12
- interferometry, tear film, 33
- internal marketing, 76
- intraocular lens exchange, 230–231
  - power calculation, 230
  - surgical technique, 231–232
- intraoperative considerations, ocular surface disease, 37
- intraoperative wavefront aberrometry, 115–122
  - astigmatism, 116
  - intraocular lens power calculations, 115–116
  - Optiwave Refractive Analysis system, 117, 121
    - data display, 120
    - error message, 120
    - image capture, 117–121
    - pseudophakic data, 121
    - reticle overlay, 120–121
    - VerifEye, 120–121

iStent/iStent Inject, micro-invasive glaucoma surgery, 143–144
iStent Supra, micro-invasive glaucoma surgery, 147–148

lactoferrin analysis, 33
laser advanced surface ablation, 240
laser platforms, femtosecond laser-assisted cataract surgery, 96–100
  imaging, 99
  patient interface, 96–99
LASIK
  excimer laser enhancement, 234–235
  promotion, 11
lens fragmentation, 101–102
light-adjustable intraocular lenses, 57–59
  preoperative testing, 57–59
limbal relaxing incisions, 102–104, 167–177
  dimensions, astigmatism, 168
  femtosecond laser-assisted cataract surgery, 175
  future of, 175–176
  instrumentation, 173
  measuring results, 175
  origin, 167–168
  patient counseling, 173
  posterior astigmatism, 169–170
  postoperative care, 174
  surgical planning, 168–169
  technique, 173
  treatment systems, 170–173
logistics, femtosecond laser-assisted cataract surgery, 104–105

management of practice, 61–74
  co-management, 67–71
  covered services, vs noncovered services, 62
  deluxe items, 64
  femtosecond lasers, 62
  financial waivers, 64–66
  problems, avoiding, 71
  professional charge, 66–67
  refractive cataract surgery, 61–62
marketing, 13–14, 75–86
  astigmatism surgery, 83–84
  budget, 76–77
  contact information, 77
  counselors, preparing, 85
  discussions, scheduling, 82
  elements of, 77
  hiring staff, 80–81
  honesty, 77
  internal marketing, 76
  laser-assisted cataract surgery, 84–85
  media placement, 77–79
    newsprint, 79
    radio, 78
    social media, 79
    television, 78–79
  medical practice, 76
  message, 76–77
  patient evaluation, 82–83
  placement, 76–77
  plan, 76–77
    message, 76–77
    placement, 76–77
  professional agency, 79–80
  reinforming patients, 77
  staff, preparing, 85
  telephone, 81–82
    rapport, 81–82
    role playing, 81
    scripting, 81
    trust issue, 81–82
  value, 77
matrix metalloproteinase-9 detectors, 32
meibomography, 33
message
  marketing, 76–77
micro-invasive glaucoma surgery, 141–156
  ab interno trabeculotomy, 144–145
  cost, 153
  CyPass, 146
  discussion with patient, 151–153
  future developments, 142–150
  Hydrus, 144
  InnFocus Micro-Shunt, 149
  iStent/iStent Inject, 143–144

iStent Supra, 147–148
Schlemm's canal, 142–146
subconjunctival space, 148–150
suprachoroidal/supraciliary space, 146–147
Trabectome, 144
trabecular bypass, 142–146
Xen implant, 149
micro-radial keratotomy, enhancement, 245–256
microincisional cataract surgery, 123–140
aberrations, 135
advantages, 124
astigmatism, 135
bimanual, 129
capsulorrhexis, 128–129
early postoperative visual acuity, 135
endothelial cell loss, 132–135
fluidics, 125–126
hyrodissection, 128–129
incision, 126–128
intraocular lenses, 132
posterior capsule opacification formation, 135–138
transitioning to, 129–131
ultrasound power modulation, 129
monovision, 177–188
compromises, 182
cost, 181–182
history of, 177–179
implementation, 183–185
patient education, 181–183
presbyopic refractive channel, 180–185
refractive orbit, 183–185
surgeon role, 182–183
multifocal implants, 189–198
contraindications, 192–193
enhancements, 197–198
intraocular lens selection, 193–195
preoperative measurements, 191–192
multifocal lens, preoperative testing, 42–43

Nd:YAG laser capsulotomy, excimer laser enhancements, 236
needs of patient, 20
newsprint, ad placement, 79
nomograms, excimer laser enhancements, 237
noncovered service, pricing, 12–13
nonsteroidal anti-inflammatory drugs, 218
NSAID. *See* Nonsteroidal anti-inflammatory drugs

ocular surface disease, 30–31
allergy, unstable tear film, 29
blepharitis, unstable tear film, 28–29
conjunctival impression cytology, 33–34
dry eye, unstable tear film, 28
history, 31
immunoglobulin E analysis, 33
intraoperative considerations, 37
lactoferrin analysis, 33
matrix metalloproteinase-9 detectors, 32
meibomography, 33
point-of-care diagnosis, 31
postoperative, 31, 37
preoperative diagnosis, 31–36
patient history, 31
postoperative considerations, 31
preparation, 27–39
preparative measurements, 30
risks, 29–30
slit-lamp examination, 34–36
tear film
interferometry, 33
osmolarity, 32
treatment, 36–37
unstable tear film, 28–29
office, equipping, 4–6
options, informing patient of, 10
Optiwave Refractive Analysis system, 117, 121
data display, 120
error message, 120
image capture, 117–121
pseudophakic data, 121
reticle overlay, 120–121
VerifEye, 120–121
ORA. *See* Optiwave Refractive Analysis system
osmolarity, tear film, 32

patient communication, 6–8, 87–92
  cost of monovision, 181–182
  counseling, 173
  education, patient, 87–92
    family members, discussion with, 88
    follow-up, 91–92
    by physician, 89–90
    technology, 87–88
  scheduling, 82
  scripting message, 186–187
  unsatisfied patients, 215–224
personality of patient, 22
photorefractive keratectomy, excimer laser enhancement, 234–235
physician education of patient, 89–90
piggyback intraocular lens, 225–230
  power calculation, 226–228
  residual astigmatism, 230
  surgical technique, 228–229
placement of advertising, 76–79
  newsprint, 79
  radio, 78
  social media, 79
  television, 78–79
point-of-care diagnosis, 31
posterior capsule opacification formation, microincisional cataract surgery, 135–138
postoperative, ocular surface disease, 37
practice management, 61–74
  co-management, 67–71
  covered services vs noncovered services, 62
  deluxe items, 64
  femtosecond lasers, 62
  financial waivers, 64–66
  problems, avoiding, 71
  professional charge, 66–67
  refractive cataract surgery, 61–62
preoperative diagnosis, ocular surface disease, 31–36
  patient history, 31
  postoperative considerations, 31
preoperative refractive error, 22
preoperative testing, 41–60
  axial length, 44
  corneal power, 45–49
  error sources, intraocular lens calculation, 52–53
  estimated lens position, 49–52
  intraocular lens calculation, 52–54
    solutions, 53–54
    sources of error, 52–53
  intraocular lens calculation formulas, 49–52
  light-adjustable intraocular lenses, 57–59
  multifocal lens, 42–43
  sources of error, intraocular lens calculation, 52–53
  toric intraocular lens, 54–57
  toric lens, 41–42
presbyopia-correcting intraocular lenses, 19–23
pricing of noncovered services, 12–13
professional agency, 79–80
professional ethics, 9–14
  advertising, 13–14
  complications, patient communication, 13
  insurance company billing, 12
  LASIK promotion, 11
  noncovered service, pricing, 12–13
  options, informing patient of, 10
  residual postoperative refractive error, 13
  upcoming technology, 10–11
prognosis, 15–25
  astigmatism correction, 17
  contraindications, 23
  dry eye, 22–23
  dysfunctional lens syndrome, 18–19
  expectations of patient, 20–22
  lens position, 19–20
  needs of patient, 20
  personality of patient, 22
  preoperative refractive error, 22
  presbyopia-correcting intraocular lenses, 19–23
  pupil size, 20

refractive cataract patient assessment, 17–18
refractive lens exchange patient assessment, 18–19
residual postoperative refractive error, 13
toric intraocular lenses, 17
pseudophakic data, Optiwave Refractive Analysis system, 121
public relations, 75–86
pupil size, 20
pupillary miosis, 110

radial keratotomy, excimer laser enhancement, 234–235
radio, ad placement, 78
rapport, during telephone advertising, 81–82
refractive cataract patient assessment, 17–18
refractive cataract surgery, 61–62
advertising, 75–86
astigmatic keratotomy, 245–256
Crystalens, 199–212
ethical issues, 9–14
exchange of intraocular lens, 225–232
excimer laser enhancement, 233–244
femtosecond laser-assisted cataract surgery, 95–60
intraoperative wavefront aberrometry, 115–122
limbal relaxing incisions, 167–177
management of practice, 61–74
micro-invasive glaucoma surgery, 141–156
micro-radial keratotomy, 245–256
microincisional cataract surgery, 123–140
monovision integration, presbyopic intraocular lens surgery, 177–188
multifocal implants, 189–198
ocular surface preparation, 27–39
patient education, 87–92
piggyback intraocular lens, 225–232
preoperative testing, 41–60
prognostic predictors, 15–25
public relations, 75–86
refractive intraocular lenses, 3–8
toric intraocular lens, 157–167
Trulign, 199–212
unsatisfied patients, 215–224
refractive intraocular lenses, 3–8
confidence, surgical, 3
defining, 1–8
office, equipping, 4–6
refractive lens exchange patient assessment, 18–19
reinforming patients, 77
relaxing incisions, limbal, 167–177. *See also* limbal relaxing incisions
residual postoperative refractive error, 13
reticle overlay, Optiwave Refractive Analysis system, 120–121
role playing, during telephone advertising, 81

Schlemm's canal, micro-invasive glaucoma surgery, 142–146
scripting, telephone marketing, 81
slit-lamp examination, 34–36
social media, ad placement, 79
solutions, calculations, 53–54
sources of error
calculations, 52–53
intraocular lens calculation, 52–53
staff
hiring, 80–81
preparing, 85
surgical confidence, 3
surgical results, prediction of
expectations of patient, 20–22
needs of patient, 20
personality of patient, 22
refractive cataract patient assessment, 17–18
refractive lens exchange patient assessment, 18–19

tear film
allergy, 29
blepharitis, 28–29

interferometry, 33
osmolarity, 32
unstable, 28–29
technology, education of patient regarding, 87–88
upcoming technology, 10–11
telephone contact, 81–82
rapport, 81–82
role playing, 81
scripting, 81
trust issue, 81–82
television, ad placement, 78–79
toric intraocular lens, 17, 54–57, 157–167
Barrett toric calculator, 162–163
corneal marking, 163–164
double-angle plots, 160–161
measurement, corneal astigmatism, 159–160
placement, 164
posterior cornea, 161–162
preoperative testing, 41–42, 54–57
residual refractive astigmatism, 164–165
single-angle plots, 160–161
surgically induced astigmatism, 162
Trabectome, micro-invasive glaucoma surgery, 144
trust issue in telephone marketing, 81–82

ultrasound power modulation, microincisional cataract surgery, 129
unsatisfied patients, 215–224
capsular opacification, 220
centration, intraocular lens, 222–223
circumference of pupil, 223
consecutive treatment, 219
cornea, ocular surface disease, 220–221
cylinder, residual refractive error, 220
cystoid macular edema, 218, 220
nonsteroidal anti-inflammatory drugs, 218
patient management, 223–224
preoperative education, 215–218
preoperative expectations, 219
unstable tear film, 28–29
upcoming technology, 10–11

VerifEye, 120–121
Optiwave Refractive Analysis system, 120–121
VISX. *See* WaveScan

wavefront aberrometry, 115–122
astigmatism, 116
intraocular lens power calculations, 115–116
Optiwave Refractive Analysis system, 117, 121
data display, 120
error message, 120
image capture, 117–121
pseudophakic data, 121
reticle overlay, 120–121
VerifEye, 120–121
WaveScan, 250

Xen implant, micro-invasive glaucoma surgery, 149